PROCEDURAL & ULTRASOUND SKILLS IN EMERGENCY MEDICINE

Procedural & Ultrasound Skills in Emergency Medicine

SLO6

MOUSSA ISSA

Moussa Issa EM Academy

MOUSSA ISSA

EM ACADEMY

ISBN-13: 978-1916029699
BISAC: Medical / Emergency Medicine
Authored by Moussa Issa
Published by: Moussa Issa EM Academy

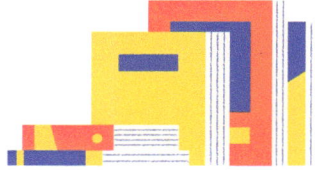

FOREWORD

The field of emergency medicine is constantly evolving; similarly, competency and skills provision is expanding too. Furthermore, each generation of emergency physicians will require additional knowledge and skills to meet the requirements of their training era. Thus, acquiring sufficient skills has become an increasingly important concept in any apprenticeship in emergency medicine.

Procedural and ultrasound skills are recognised as particularly useful by the Royal College of Emergency Medicine (RCEM) and form an integral part of all assessments run by the College. This growing importance is mainly due to increased attention to patient safety and more rigorous standards in the accreditation of training programs.

With the rise of technology and the plenitude of ultrasound machines in many emergency departments, point of care ultrasound (POCUS) has evolved as "the skill to acquire" by any emergency physician. If performed correctly, POCUS offers substantial advantages in procedures' preciseness and reduces several complications. Therefore, it is necessary to attain a certain level of dexterity to perform ultrasound correctly and prevent patient complications.

RCEM has published a comprehensive list of skills that an ED physician should comprehend. Furthermore, ED clinicians must be familiar with every procedure's indications, contraindications, landmarks, and potential complications. In addition to providing a detailed understanding of emergency procedures, this textbook is a perfect resource for medical students and emergency clinicians. In this book, Emergency physicians will encounter a wealth of information about established and emerging procedural and ultrasound skills issues.

Dr Ismat AbdelRhman AlBorhan

PREFACE

As the author of this new edition, I am thrilled about introducing the latest edition of the new Emergency Medicine manual. Anyone who has gone through the new RCEM curriculum will agree that it can be daunting navigating through the various SLOS. We have been used to looking for topics and headers, whereas the new curriculum only deals with outcomes. The outcomes can cover a wide range of topics, and given the broad non-exhausting field of emergency medicine, it can be challenging for one studying for an exam to know what to look for under a certain SLO.

To address this very issue, I began work on the new textbook. What began as work to cover the new RCEM curriculum has turned into a comprehensive textbook for Emergency medicine. This book can be used by one starting as an SHO/ACCS trainee in emergency medicine to any HST trainee to learn, fill in the knowledge gaps, and have a solid theoretical base for the exams. With this book in hand, you will find navigating the RCEM curriculum and the various SLOS more stream-lined to what you need to be learning.

Unlike previous editions where I worked with a limited team of colleagues, a team of doctors, all with a passion for learning, have come together to research journals and write and cross-reference articles. So what you will find is an amalgamation of a lot of hard work and dedication by some brilliant doctors with the final editing done by myself.

I hope you will find this manual helpful, and I look forward to your feedback on this new edition.

Dr Moussa Issa
MBBS, MRCEM, FRCEM, MSc, PhD candidate
Consultant Emergency Medicine

LIST OF CONTRIBUTORS

Amjad Alkanas,
Ashraf Ahmed,
Babar Ali,
Crispin Kibamba,
Dhileeban, Suchitra,
Diana George,
Eric Zogo,
Ismat AbdelRhman AlBorhan,
Malika Kefi,
Manitheepan Kandiah,
Mena-Wisdom Ewhrudjakpor,
Mohammed Dahab,
Mohammed H. Faheem,
Mohammed Oseni,
Mohanad Abdelmagid,
Muhammad Yasir,
Neha Hudlikar,
Qazi Zia Ullah,
Saba Masud,
Sarah Abdallah,
Sharvani Dhandibothla.
Taposim Nath,
Vijaya Manu Mohan,
Waballah Abdallah.

ACKNOWLEDGEMENT

To my wife and children: Marlene, Tatiana, Kevin, Ryan, and Brandon. I continue to thank you for your love and support. You've always been by my side and never complained, watching me working on my books when you needed me the most.

To my co-Editors: Tina Cardoza, Babar Ali, Ashraf Ahmed, Amjad Alkanas, Crispin Kibamba, Eric Zogo, Malika Kefi, Mena-Wisdom Ewhrudjakpor, Mohammed Dahab, Mohammed H. Faheem, Muhammad Yasir, Mohammed Oseni, Sasha Preskey, Ash Darmalingam, Dhileeban, Suchitra, Waballah Abdallah, Sarah Abdallah, Manitheepan Kandiah, Saba Masud, Sagar Kakad, Vijaya Manu Mohan, Taposim Nath and Sharvani Dhandibothla. **Special thanks** to Diana George, Neha Hudlikar, Mena-Wisdom Ewhrudjakpor, Qazi Zia Ullah, Ismat AbdelRhman Al-Borhan and Mohanad Abdelmagid. You are fantastic co-authors, hard workers and, the kind of collaborators everyone will dream of having; thank you, and I appreciate your contribution more than you'll ever know.

To all my clients and Colleagues: Your continued patronage has enabled me to keep this book running. For this, I never mind arthritis on my writing hand. We have ventured many roads together, some new and some well-travelled, but we have continued to sharpen each other with patience, perception, and perseverance. Thanks to you, the pain cannot overcome the happiness I am feeling right now.

To you: The only thing that can stop you from showing the best results is being so highly nervous. There's no need to be scared, buddy. You are ready to show everyone that you are the brightest fella in the world. Good luck!

I feel blessed that social media have given me the chance to reconnect or stay connected with many colleagues worldwide. I am grateful to you all and wish you success throughout your exams.

An exam is not a game, It's a background for your future. So, I wish you to pass all exams!

Dr Moussa Issa - MBBS, MRCEM, FRCEM, MSc, PhD Candidate

DEDICATION

To some other important people:
Dr Arnold Mangala and Dr Arsene Kambale,
Albert Muya Dibaya, Ambroise Manika, Cathy Kalombo, Crispin Kibamba, Diulu Kabongo, Eric Zogo, Freddy Kibambi, Jody Mbuilu, Ken Diango, Louise Lalu, Peter Ndjadi, Polycarpe Makinga, Serge Kalombo, Stanys Lumeya, Stephane Tshitenge, Suzan Mukonkole, Valery Tshilombo, William Kabeya, and others with whom we are working endlessly to enhance the healthcare system and medical education in low and middle-income African countries, I salute your dynamism.

To my colleagues with whom we have come a long way:
Aimee Meno, Alain Kabongo, Alain M. Mukendi, Allen Bamuamba, Andy M. Muela, Ange Mampuya, Baby Mpiana, Bibi Onoya, Bijou Muke, Bruno Numu, Cami Bilo, Chirac Malonda, Christian K. Kayembe, Clement Balilo, Clovis Kalobu, Daddy Dionso, Danny Balayi, Danny Irung, Davin L. Isenge, Delphin Okesha, Dieudonné Mvumbi, Didier Kasay, Esperance Mawana, Eugene Bokila, Faustin Katumba, Fiston Kambi, France Botale, Francis Kiese, Francis Nzakimuena, Tathy Mvumbi, Geoffrey Belanganay, Gervais Suaka, Gina Engumba, Gloria Bugugu, Hergy Diebo, James Lamoury, JL Mangwele, JP Omana, JR Mobando, Jimmy Amsini, Jimmy Kilembe, John Otomba, Jose Mbikayi, Junior Matangila, Kesh Mobumba, Lino Luboya, Louise Hanyane, Louison M. Lutete, Maurice Biduaya, Mays JP K. Kisala, Michaux Fwankenda, Nancy Ntatukidi, Nelly Kabedi, Olivier mangeli, Papy Bukasa, Papy Lofembe, Papy Lundoluka, Papy Mabutuayau, Patou Ngida, Patrick Kankwanda, Patrick Ntalaja, Pitshou Miansi, Placide Mbala, René Tshimanga, Sabin Baza, Sandra Kilombo, Serge Katshunga, Shadrack Mbembele, Solange Tshimbalanga, Sylvain Kalonji, Taty Takoy, Tony Wawina, Vanhove Kashama, Verone Masudi, Yves Mutiri, Zacharie Tshibangu, Zeny Modjo. Thank you for your continued support and uplifting messages.

In memory of Dr Patrice Lomalisa, Dr Jean Bruno Kingiela, Dr Dedie Bandubola, Dr Kitenge Nungu and Dr Felly Kapanga,
"I am better for knowing you, better for loving you, better for having met you. May you be as blessed in the next life, dear brothers, as I was in this one by knowing you."
Gone too soon!

CONTENTS

Foreword   v

Preface   vii

PART ONE: PROCEDURAL SKILLS IN EMERGENCY MEDICINE

1	Abdominal Paracentesis	2
2	Bag Valve Mask Ventilation	12
3	Blood Gas Sampling - Arterial	18
4	Cannulation - Arterial	24
5	Cannulation - Peripheral Venous	31
6	Cannulation – Intraosseous	39
7	Cannulation - Central Venous	48
8	Cardioversion & Pacing	59
9	Cricothyroidotomy	77
10	End-Tidal Capnography	91

11	Escharotomy	104
12	Fasciotomy	110
13	Large Joint Clinical Examination	116
14	Large Joint Aspiration	163
15	Lateral Canthotomy & Cantholysis	167
16	Lumbar Puncture	173
17	Non-Invasive Ventilation	184
18	Invasive Mechanical Ventilation	196
19	Pericardiocentesis	210
20	Procedural Sedation	219
21	Rapid Sequence Intubation	234
22	Reduction of Dislocation/Fracture	250
23	Regional Nerve Block	290
24	Resuscitative Hysterotomy	333
25	Tracheostomy Tube Displaced	343

26   Tracheal Tube Displaced   347

27   Thoracentesis   349

28   Thoracostomy – Needle Decompression   356

29   Thoracostomy – Chest Drain   361

30   Thoracostomy - Seldinger Technique   369

31   Thoracotomy - Emergency   375

PART TWO: POINT OF CARE ULTRASOUND "POCUS" IN EMERGENCY MEDICINE

32   Ultrasound Physics   380

33   e-FAST Examination   394

34   Ultrasound of the Abdominal Aorta & IVC   407

35   Ultrasound Guided Vascular Access   419

36   Ultrasound Guided Femoral Nerve Block   433

37   Deep Vein Thrombosis Ultrasound   439

38   Echo in Life Support   451

39   RUSH Protocol   477

The New Moussa Issa EM Academy

Preparing for such high-level exams requires participants to retrieve several up-to-date publications, books, and guidelines. This task is time-consuming! Thus, we have accomplished that challenging part of the job by bringing you the most updated recommendations and guidance.

You need to grab the book, sit down, read it, and clear it!

www.moussaissabooks.com

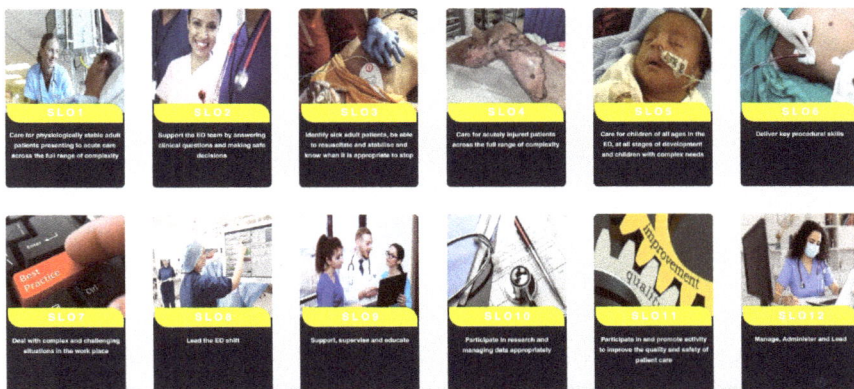

eLearning Modules

To read books online: *www.moussaissabooks.com/elearning*

To browse the SLOs: *www.moussaissabooks.com/slos*

Read anytime, anywhere and on any device!

SLO1 - Endocrinological Emergencies
182 Days

Free

SLO5 - Paediatric Emergency Medicine
182 Days

Free

SLO6 - Procedural Skills in Emergency Medicine
182 Days

2 Plans Available

PART ONE: PROCEDURAL SKILLS IN EMERGENCY MEDICINE

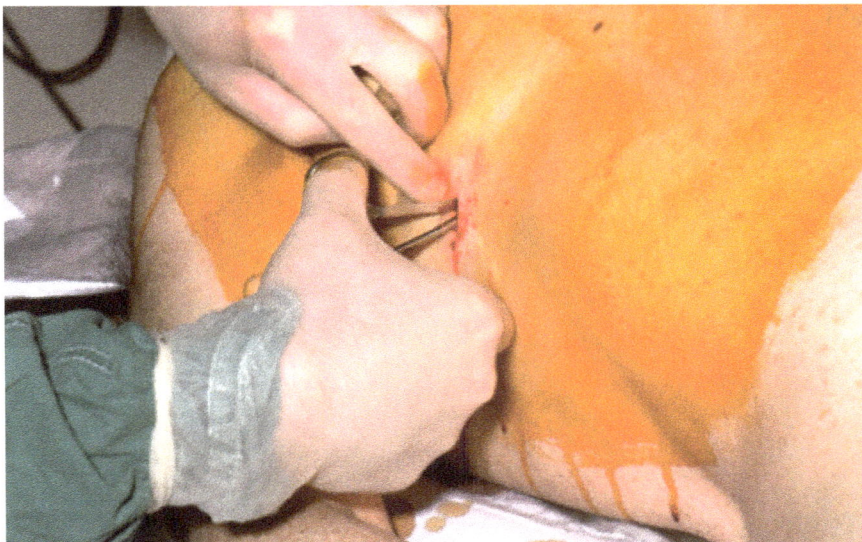

| 1 |

Abdominal Paracentesis

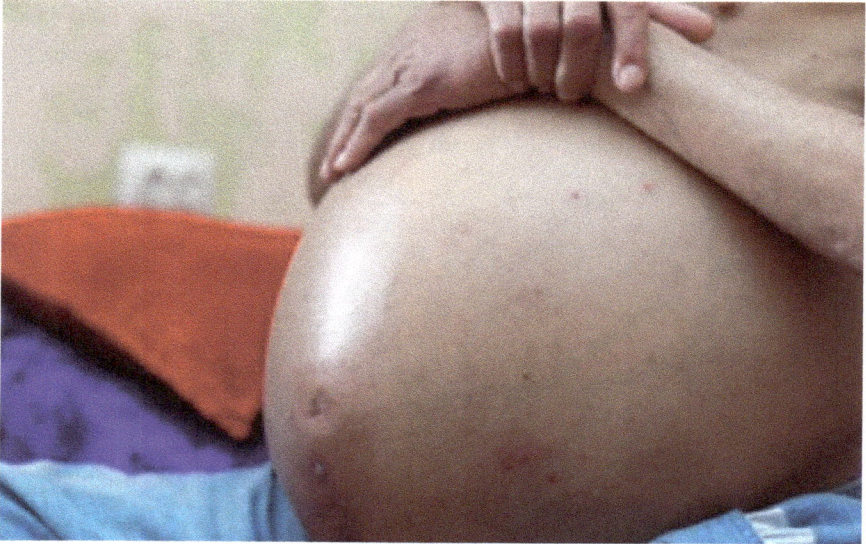

Overview

Ascites is a collection of fluid within the peritoneal cavity of the abdomen and can occur in association with various diseases such as cancer, cirrhosis of the liver, congestive cardiac failure, and protein depletion. *Abdominal paracentesis* is a simple bedside or clinic procedure in which a needle is inserted into the peritoneal cavity, and ascitic fluid is removed. Ascites may be noticed on clinical examination as abdominal distention and the presence of a fluid wave.

Therapeutic paracentesis is indicated to relieve respiratory difficulty due to increased intra-abdominal pressure caused by ascites (Mayeaux, 2021). Diagnostic paracentesis refers to removing a small quantity of fluid for testing.

Objectives

- By the end of this chapter, you should be able to:
  - Explain the indications and contraindications for ascitic-tap paracentesis.
  - Describe the technique involved in ascitic-tap paracentesis.
  - Review the common complications of ascitic-tap paracentesis.

Causes

- *Causes of transudative ascites include the following:*
  - Heart failure
  - Hepatic cirrhosis
  - Alcoholic hepatitis
  - Fulminant hepatic failure
  - Portal vein thrombosis
- **Causes of exudative ascites include the following:**
  - Peritoneal carcinomatosis
  - Inflammation of the pancreas or biliary system
  - Nephrotic syndrome
  - Peritonitis
  - Ischemic or obstructed bowel

Indications

- **Diagnostic tap is used for the following:**
  - New-onset ascites - Fluid evaluation helps to determine aetiology, differentiate transudate versus exudate, detect the presence of cancerous cells, or address other considerations.
  - Suspected spontaneous or secondary bacterial peritonitis
- **Therapeutic tap is used for the following:**
  - Respiratory compromise secondary to ascites

○ Abdominal pain or pressure secondary to ascites (including abdominal compartment syndrome

Contraindications

- **Absolute:**
  - ○ An acute abdomen that requires surgery
  - ○ Overlying infection or Abdominal wall cellulitis- chose another site
- **Relative:**
  - ○ An acute abdomen that requires surgery
  - ○ Severe thrombocytopenia
  - ○ Coagulopathy
  - ○ Pregnancy
  - ○ Distended urinary bladder
  - ○ Distended bowel
  - ○ Intra-abdominal adhesions

Consent

According to the GMC, the consent can be (GMC, 2019):

- *Informed consent*: the patient should be provided with all the information about what the procedure involves, including the benefits and risks, whether there are reasonable alternative treatments, and what will happen if the procedure fails.
- *Verbal consent*: The patient says they're happy to have the procedure done
- *Implied consent*: Assuming that the patient has voluntarily exposed the abdomen for the procedure.
- *Voluntary:* the decision to either consent or not to consent to the procedure must be made by the patient and must not be influenced by pressure from medical staff, friends, or family.

All adults are presumed to have sufficient capacity to decide on their own medical treatment unless there's significant evidence to suggest otherwise (GMC, 2019).

- *Capacity:* the patient must be capable of giving consent, which means they understand the information given to them and can use it to make an informed decision.
- In case of emergency or if a person **does not have the capacity** to decide about their treatment and they have not appointed a lasting power of attorney (LPA), emergency physicians should go ahead with the procedure if they believe it's in the person's best interests.
- If children are able to consent, they usually consent themselves. But someone with parental responsibility may need to give consent for a child up to the age of 16 to have treatment.

Equipment
- Ultrasound (ideally)
- Dressing trolley & sharps bin
- Antiseptic swab sticks
- Fenestrated drape
- Lidocaine 1%, 5-mL ampule
- Syringes 10 mL & 60 mL
- 2-inch-long injection needle
- 11 blade scalpel
- 14-gauge catheter over 17-gauge × 6-inch needle with three-way stopcock or one-way valve, self-sealing valve, and a 5-mL Luer Lock syringe
- Tubing set with roller clamp
- Drainage bag or vacuum container
- Specimen containers
- Blood culture bottles
- Dressing

Pre-procedure

- Consent patient and explain the procedure: Consent for infection, bleeding, pain, failure, damage to surrounding structures (especially bowel perforation – rare), leakage
- Positioning: Lie patient flat and examine clinically to confirm ascites.
- Use the ultrasound machine to identify the insertion site.
- Define landmarks: Aim for 1/3 to ½ of the way between the anterior superior iliac spine and the umbilicus avoiding vessels and scars.

Procedure for ascitic tap

- Position the patient supine in the bed with their head resting on a pillow.
    - Select an appropriate point on the abdominal wall in the right or left lower quadrant, lateral to the rectus sheath.
    - If a suitable site cannot be found with palpation and percussion, consider using ultrasound to mark a spot.
    - Clean the site and surrounding area with 2% Chlorhexidine and apply a sterile drape.
    - Anaesthetise the skin with Lidocaine using the orange needle. Anaesthetise deeper tissues using the green needle, aspirating as you insert the needle to ensure you are not in a vessel before infiltrating with lidocaine.
    - Use a maximum of 10mls of Lidocaine.
    - Take a clean green needle and 20ml syringe and insert through the skin advancing and aspirating until fluid is withdrawn
    - Aspirate 20ml then remove the needle and apply a sterile dressing

Technical Considerations

Depending on the clinical situation, fluid may be sent for the following laboratory tests:

- Gram stain
- Cell count (elevated counts may suggest infection)
- Bacterial culture
- Total protein level
- Triglyceride levels (elevated in chylous ascites)
- Bilirubin level (maybe elevated in bowel perforation)
- Glucose level
- Albumin level, used in conjunction with serum albumin levels obtained the same day (used to calculate SAAG; see the Ascites Albumin Gradient calculator)
- Amylase level (elevation suggests pancreatic source)
- Lactate dehydrogenase (LDH) level
- Cytology

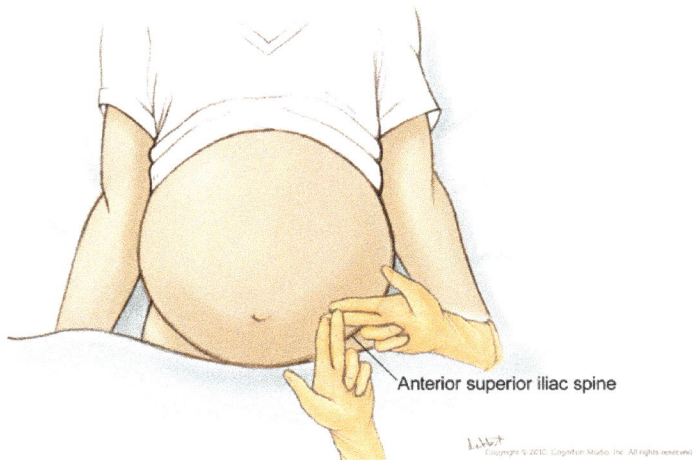

Fig. 1.1.1. Paracentesis site
Hepatitis C Online

To identify the preferred region for paracentesis in the left lower quadrant, first, locate the anterior superior iliac spine. Then, mark a spot 2 fingerbreadths (3 cm) cephalad and 2 fingerbreadths (3 cm) medial to the anterior superior iliac spine.

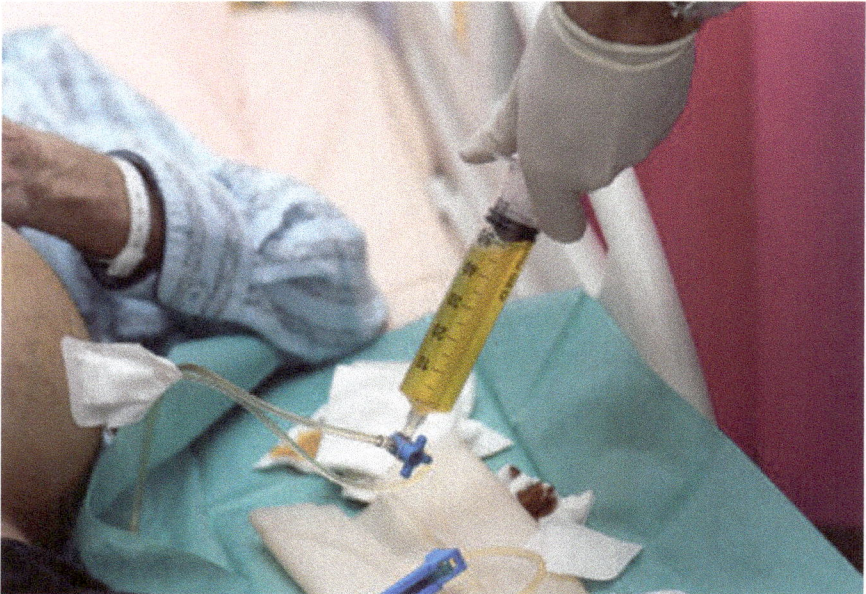

Fig. 1.1.2. Paracentesis fluid collection

Complications

- Persistent leakage from the needle insertion site
- Abdominal wall hematoma
- Bowel perforation
- Introduction of infection
- Hypotension (after a large-volume paracentesis)
- Dilutional hyponatremia
- Hepatorenal syndrome
- Bleeding
- Post paracentesis circulatory dysfunction

Serum-Ascites Albumin Gradient (SAAG)

- The serum ascites albumin gradient (SAAG) can be used to identify the cause of the ascites.
- It is calculated by subtracting the albumin concentration in the Ascites from the albumin concentration in the serum.

SAAG = serum albumin – ascites albumin

A high gradient (>1.1 g/dL) suggests portal hypertension. Such conditions may include the following:

- Cirrhosis
- Fulminant hepatic failure
- Veno-occlusive disease
- Congestive heart failure
- Portal hypertension
- Nephrotic syndrome
- Hepatic vein obstruction (i.e., Budd-Chiari syndrome)
- Myxoedema
- Malignancy
- Ovarian tumours
- Pancreatic
- Biliary ascites
- Trauma

A low gradient (SAAG < 1.1 g/dL) indicates nonportal hypertension and suggests a peritoneal cause of ascites. Such conditions may include the following:

- Primary peritoneal mesothelioma
- Secondary peritoneal carcinomatosis
- Tuberculous peritonitis
- Sarcoidosis
- Systemic Lupus Erythematosus
- Henoch-Schönlein purpura
- Eosinophilic gastroenteritis
- Whipple disease
- Endometriosis

- Fungal and parasitic infections (e.g., Candida, Histoplasma, Cryptococcus, Schistosoma mansoni, Strongyloides, Entamoeba histolytica)

Pearls and Pitfalls

- **Pearls**
  - The preferred site of entry is in the midline of the abdomen, below the umbilicus.
  - Post-paracentesis circulatory dysfunction (PPCD) occurs secondary to hypovolemia after large-volume paracentesis (>4 L) in cirrhotic patients. It is associated with worsening hyponatremia, renal dysfunction, shorter time to ascites recurrence, and increased mortality.
  - Prevention of PPCD has been demonstrated with the administration of 6–8 g of albumin per litre of Ascites removed.
- **Pitfalls**
  - Polymorphonuclear lymphocyte (PMN) count greater than 250/mm³ is diagnostic of spontaneous bacterial peritonitis.

Spontaneous Bacterial Peritonitis

Spontaneous bacterial peritonitis (SBP) is the infection of ascitic fluid in the absence of any contiguous source of infection (Runyon, 2004). Despite the amelioration of mortality from SBP, with prompt diagnosis and treatment, the related incidence in patients with ascites ranges between 7–30% annually (Wong, 2005). According to the British Society of Gastroenterology (BSG) guidelines on the management of ascites in cirrhosis (Moore & Aithal, 2006), a prompt diagnosis and timely management can lead to an in-hospital mortality reduction from 90% to less than 20% (Garcia-Tsao, 2001). The commonest organisms isolated in patients with SBP include Escherichia coli, gram-positive cocci (mainly streptococcus species) and enterococci. Five days of treatment with cefotaxime is as effective as 10-day therapy, and the low dose (2 g twice daily) is similar in efficacy to the higher doses (2 g four times daily). Other cephalosporins, such as ceftriaxone and ceftazidime as well as co-amoxiclav (amoxicillin plus clavulanic acid), are as effective as cefotaxime in resolving SBP.

Further reading

Medscape- paracentesis: https://emedicine.medscape.com/article/80944-overview

References

Garcia-Tsao, G. (2001). Current management of the complications of cirrhosis and portal hypertension: variceal hemorrhage, ascites, and spontaneous bacterial peritonitis. Gastroenterology, 120(3), 726-748. https://doi.org/10.1053/gast.2001.22580

GMC. (2019). Consent for treatment. General Medical Council UK. https://www.nhs.uk/conditions/consent-to-treatment/

Mayeaux, E. J. (2021). Abdominal Paracentesis. 5minuteConsult. Retrieved 01 Dec. 2021 from https://5minuteconsult.com/collection-content/30-156350/procedures/abdominal-paracentesis

Moore, K. P., & Aithal, G. P. (2006). Guidelines on the management of ascites in cirrhosis. Gut, 55 Suppl 6(Suppl 6), vi1-12. https://doi.org/10.1136/gut.2006.099580

Runyon, B. A. (2004). Early events in spontaneous bacterial peritonitis. Gut, 53(6), 782-784. https://doi.org/10.1136/gut.2003.035311

Wong, F. (2005). Volume expanders for spontaneous bacterial peritonitis: Are we comparing oranges with oranges? Hepatology, 42(3), 533-535. https://doi.org/10.1002/hep.20862

| 2 |

Bag Valve Mask Ventilation

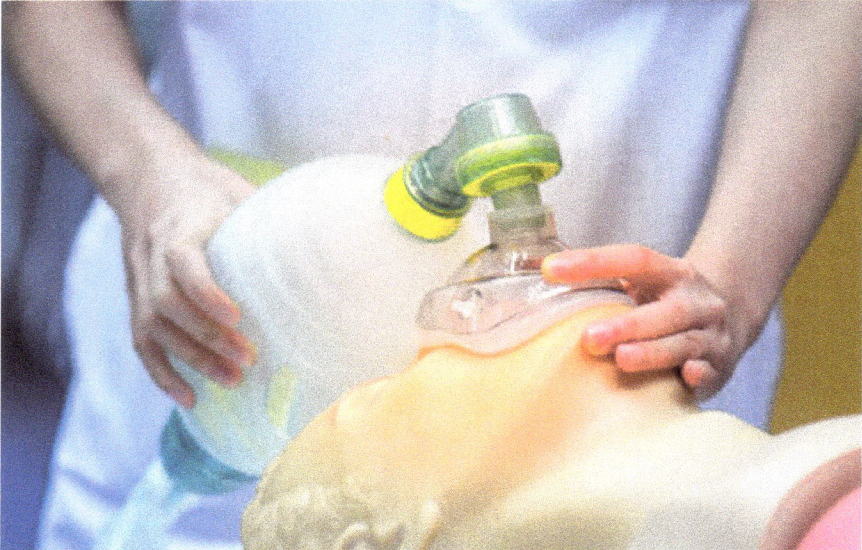

Overview

Bag valve mask (BVM) ventilation is a skill of the highest interest for any emergency physician but remains one of the most challenging skills to acquire (Bucher et al., 2021). Of all the fundamental skills applied by emergency physicians, few are more critical than the ability to ventilate a critically ill patient. The BVM is perhaps one of the most effective equipment in saving the patient's life. However, unfortunately, it is very often used with little to no training and, consequently, not very effectively (Levitan, 2004). When a patient cannot breathe, the BVM enables emergency practitioners working within any setting or location to address the lack of oxygenation to a patient. Provided there is an adequate gas exchange at the alveolar level and adequate circulation to the tissues, artificial ventilation via the BVM in the hands of a skilled practitioner can keep a patient alive indefinitely. However, if BVM ventilation is incorrectly performed, it can expedite hypoxia and worsen the airway obstruction that naturally occurs during deeply depressed levels of consciousness, leading to severe injury or death (Rock, 2014). In addition, there is nothing more likely to cause a degree of panic in a stressful position than if the physician managing the airway cannot ventilate the patient.

Objectives
- By the end of this chapter, you should be able to:
  - Outline the anatomy of the airway.
  - Review the indications for bag valve mask ventilation.
  - Learn the technique of bag valve mask ventilation.
  - Understand the challenges of bag-valve ventilation in critically ill patients.

Indications
- Altered mental status with the inability to protect the airway
- Apnoea
- Hypercapnic respiratory failure
- Hypoventilation
- Hypoxic respiratory failure
- Rescue manoeuvre if failed intubation

Contraindications
- **Absolute**
  - Inability to ventilate due to lack of seal (thick beard, deforming facial trauma)
  - Inability to ventilate secondary to complete upper airway obstruction
  - Active, adequate spontaneous ventilation
- **Relative**
  - Full stomach (aspiration risk)

○ After induction and paralysis during rapid sequence intubation (aspiration risk)

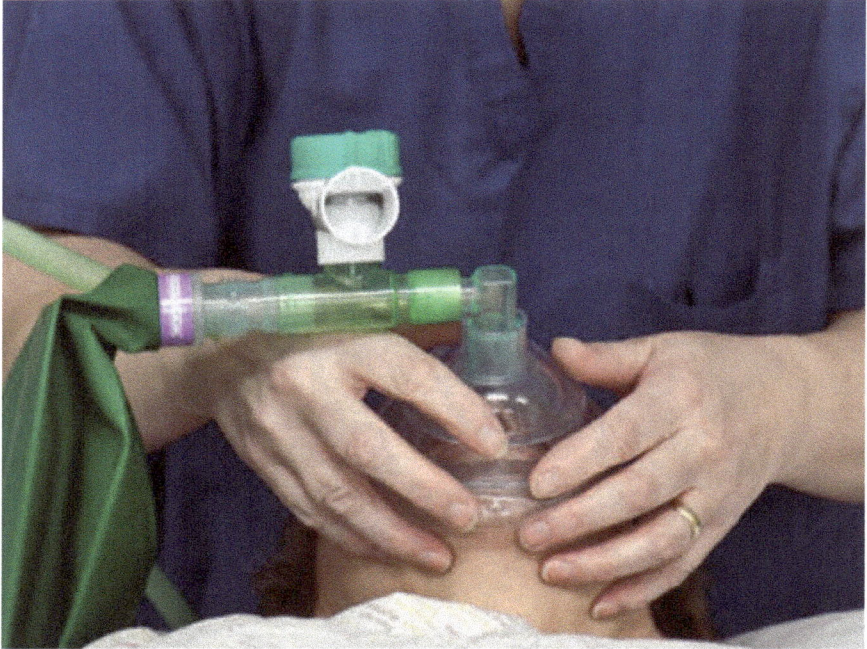

Fig. 1.2.1. Bag Valve Mask holding technique

Equipment

- Universal precautions: Gloves, mask, gown, and eye protection
- Bag valve mask (BVM) with reservoir
- PEEP valve
- Oxygen connector tubing
- Lubricant jelly
- Adequate size ventilation face masks
- Pulse oximeter
- Capnography equipment
- Oropharyngeal airways
- Nasopharyngeal airways
- Oxygen source (100% oxygen, 15 L/minute)
- Nasogastric tube
- Suctioning apparatus and Yankauer catheter

- Magill forceps

Procedure

- Position patient in "sniffing" position.
- Open the airway with chin-lift/head-tilt or jaw thrust manoeuvres.
- Place airway adjuncts to maintain airway patency.
  - Use oral airway in unconscious patients.
  - Use nasal airway in semi responsive patients.
    - Attach oxygen tubing to high-flow oxygen (15 L/min).
    - Place appropriately sized mask on patient's face covering the nose and mouth.
  - For the one-handed technique, use a non-dominant hand to make a "C" with index finger and thumb on top of the mask and form an "E" with the rest of the fingers using them to pull up on the mandible (E–C technique). Use the dominant hand to provide bag ventilations.
  - For the two-handed, two-person technique (preferred), make two semicircles with index fingers and thumbs of both hands on top of the mask and use the rest of the fingers to pull up on the mandible.
    - Consider the Sellick manoeuvre (cricoid pressure) to compress the oesophagus against the cervical vertebrae, preventing gastric insufflation.
    - Ventilate patient providing reduced tidal volume breaths (500 mL) at a rate of 10–12 breaths per minute.
    - Give each breath gently over 1–1.5 s to avoid high peak pressures, avoiding gastric insufflation.
    - Prepare for definitive airway as dictated by the clinical scenario.

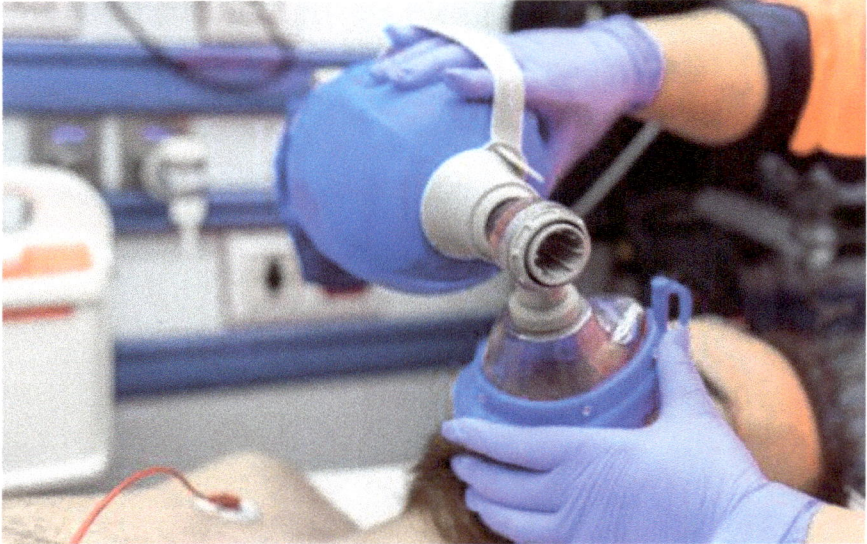

Fig. 1.2.2-6. BVM ventilation

Complications

- Stomach inflation may lead to vomiting and aspiration.
- Increased positive thoracic pressure may cause decreased pre-load, worsening cardiac output, and/or hypotension.
- Hypoventilation (inadequate O2 tidal volume, airway patency, or mask seal).

Post-procedure care

- Continue with the patient's resuscitation according to the life support guidelines by applying ABCDE principles.
- Seek help as soon as possible.
- Regularly reassess the airway and the ability of the patient to control his airway
- Measure arterial blood oxygen saturation as soon as practical by ABG sampling and/or pulse oximetry and titrate inspired oxygen to keep a blood arterial oxygen saturation between 94% to 98% (Soar et al., 2021).
- If the patient's Glasgow Coma Scale (GCS) is 8 or lower, consider a definitive airway with an endotracheal tube.

Further Reading

Life in The Fast lane- Bag-Valve-Mask (BVM) Ventilation: https://litfl.com/bag-valve-mask-bvm-ventilation/

References

Bucher, J. T., Vashisht, R., Ladd, M., & Cooper ., J. S. (2021). Bag Mask Ventilation. StatPearls. Retrieved 02 Dec. 2021 from https://www.ncbi.nlm.nih.gov/books/NBK441924/

Levitan, R. (2004). Airway CAM Guide to Intubation and Practical Emergency Airway Management.

Rock, M. (2014). The Dos and Don'ts of Bag-Valve Mask Ventilation. JEMS. Retrieved 01 Dec. 2021§ from https://www.jems.com/patient-care/dos-and-don-ts-bag-valve-mask-ventilatio/

Soar, J., Böttiger, B. W., Carli, P., Couper, K., Deakin, C. D., Djärv, T., . . . Nolan, J. P. (2021). European Resuscitation Council Guidelines 2021: Adult advanced life support. Resuscitation, 161, 115-151. https://doi.org/10.1016/j.resuscitation.2021.02.010

| 3 |

Blood Gas Sampling - Arterial

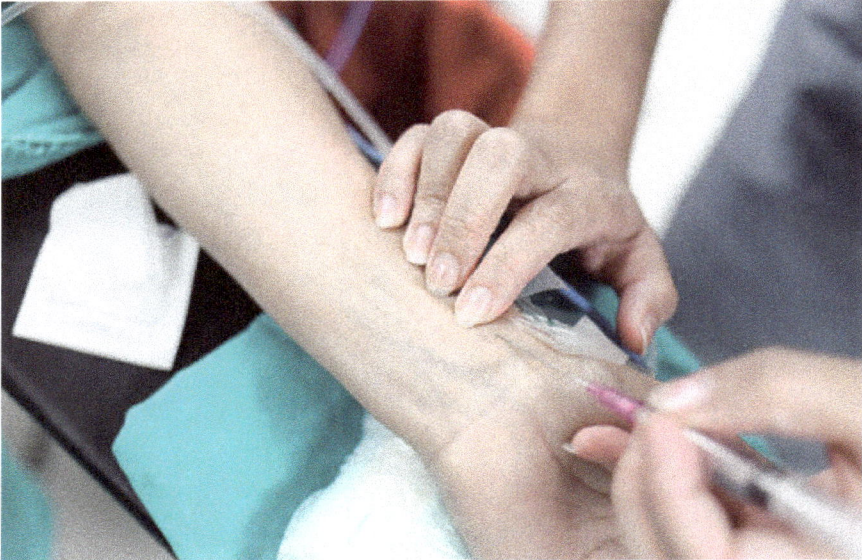

Overview

Phlebotomy has been practised for centuries and is still one of the most common invasive healthcare procedures. Every move in the phlebotomy process influences the quality of the specimen and is thus crucial for limiting laboratory error, patient harm and even death (WHO, 2010).

Objectives

- By the end of this chapter, you should be able to:
    ○ Outline the indications for arterial blood gas.
    ○ Explain the contraindications of arterial blood gas.

- highlight the complications following an arterial blood gas sampling
- Describe the technique of performing an arterial blood gas sampling.

Indications

- To interpret oxygenation levels
- To assess for potential respiratory derangements
- To assess for potential metabolic derangements
- To monitor the acid-base status
- To assess carboxyhaemoglobin in CO poisoning
- To assess lactate
- To gain preliminary results for electrolytes and Haemoglobin
- Can be conducted as a one-off sample or repeated sampling to determine response to interventions

Contraindications

- **Absolute:**
  - Absent pulse
  - Thromboangiitis obliterans (Buerger's disease)
  - Full-thickness burns over the cannulation site
  - Inadequate circulation to the extremity
  - Raynaud syndrome
- **Relative:**
  - Anticoagulation
  - Coagulopathy
  - Atherosclerosis
  - Inadequate collateral flow
  - Infection at the cannulation site
  - Partial-thickness burn at the cannulation site
  - Previous surgery in the area
  - Synthetic vascular graft

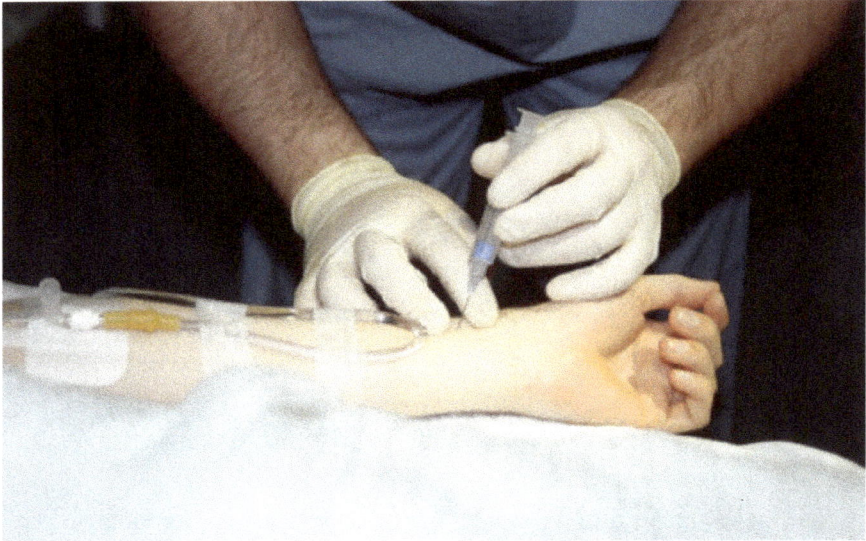

Fig. 1.3.1. ABG sampling

Consent

According to the GMC, the consent can be (GMC, 2019):

- *Informed consent:* the patient should be provided with all the information about what the procedure involves, including the benefits and risks, whether there are reasonable alternative treatments, and what will happen if the procedure fails.
- *Verbal consent:* The patient says they're happy to have the procedure done
- *Implied consent:* Assuming that the patient has extended the arm or voluntarily exposed the wrist for the puncture.
- *Voluntary:* the decision to either consent or not to consent to the procedure must be made by the patient and must not be influenced by pressure from medical staff, friends, or family.

All adults are presumed to have sufficient capacity to decide on their own medical treatment unless there's significant evidence to suggest otherwise (GMC, 2019).

- **Capacity**: the patient must be capable of giving consent, which means they understand the information given to them and can use it to make an informed decision.
- In case of emergency or if a person **does not have the capacity** to decide about their treatment and they have not appointed a lasting power of attorney (LPA), emergency physicians should go ahead with the procedure if they believe it's in the person's best interests.
- If children are able to consent, they usually consent themselves. But someone with parental responsibility may need to give consent for a child up to the age of 16 to have treatment.

Equipment

- Gloves
- Apron
- Pre-heparinised arterial blood gas syringe and bung or cap
- Arterial blood gas needle (23 G)
- Alcohol wipe (70% isopropyl)
- Gauze or cotton wool
- Tape
- Lidocaine 1% (1 mL)
- Subcutaneous needle (25-27 G)
- Small syringe for lidocaine (1-2 ml)
- Sharps container

Procedure

- Check if the patient has an allergy to local anaesthetic(e.g., lidocaine).
- Consent the patient verbally after explaining the procedure
- Set up a tray with a sharps bin
- Expel excess heparin from ABG syringe
- Palpate for radial pulse
- Transfix artery between forefinger and middle finger

- Insert ABG syringe into the palpated artery
- Depending on the syringe it may self-fill or you may need to withdraw the plunger carefully.
- Remove needle and syringe after sample gained (only 1-2ml required)

Considerations

How oxygen therapy impacts ABG results:

- **PaO2**should be **greater than 10 kPa** when oxygenating on room **air** in a healthy patient.
- If the patient is receiving **oxygen therapy** their **PaO2** should be approximately **10kPa less than** the % **inspired concentration FiO2** (so a patient on 40% oxygen would be expected to have a PaO2 of approximately 30kPa

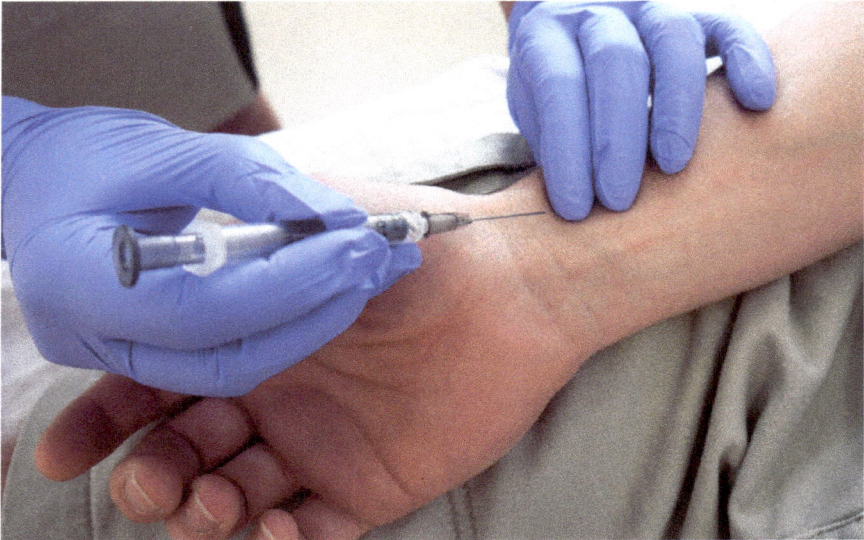

Fig.1.3.2. ABG sampling technique

Post-procedure care

- Apply pressure to the area with gauze and tape.
- Advise patient to continue giving pressure for 5-10 minutes

- Take the sample to the analyser as soon as possible
- Ensure the result is labelled with the patient's details and documented in the notes
- Ensure inspired oxygen concentration is clearly documented
- In the event of failure, call for senior help

Complications

- Haemorrhage
- Hematoma (at puncture site)
- Infection (at the insertion site or systemic)
- Thrombosis
- Arteriovenous fistula
- Pseudoaneurysm formation
- Exsanguination (secondary to dislodgement of the catheter)
- Cerebrovascular accident (CVA; secondary to air embolism)

Further reading

Medscape- Arterial Blood Gas Sampling Technique: https://emedicine.medscape.com/article/1902703-technique

References

GMC. (2019). Consent for treatment. General Medical Council UK. https://www.nhs.uk/conditions/consent-to-treatment/

WHO. (2010). WHO guidelines on drawing blood: best practices in phlebotomy. World Health Organization. Retrieved 26 Nov. 2021 from http://apps.who.int/iris/bitstream/handle/10665/44294/9789241599221_eng.pdf?sequence=1

| 4 |

Cannulation - Arterial

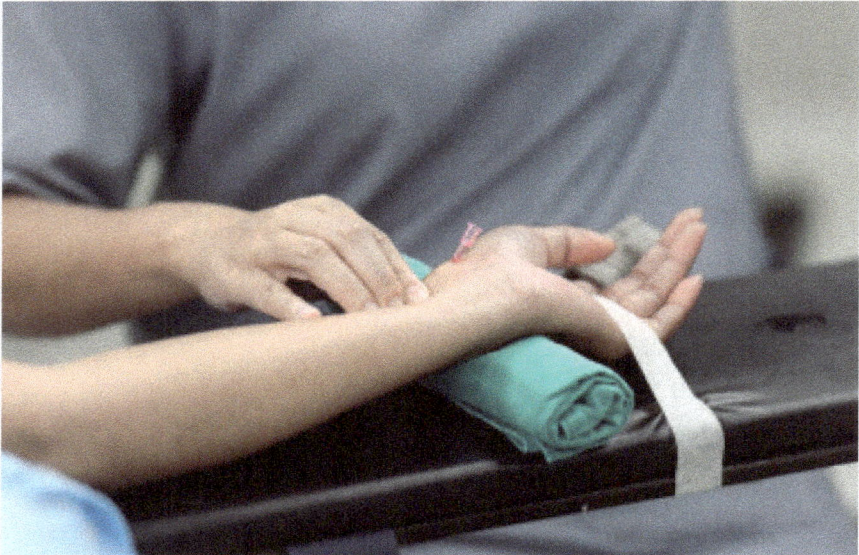

Overview

Arterial cannulation is a procedure commonly performed in acute and critical care settings. It gives precise blood pressure and the mean arterial pressure measurements than non-invasive means. Therefore, it provides instant recognition of clinical changes, thus enabling more active intervention and stabilization of a patient (Hager & Burns, 2021)

Objectives
- By the end of this chapter, you should be able to:
  - Outline the indications for inserting arterial lines.
  - Recall the contraindications of arterial cannulation

- Evoke the complications following an arterial line insertion.
- Describe the technique of inserting arterial lines.

Indications

- Continuous monitoring of blood pressure in acute illness or major surgery
- Serial sampling of arterial blood during resuscitation
- Inability to use non-invasive blood pressure monitoring (g., burns, morbid obesity)
- Continuous infusion of vasoactive inotropes (g., phentolamine for reversal of local anaesthesia)
- Angiography
- Embolization

Contraindications

- **Absolute**
  - Circulatory compromise in the extremity
  - Full-thickness burns of the extremity
  - Raynaud's syndrome
  - Thromboangiitis obliterans (Buerger's disease)
- **Relative**
  - Recent surgery in the extremity
  - Local skin infection
  - Abnormal coagulation
  - Insufficient collateral circulation
  - Superficial and partial thickness burns of the extremity
  - Arteriosclerosis

Equipment

- Skin prep solution such as povidone-iodine or chlorhexidine
- Sterile gloves and drapes
- A 20-ga length appropriate catheter

- Five ml 1% lidocaine without epinephrine
- A 3 ml syringe with 25ga or 27ga needle for subcutaneous administration of lidocaine
- 11 blade scalpel
- A 4-0 nylon suture
- Adhesive tape
- A 3-way stopcock
- Transducer kit
- Pressure tubing
- Size appropriate arm board (for radial artery access)
- Needle holder
- Intravenous (IV) tubing T-connector
- Ultrasound machine

Consent

According to the GMC, the consent can be (GMC, 2019):

- *Informed consent*: the patient should be provided with all the information about what the procedure involves, including the benefits and risks, whether there are reasonable alternative treatments, and what will happen if the procedure fails.
- *Verbal consent*: The patient says they're happy to have the procedure done
- *Implied consent*: Assuming that the patient has extended the arm or voluntarily exposed the wrist for the puncture.
- *Voluntary:* the decision to either consent or not to consent to the procedure must be made by the patient and must not be influenced by pressure from medical staff, friends or family.

All adults are presumed to have sufficient capacity to decide on their own medical treatment unless there's significant evidence to suggest otherwise (GMC, 2019).

- *Capacity:* the patient must be capable of giving consent, which means they understand the information given to them and can use it to make an informed decision.
- In case of emergency or if a person ***does not have the capacity*** to decide about their treatment and they have not appointed a lasting power of attorney (LPA), emergency physicians should go ahead with the procedure if they believe it's in the person's best interests.
- If children are able to consent, they usually consent themselves. But someone with parental responsibility may need to give consent for a child up to the age of 16 to have treatment.

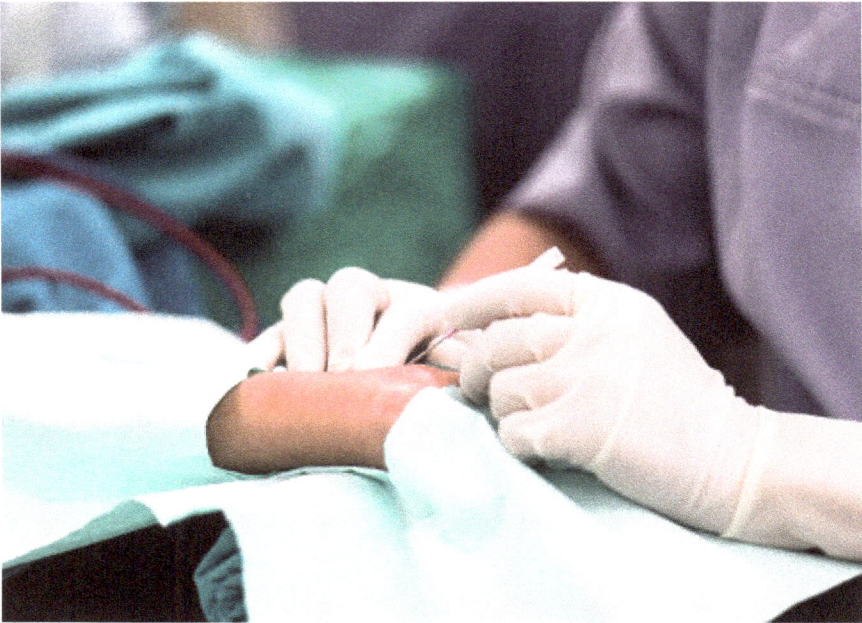

Fig. 1.4.1. Arterial cannulation

Anatomical Considerations

- After gaining consent for the procedure or assuming that this is a life-threatening emergency, the initial step in preparing for arterial cannulation is to locate the area for insertion and appropriately position it.

- The radial artery is situated between the brachioradialis tendons and flexor carpi radialis tendons, around 1-2 cm from the wrist.
- The artery lies medial to the bony head of the distal radius (Liu, 2020b).
- The initial puncture site should be as distal as possible (approximately 1 cm proximal to the styloid process), to prevent puncture of the retinaculum flexorum and the small superficial branch of the radial artery.
- Before radial artery cannulation, many experts recommend the performance of **Allen's test.**

Procedure
- Locate the radial artery with gentle pressure
- Angle the needle 45 degrees toward the arm
- Pierce the skin distal to palpated artery position
- Gradually advance the needle until spontaneous blood enters
- Advance the guidewire into the artery
- Withdraw needle
- Push flushed plastic cannula over top of the guidewire
- Connect the Heparinised saline syringe
- Re-flush cannula with 2 ml Heparinised saline
- Seal the artery
- Attach the transducer and high-pressure infusion set
- Remove pad under the wrist and secure the arm board

Allen's Test

This procedure assesses for adequate collateral circulation to the hand via the ulnar artery.

- Raise the hand and ask the patient to make a fist for 30 seconds while applying simultaneous pressure to the ulnar and the radial arteries to occlude them.

- Instruct the patient to repeatedly clench the fist tightly to exsanguinate the hand while occlusion of the arteries is maintained. Without releasing digital pressure on arteries, instruct the patient to extend fingers and observe the palmar surface to confirm blanching of skin.
- Release pressure on ulnar artery only and observe palmar surface for reperfusion:
  - If reperfusion of the hand does not occur within 5–10s, ulnar arterial blood flow may be compromised, and radial artery cannulation should not be attempted.
  - If reperfusion is brisk, repeat the test releasing pressure on the radial artery only and observing the palmar surface for reperfusion.
  - If the return of rubor takes longer than 5–10 s, radial artery puncture should not be performed.

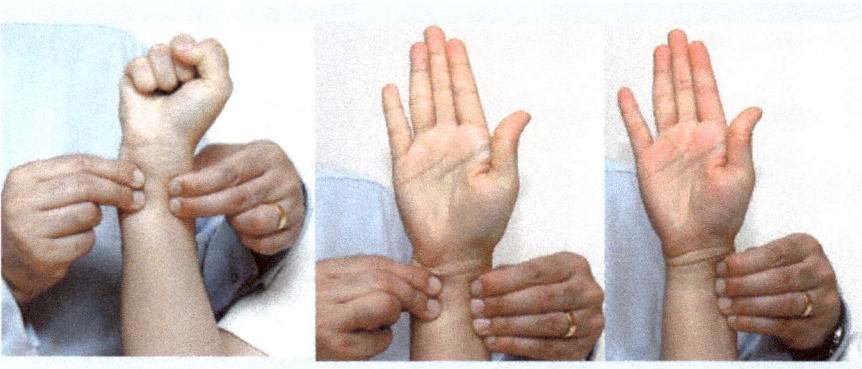

Fig. 1.4.3. Allen's test
Credit - Learn from Doctor

Allen test Normal (positive): The patient's hand quickly becomes warm and returns to its normal colour. This means that one artery alone will be enough to supply blood to the hand and fingers.

Allen test Abnormal (negative): The patient's hand remains pale and cold. This means that one artery is not enough to supply blood to the hand and fingers. Blood will not be collected from an artery in this hand.

Complications

- Haemorrhage
- Hematoma (at puncture site)
- Infection (at the insertion site or systemic)
- Thrombosis
- Arteriovenous fistula
- Pseudoaneurysm formation
- Exsanguination (secondary to dislodgement of the catheter)
- Cerebrovascular accident (CVA; secondary to air embolism)

Further reading

Medscape-Arterial line placement: https://emedicine.med-scape.com/article/1999586-overview

References

GMC. (2019). Consent for treatment. General Medical Council UK. https://www.nhs.uk/conditions/consent-to-treatment/

Hager, H., & Burns, B. (2021). Arterial Cannulation. Statpearls. https://www.ncbi.nlm.nih.gov/books/NBK482242/

Liu, Y. T. (2020b). How To Do Radial Artery Cannulation. MSD Manual. Retrieved 25 Nov. 2021 from https://www.msdmanuals.com/en-gb/professional/critical-care-medicine/how-to-do-peripheral-vas-cular-procedures/how-to-do-radial-artery-cannulation

| 5 |

Cannulation - Peripheral Venous

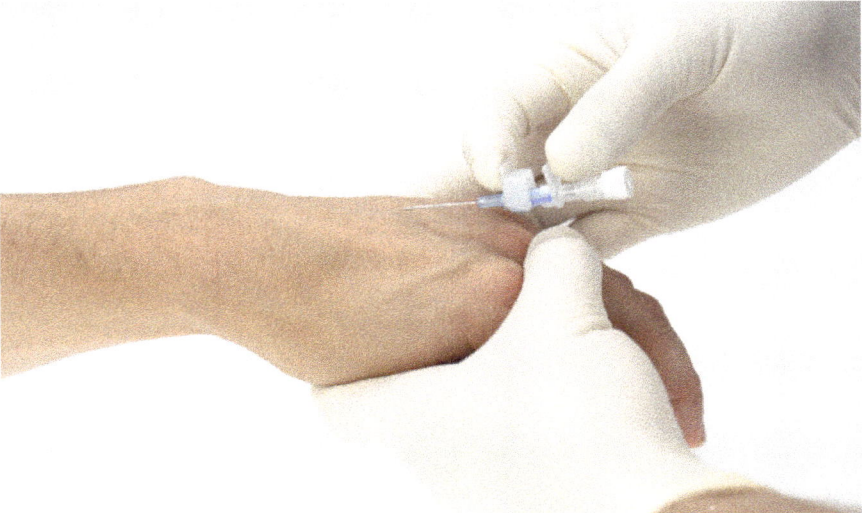

Overview

Peripheral venous cannulation is the process of inserting a small hollow catheter over a needle into a peripheral vein. It is an invasive procedure that suitably trained practitioners should entirely carry out. Nevertheless, the insertion of peripheral venous cannulas is one of the most frequently performed procedures in the Emergency department (ED). It facilitates the administration of intravenous fluids and medication, nutrition, and haemodynamic monitoring. In the UK, more than 30% of patients will have at least one cannula inserted during their stay in the ED.

Objectives

- By the end of this chapter, you should be able to:
    - Outline the indications for inserting a peripheral venous cannula.
    - Highlight the contraindications of a peripheral venous cannula insertion
    - Evoke the complications following a peripheral venous cannula insertion
    - Describe the technique of inserting a peripheral venous cannula.

Indications

- Administration of intravenous medicines.
- Transfusions of blood or blood components.
- Maintenance or correction of hydration levels if unable to tolerate oral fluids.
- Potential venous access.

Contraindications

- **Absolute**
    - None
- **Relative**
    - Extremities that have massive oedema,
    - Burns or injury
    - The presence of infection as suggested by inflammation, phlebitis, cellulitis.
    - The presence of injury or damage (e.g., fracture, Stroke, oedema, lymphadenopathy).
    - Ipsilateral mastectomy or lymph node dissection
    - Veins that are mobile or tortuous, or sited near a bony prominence.
    - If intravenous therapy is predicted to be long-term.
    - Continuous infusions or therapies which are vesicant or have a pH of 9.

Equipment

- A cannula itself
- Cleansing materials: Alcohol, chlorhexidine, or povidone-iodine swabs or wipes
- Nonsterile gloves
- A gauze,
- A needle-free bung,
- A prepared flush of sterile normal saline,
- Tourniquet, single use
- IV catheter: 18- or 20-gauge routinely for adults, 14- or 16-gauge for high-volume infusion and 22- or 24-gauge in infants and small children
- IV infusion set: IV solution bag, hanger, tubing or saline lock
- Dressing materials: tape, gauze, scissors, transparent occlusive dressing

Optional equipment:

- Local anaesthetic agents
- A topical ointment containing local anaesthetic
- An ultrasound machine (Schoenfeld et al., 2011)
- Vein-finder device (e.g., infrared vein viewer, ultrasonography device)

Consent

According to the GMC, the consent can be (GMC, 2019):

- *Informed consent*: the patient should be provided with all the information about what the procedure involves, including the benefits and risks, whether there are reasonable alternative treatments, and what will happen if the procedure fails.
- *Verbal consent*: The patient says they're happy to have the procedure done

- *Implied consent*: Assuming that the patient has extended the arm or voluntarily exposed the elbow for the puncture.
- *Voluntary:* the decision to either consent or not to consent to the procedure must be made by the patient and must not be influenced by pressure from medical staff, friends, or family.

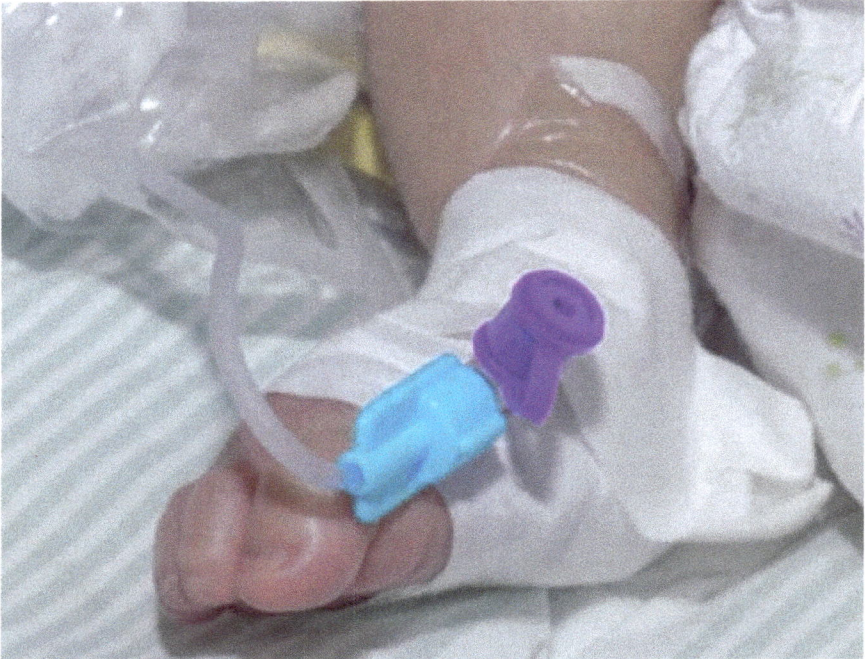

Fig.1.5.1. Paediatric peripheral venous cannulation

All adults are presumed to have sufficient capacity to decide on their own medical treatment unless there's significant evidence to suggest otherwise (GMC, 2019).

- *Capacity:* the patient must be capable of giving consent, which means they understand the information given to them and can use it to make an informed decision.
- In case of emergency or if a person **does not have the capacity** to decide about their treatment and they have not appointed a lasting power of attorney (LPA), emergency physicians should go

ahead with the procedure if they believe it's in the person's best interests.

- If children are able to consent, they usually consent themselves. But someone with parental responsibility may need to give consent for a child up to the age of 16 to have treatment.

Peripheral IV sites

- The preferred site in the emergency department is the veins of the forearm, followed by the median cubital vein that crosses the antecubital fossa.
- In trauma patients, it is common to go directly to the median cubital vein as the first choice because it will accommodate a large-bore IV and it is generally easy to catheterize.
- In circumstances where the veins of the upper extremities are inaccessible, the veins of the dorsum of the foot or the saphenous vein of the lower leg can be used. In circumstances in which no peripheral IV access is possible a central IV can be started.

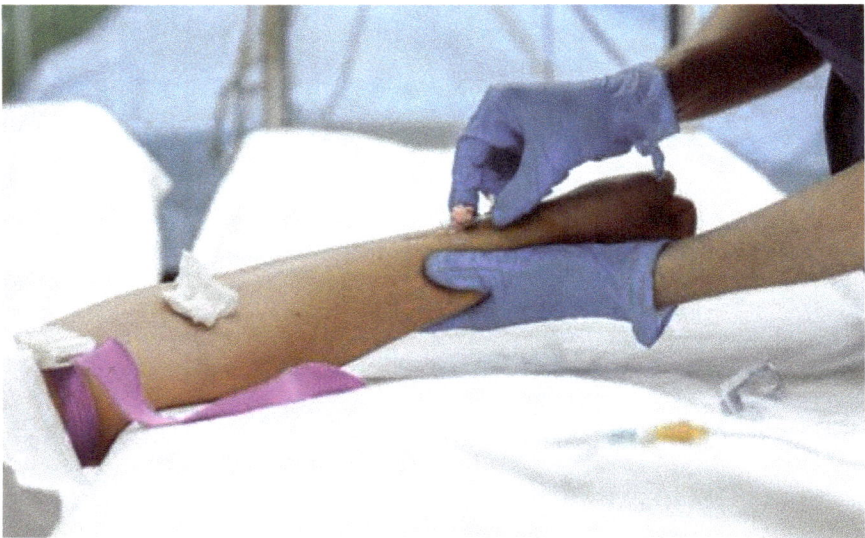

Fig.1.5.2. Inserting a cannula

Procedure

- Prior to beginning the procedure, wash your hands following your local policy and use an alcohol rub/gel.
- Don sterile gloves and apron
- Prepare the site by wiping with an appropriate skin preparation/ alcohol swab and allow to dry naturally before proceeding.
- Do not re-palpate after preparing the skin.
- Apply tourniquet above the insertion site.
- The tourniquet should not be applied for longer than 1 minute.
- Notify the patient that an injection/scratch is imminent.
- Secure the vein by applying manual traction on the skin a few centimetres below the proposed cannulation site
- With the bevel of the cannula facing upwards, insert the needle (and cannula) into the vein.
- Wait for the first flashback of blood in the flashback chamber of the needle and as soon as the blood is visible in the cannula advance the cannula over the needle into the vein.
- Retract the needle slightly and the second flashback of blood will be seen along the shaft of the cannula.
- Keeping skin traction with the non-dominant hand, and using the dominant hand, slowly push the cannula off the needle into the vein.
- At this point, release the tourniquet and apply pressure to the vein above the cannula tip and withdraw the needle from the cannula and apply a connector/adapter.
- Secure the hub of the cannula in place with a semi-occlusive or transparent dressing.

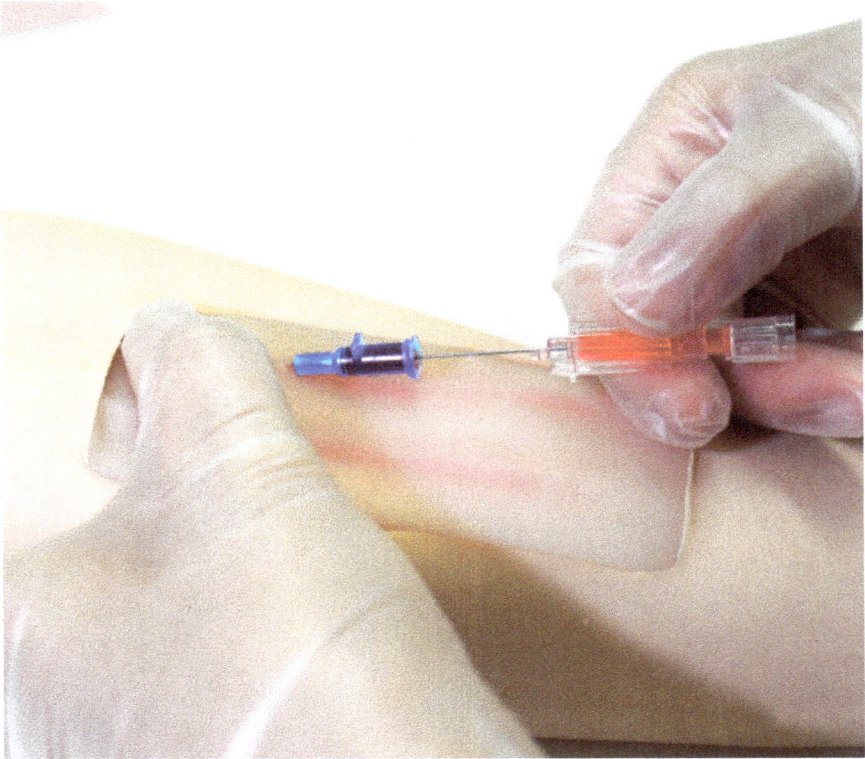

Fig.1.5.3. Inserting a 22G cannula

Complications
- Failure of the procedure
- Damage to arteries or nerves
- Hematoma or bleeding at the insertion site
- Thrombophlebitis (Mbamalu & Banerjee, 1999)
- Leakage
- Anaphylaxis (rare): Usually due to the medication rather than the line
- Vasovagal syncope

Post-Procedure care

- Tell the patient to notify the nursing staff if (TeachMe Surgery, 2018):
- The cannula site becomes painful, red, hot, or swollen
- The area around the cannula feels wet or the dressing is coming loose
- The cannula is limiting their self-care
- Thank the patient and leave the patient's bedside.
- Ensure the correct cannula insertion documentation is filled out completely and placed in the patient's notes.
- Inform the nursing staff and place any cannula care pathway stickers into the nursing notes
- Ideally, the cannula should be checked and flushed 3 times a day and should be removed after 72hrs.

Further reading

Medscape- Intravenous Cannulation: https://emedicine.medscape.com/article/1998177-overview

References

GMC. (2019). Consent for treatment. General Medical Council UK. https://www.nhs.uk/conditions/consent-to-treatment/

Mbamalu, D., & Banerjee, A. (1999). Methods of obtaining peripheral venous access in difficult situations. Postgrad Med J, 75(886), 459-462. https://doi.org/10.1136/pgmj.75.886.459

Schoenfeld, E., Shokoohi, H., & Boniface, K. (2011). Ultrasound-guided peripheral intravenous access in the emergency department: patient-centered survey. West J Emerg Med, 12(4), 475-477. https://doi.org/10.5811/westjem.2011.3.1920

TeachMe Surgery. (2018). Intravenous Cannulation. TeachMe Surgery. Retrieved 25 Nov. 2021 from https://teachmesurgery.com/skills/clinical/cannulation/

| 6 |

Cannulation – Intraosseous

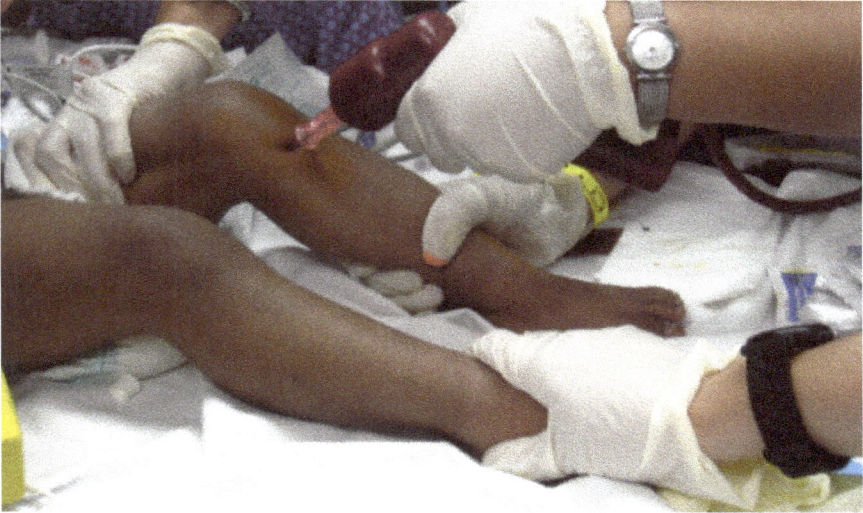

Overview

Intraosseous (IO) cannulation is the insertion of a firm needle through cortical bone and into the medullary cavity (Liu, 2020a). IO cannulation is a fast and reliable intervention to secure vascular access in a critically ill or injured patient when peripheral or central venous access is challenging or delayed (Whitney & Langhan, 2017). Any fluid or substance routinely administered via IV (including medication and blood products) may be given by intraosseous infusion (Liu, 2020a).

Objectives

- By the end of this chapter, you should be able to:
    - Describe the indications of IO cannulation.
    - Evoke contraindications of IO cannulation

○ Recall the complications following IO cannulation

○ Describe the technique of performing IO cannulation

Indications

- Urgent venous access is required after 3 failed attempts at venous cannulation
- Difficulty in establishing venous access, as in the following settings: Burns, Obesity, Oedema, Seizures
- Condition necessitating rapid high-volume fluid infusion, such as the following: Hypovolemic shock, Burns
- Afford access to the systemic venous circulation, as with the following: Cardiopulmonary arrest, Burns, Blood draws, Local anaesthesia, and Medication infusion.

Contraindications

- Fracture in the target bone
- Previous, significant orthopaedic surgery at the insertion site, prosthetic limb or joint.
- IO in past 48 hours in the target bone
- Infection at the area of insertion
- Excessive tissue (severe obesity) and/or absence of adequate anatomical landmarks

Equipment

- Antiseptic solution (e.g., chlorhexidine, povidone-iodine, alcohol)
- Towels (rolled up)
- Gloves
- Intraosseous needles and sometimes insertion device
- Syringes, 5 to 60 mL, based on anticipated need
- Sterile saline, for flushes
- Sterile gauze (eg, 10 cm × 10 cm squares)
- IV connection tubing and fluids

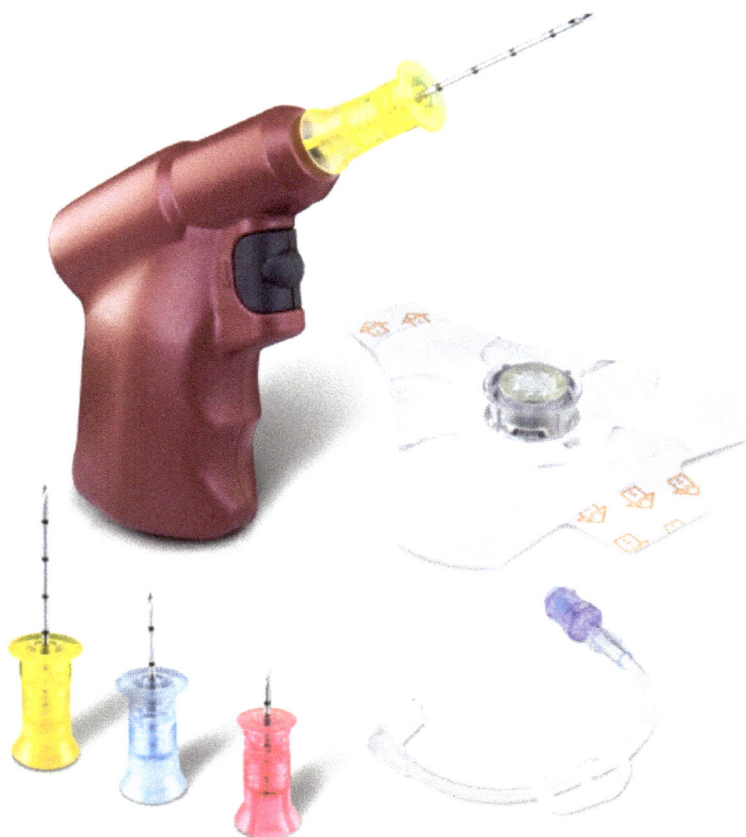

Fig1.6.1. Drill and IO needles different sizes

- *Optional equipment (if the patient is conscious)* **(Liu, 2020a):**
    - Local anaesthetic (1% lidocaine without epinephrine, a 25- or 22-gauge needle, a 3- or 5-mL syringe)
    - Intramedullary anaesthetic (2% lidocaine, preservative-free IV solution)
- *EZ-IO Needle selection (based on the weight of the patient):*
    - Pink 15mm (3-39kg)
    - Blue 25mm (40kg and above)
    - Yellow 45mm (excessive tissue or humerus)

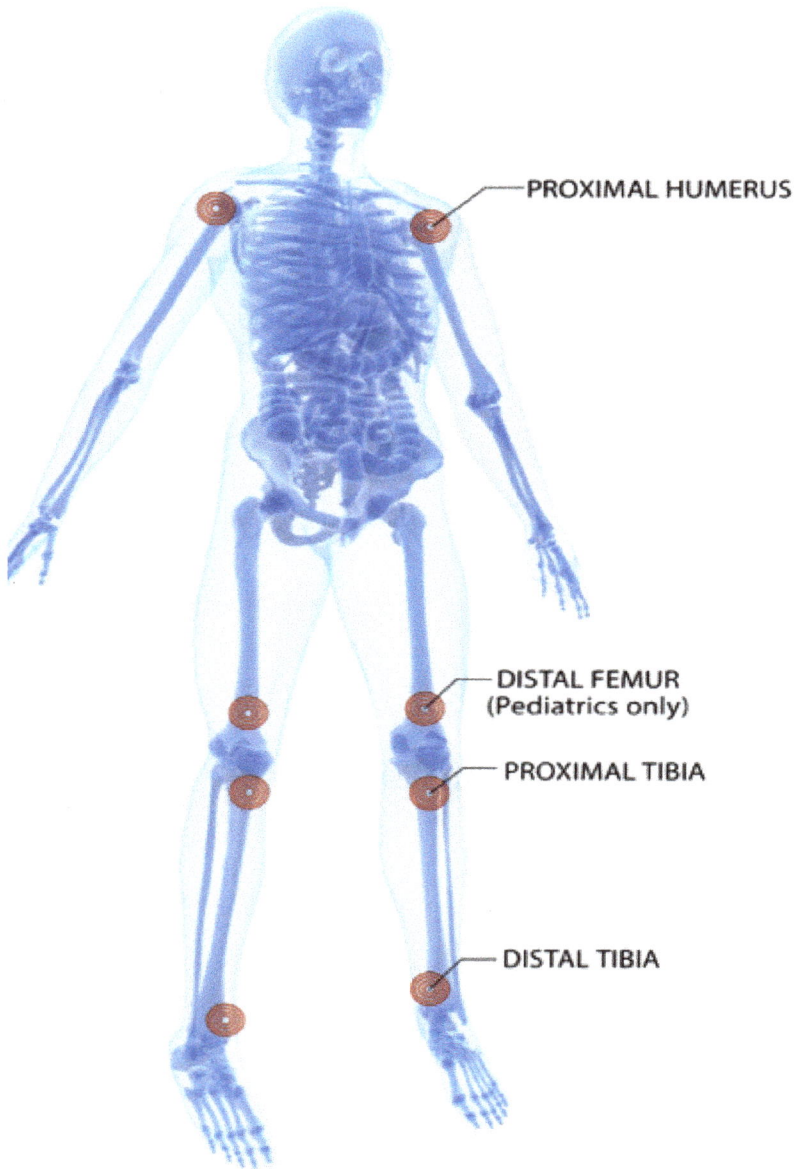

Fig.1.6.2. Landmarks for intraosseous cannulation

Landmarks

If possible, avoid areas of burns or of skin infection.

- Proximal tibia: Anteromedial surface, 2-3 cm below the tibial tuberosity
- Distal tibia: Proximal to the medial malleolus
- Distal femur: Midline, 2-3 cm above the external condyle
- Sternum, Deltoid, Iliac crest

Consent

According to the GMC, the consent can be (GMC, 2019):

- *Informed consent*: the patient should be provided with all the information about what the procedure involves, including the benefits and risks, whether there are reasonable alternative treatments, and what will happen if the procedure fails.
- *Verbal consent*: The patient says they're happy to have the procedure done
- *Implied consent*: Assuming that the patient has extended the limb or voluntarily exposed the area for the puncture.
- *Voluntary:* the decision to either consent or not to consent to the procedure must be made by the patient and must not be influenced by pressure from medical staff, friends, or family.

All adults are presumed to have sufficient capacity to decide on their own medical treatment unless there's significant evidence to suggest otherwise (GMC, 2019).

- **Capacity**: the patient must be capable of giving consent, which means they understand the information given to them and can use it to make an informed decision.

- In case of emergency or if a person **does not have the capacity** to decide about their treatment and they have not appointed a lasting power of attorney (LPA), emergency physicians should go ahead with the procedure if they believe it's in the person's best interests.
- If children are able to consent, they usually consent themselves. But someone with parental responsibility may need to give consent for a child up to the age of 16 to have treatment.

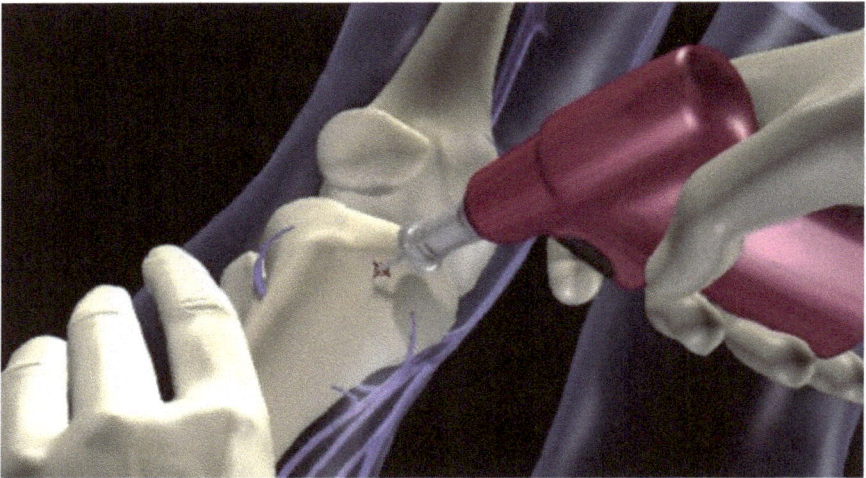

Fig.1.6.3. Proximal tibia IO insertion site

Procedure

- Identify landmarks
- Clean skin
- Place the relevant needle on a drill and remove the safety cap
- Progress needle through the skin to bone
- 5 mm of the catheter (at least one black line) must be visible outside the skin.
- Drill needle perpendicular into the bone at the site with gentle, constant pressure
- When needle tip contacts bone there should be 5mm of catheter visible outside of the skin (if not you may need a longer needle)

- Continue drilling through bone until "give" or "pop" occurs, and needle tip enters medullary space
- Remove stylet (caution: stylet is extremely sharp - place in a sharps container)
- Attach the manufacturer's extension set (helpful if this is pre-flushed with saline and/or lidocaine)
- Aspirate blood/marrow to confirm placement
- If the patient is awake, slowly infuse 2% lidocaine (cardiac lidocaine) 2-3mL through the IO line (IO infusion is painful as the marrow cavity expands)
- Flush saline through extension set to expand marrow cavity (helps ensure adequate flow rates)
- Apply the dressing

Considerations

- Any lab can be sent from an IO blood sample
- It is important to be cognizant of the correlation between certain labs when obtained via IO vs IV.
- There is no reliable correlation with Sodium, Potassium, CO_2, and calcium levels (Miller et al., 2010).
- Potassium is often elevated due to haemolysis
- WBCs are higher and platelet counts are lower
- Only need to discard 2mL of blood before sending it to the lab
- Any medication that can be given in peripheral IV can be given through IO.
- RSI medications can be given through IO with the same efficacy using the same doses as IV medications.
- Drips or IV fluids should be dispensed with a pressure bag or infusion pump.

Complications

- Failure to enter the bone marrow, with extravasation or subperiosteal infusion
- Through and through penetration of the bone

- Osteomyelitis (rare in short term use)
- Growth plate injury
- Local infection,
- Skin necrosis,
- Pain
- Compartment syndrome,
- Fat and bone microemboli have all been reported (rare)

Post-procedure care

- Intraosseous infusion should be limited to emergency resuscitation of the child and discontinued as other venous access has been obtained.
- All IO lines should be removed within 24 hours of the insertion time or earlier if there is any sign of extravasation (i.e., progressive pain or swelling at the insertion site).

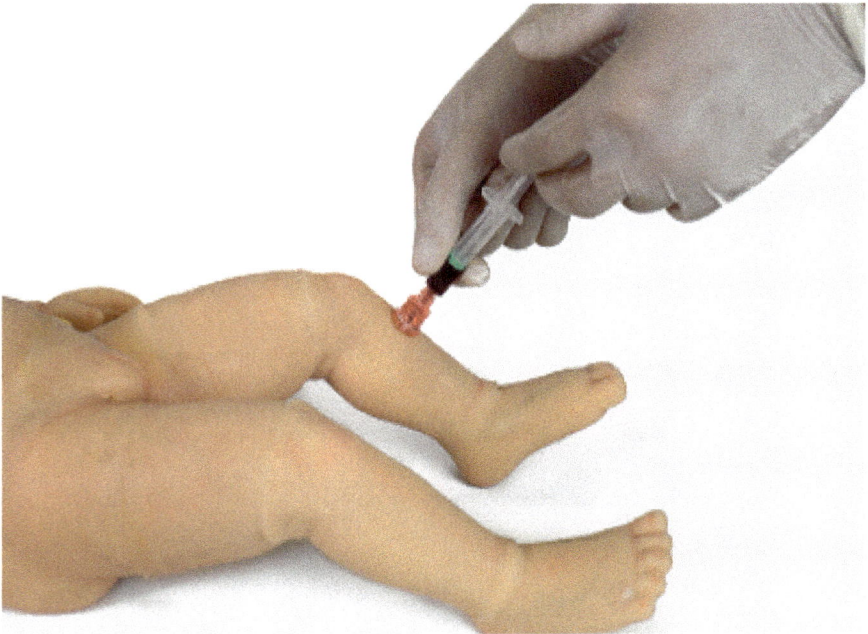

Fig.1.6.4. Blood aspiration from IO needle

Further reading

ATLS® - Advanced Trauma Life Support, 10th Edition - Student Course Material - Copyright© 2018 American College of Surgeons.

References

GMC. (2019). Consent for treatment. General Medical Council UK. https://www.nhs.uk/conditions/consent-to-treatment/

Liu, Y. T. (2020a). How To Do Intraosseous Cannulation, Manually and With a Power Drill. MSD Manuals. Retrieved 26 Nov. 2021 from https://www.msdmanuals.com/en-gb/professional/critical-care-medicine/how-to-do-peripheral-vascular-procedures/how-to-do-intraosseous-cannulation,-manually-and-with-a-power-drill

Miller, L. J., Philbeck, T. E., Montez, D., & Spadaccini, C. J. (2010). A new study of intraosseous blood for laboratory analysis. Arch Pathol Lab Med, 134(9), 1253-1260. https://doi.org/10.5858/2009-0381-oa.1

Whitney, R., & Langhan, M. (2017). Vascular Access in Pediatric Patients in the Emergency Department: Types of Access, Indications, and Complications. Pediatr Emerg Med Pract, 14(6), 1-20.

| 7 |

Cannulation - Central Venous

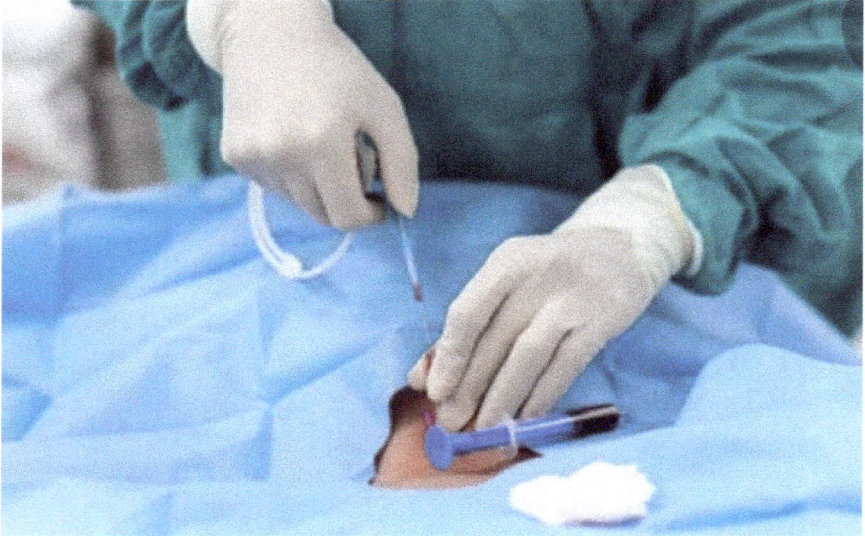

Overview

Central venous catheter insertion is an essential procedure commonly performed for the care of critically ill patients (Kolikof et al., 2021). A central line is typically inserted applying a sterile procedure unless a patient is unstable, in which case sterility may be a secondary concern. In 1994, around 200,000 central venous catheters were inserted in the United Kingdom, and the number is presumably higher today (Smith & Nolan, 2013). In practice, they are three potential sites for CVL insertion in the adult patient (internal jugular vein, femoral vein, and subclavian vein).

The right internal jugular vein and left subclavian vein are the most straightforward routes to the right atrium via the superior vena cava. The femoral veins are compressible sites, and they are suitable for coagulopathic patients. The subclavian vein approach is at higher risk for pneumothorax than the internal jugular vein approach. Ultrasound guidance can benefit all approaches and is the recommended approach (Smith & Nolan, 2013).

Objectives

- By the end of this chapter, you should be able to:
    - Explain the indications and contraindications for central venous catheter insertion.
    - Describe the technique involved in central venous catheter insertion.
    - Review the common complications of central venous catheter insertion.

Indications for CVC

- **Access for drugs**
    - Infusion of irritant drugs—for example, chemotherapy
    - Total parenteral nutrition
    - Poor peripheral access
    - Long term administration of drugs, such as antibiotics
- **Access for extracorporeal blood circuits**
    - Renal replacement therapy
    - Plasma exchange
- **Monitoring or interventions**
    - Central venous pressure
    - Central venous blood oxygen saturation
    - Pulmonary artery pressure
    - Temporary transvenous pacing
    - Targeted temperature management
    - Repeated blood sampling

Contraindications to CVC

- **Absolute:**
  - Infection overlying insertion site
  - Ipsilateral indwelling central vascular devices
  - Ipsilateral Haemothorax or Pneumothorax
  - Distortion of landmarks by congenital anomalies or trauma.
  - Any vascular injury proximal or distal to the insertion site (traumatic injuries).
  - Vessel thrombosis, Stenosis, or Disruption
- **Relative:**
  - Coagulopathy
  - Thrombocytopenia, which seems to correlate with a greater risk of adverse events.
  - Uncooperative awake patient.
  - Morbid obesity

Consent

According to the GMC, the consent can be (GMC, 2019):

- *Informed consent:* the patient should be provided with all the information about what the procedure involves, including the benefits and risks, whether there are reasonable alternative treatments, and what will happen if the procedure fails.
- *Verbal consent:* The patient says they're happy to have the procedure done
- *Implied consent:* Assuming that the patient has voluntarily exposed the site for the insertion of the CVC.
- *Voluntary:* the decision to either consent or not to consent to the procedure must be made by the patient and must not be influenced by pressure from medical staff, friends, or family.

All adults are presumed to have sufficient capacity to decide on their own medical treatment unless there's significant evidence to suggest otherwise (GMC, 2019).

- *Capacity:* the patient must be capable of giving consent, which means they understand the information given to them and can use it to make an informed decision.
- In case of emergency or if a person **does not have the capacity** to decide about their treatment and they have not appointed a lasting power of attorney (LPA), emergency physicians should go ahead with the procedure if they believe it's in the person's best interests.
- If children are able to consent, they usually consent themselves. But someone with parental responsibility may need to give consent for a child up to the age of 16 to have treatment.

Equipment for CVC

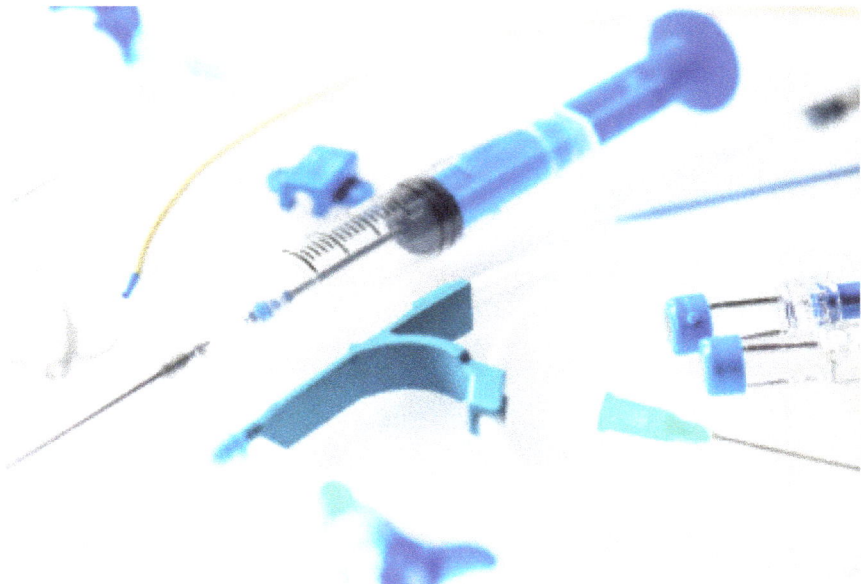

Fig.1.7.1. Central venous catheterisation kit

- Ultrasound and sterile ultrasound sheath
- Sterile trolley
- Sterile field, gloves, gown and mask
- Seldinger central line kit
- Saline flush
- Chlorhexidine
- Lignocaine (4ml (2 vials) of 2% is reasonable)
- Suture
- Scalpel
- Sterile dressing
- Pressure bag to attach to monitoring

Procedure

The steps are as follows:

- Obtain consent as above
- Wash hands and don sterile gown and gloves
- Clean the field and use a sterile area.
- Ensure that you have spare gauze swabs ready.
- Apply sterile sheath to the ultrasound probe
- Confirm anatomy
- Infiltrate the skin with 1% lidocaine next to the insertion site.
- If using landmarks for the subclavian vein CVL, the needle should be inserted roughly 1 cm inferior to the junction of the middle and medial third of the clavicle.
- If using landmarks for the femoral line CVL, the needle insertion site should be positioned almost 1 cm to 3 cm below the inguinal ligament and 0.5 cm to 1 cm medial to where the femoral artery is pulsated.
- For the subclavian CVL, the needle can be inserted at an angle as close to parallel to the skin as possible until contact is made with the clavicle, then advanced under and along the inferior aspect of the clavicle.

- Next, direct the tip of the needle towards the suprasternal notch until venous blood is aspirated.
- Insert the introducer needle with negative pressure until venous blood is aspirated, then stop advancing the needle.
- Meticulously withdraw the syringe and thread the guidewire through the introducer needle hub.
- While still holding the guidewire in place, remove the introducer needle hub.

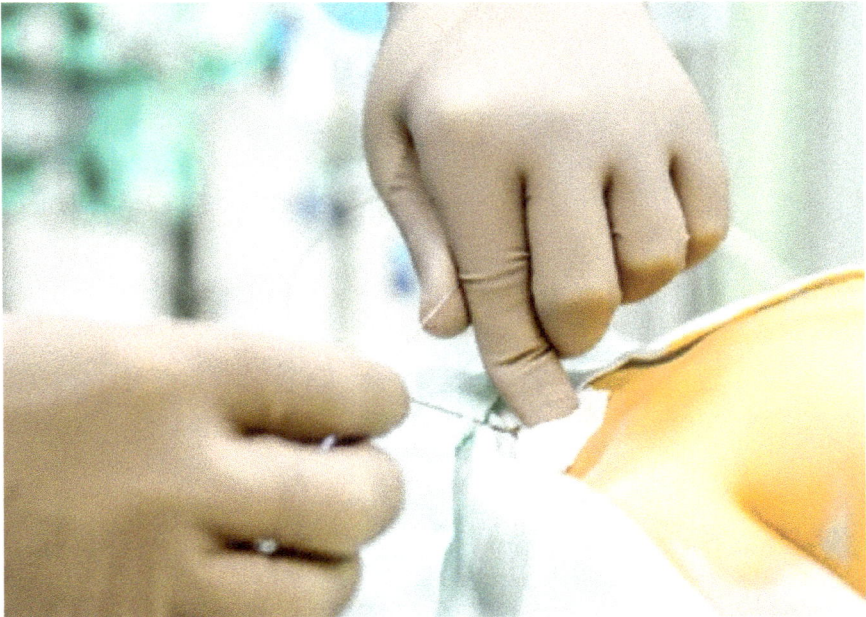

Fig.1.7.2. Insertion of the subclavian central catheter

- If possible, utilise the ultrasound to verify the guidewire insertion in the vessel in two different views.
- Next, handle the scalpel tip to create a little stab in the skin against the wire to accommodate the dilator which is inserted using a twisting motion.
- Remove the dilator and thread the catheter over the Seldinger wire.

- Do not advance the line until you have hold of the end of the wire
- Once the central line is in place, remove the wire
- Aspirate and flush all lumens and re-clamp and apply lumen caps
- Suture the line to allow 4 points of fixation
- Dress with a clear dressing so the insertion point can be seen

Advantages and disadvantages of CVC:

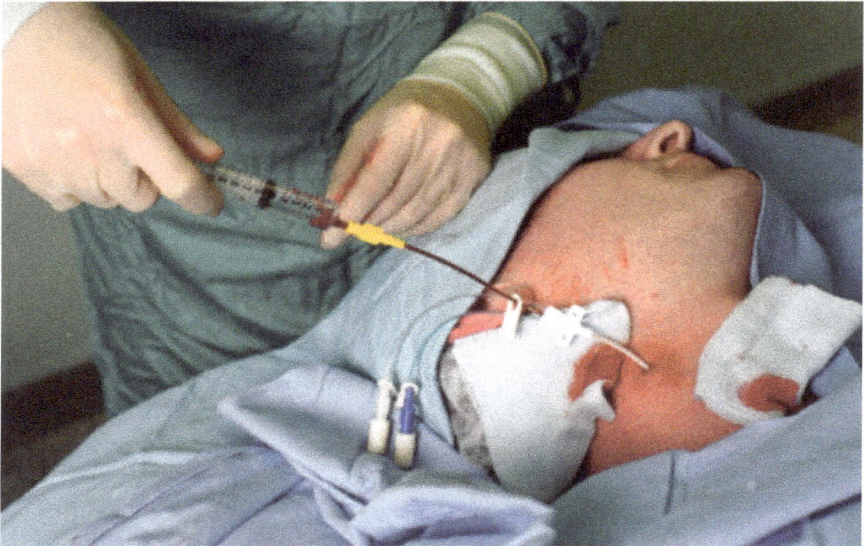

Fig.1.7.3. Central venous catheter insertion

1. External jugular:

Advantages:

- Superficial vessel that is often visible
- Coagulopathy not prohibitive
- Minimal risk of pneumothorax (especially with US guidance)
- Head-of-table access
- Prominent in elderly patients
- Rapid venous access

Disadvantages:

- Not ideal for prolonged venous access
- Poor landmarks in obese patients
- High rate of malposition
- The catheter may be difficult to thread

2. Internal jugular:

Advantages:

- Minimal risk of pneumothorax (especially with US guidance)
- Head-of-table access
- Procedure-related bleeding amenable to direct pressure
- Lower failure rate with novice operator
- Excellent target using US guidance

Disadvantages:

- Uncomfortable
- Not ideal for prolonged access
- Risk of carotid artery puncture
- Thoracic duct injury possible on left
- Dressings and catheters difficult to maintain
- Poor landmarks in obese/oedematous patients
- Potential access and maintenance issues with concomitant tracheostomy
- Vein prone to collapse with hypovolemia
- Difficult access during emergencies when airway control being established

3. Subclavian:

Advantages:

- Easier to maintain dressings

- More comfortable for the patient
- Better landmarks in obese patients
- Accessible when airway control is being established

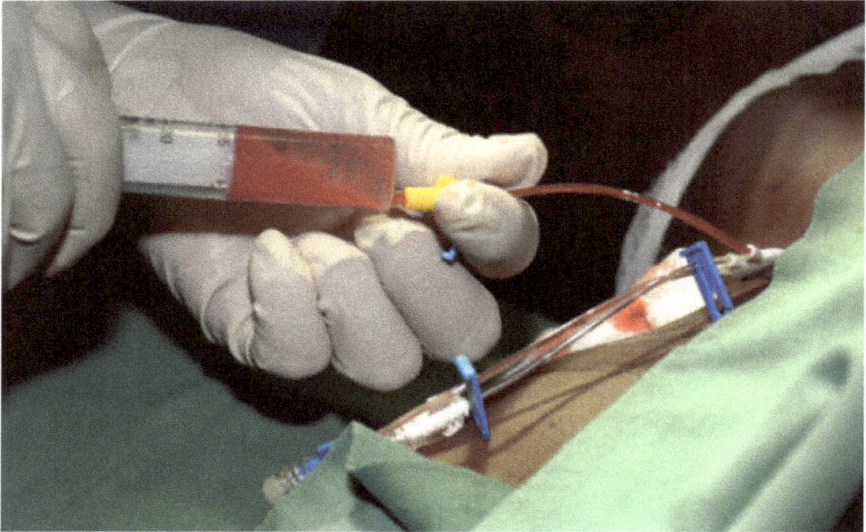

Fig.1.7.4. Flushing of the central line immediately after insertion

Disadvantages:

- Increased risk of pneumothorax
- Procedure-related bleeding less amenable to direct pressure
- Decreased success rate with inexperience
- Longer path from skin to the vessel
- Catheter malposition is more common (especially right SCV)
- Interference with chest compressions

4. Femoral:

Advantages:

- Rapid access with a high success rate
- Does not interfere with CPR
- Does not interfere with intubation
- No risk of pneumothorax

  • Trendelenburg position not necessary during insertion

Disadvantages:

  • Delayed circulation of drugs during CPR
  • Prevents patient mobilization
  • Difficult to keep site sterile
  • Difficult for PA catheter insertion
  • Increased risk of iliofemoral thrombosis

Complications

Immediate

  • Bleeding
  • Pneumothorax
  • Haemothorax
  • Arterial puncture
  • Lesions of lymphatic vessels
  • Lesions of the brachial plexus
  • Arrhythmia
  • Air embolism
  • Thoracic duct injury (with left SC or left IJ approach)
  • Catheter malposition

Delayed

  • Infection
  • Venous thrombosis
  • Pulmonary emboli
  • Catheter migration
  • Catheter embolization
  • Myocardial perforation
  • Nerve injury

Post-procedure care

A chest x-ray is needed to confirm that the tip of a jugular (or sub-clavian) CVC lies in the superior vena cava near its junction with the right atrium (the catheter can be advanced or retracted if not in the appropriate position) and to confirm that pneumothorax has not occurred (Ferrada, 2020).

Further reading

Michael Bannon et al. -Anatomic considerations for central venous cannulation: https://www.ncbi.nlm.nih.gov/pmc/articles/PMC3270925/

References

Ferrada, P. (2020). How To Do Internal Jugular Vein Cannulation. MSD Manual. https://www.msdmanuals.com/en-gb/professional/critical-care-medicine/how-to-do-central-vascular-procedures/how-to-do-internal-jugular-vein-cannulation

GMC. (2019). Consent for treatment. General Medical Council UK. https://www.nhs.uk/conditions/consent-to-treatment/

Kolikof, J., Peterson, K., & Baker, A. M. (2021). Central Venous Catheter. Statpearls. Retrieved 25 Nov. 2021 from https://www.ncbi.nlm.nih.gov/books/NBK557798/

Smith, R. N., & Nolan, J. P. (2013). Central venous catheters. BMJ, 347. https://doi.org/10.1136/bmj.f6570

Tse, A., & Schick, M. A. (2021). Central line placement. Statpearls. Retrieved 25 Nov. 2021 from https://www.ncbi.nlm.nih.gov/books/NBK470286/

| 8 |

Cardioversion & Pacing

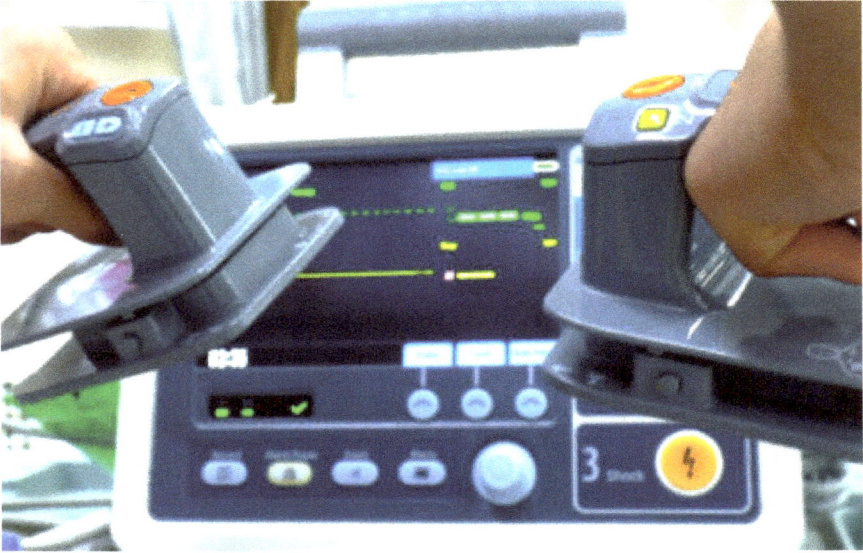

Unsynchronized Cardioversion or Defibrillation is the therapeutic act of administering a transthoracic electrical current to depolarise the myocardium so coordinated contractions can occur. The procedure is usually indicated to a person experiencing one of the two lethal ventricular dysrhythmias, ventricular fibrillation (VF) or pulseless ventricular tachycardia (VT) (Goyal et al., 2021). Under Advanced Cardiac Life Support (ACLS) guidelines, pulseless VT and VF are treated the same.

Synchronize Cardioversion or Electrical Cardioversion, or Cardioversion is the application of electricity to convert a still perfusing rhythm (e.g., ventricular tachycardia with a pulse, supraventricular tachycardias including atrial arrhythmias) to allow a normal sinus rhythm to restart. It is indicated for hemodynamically unstable patients who present in ventricular tachycardia (VT), supraventricular tachycardia (SVT), atrial flutter, and atrial fibrillation (AF). Cardioversion and pharmacologic cardioversion may also be considered for stable patients with these dysrhythmias.

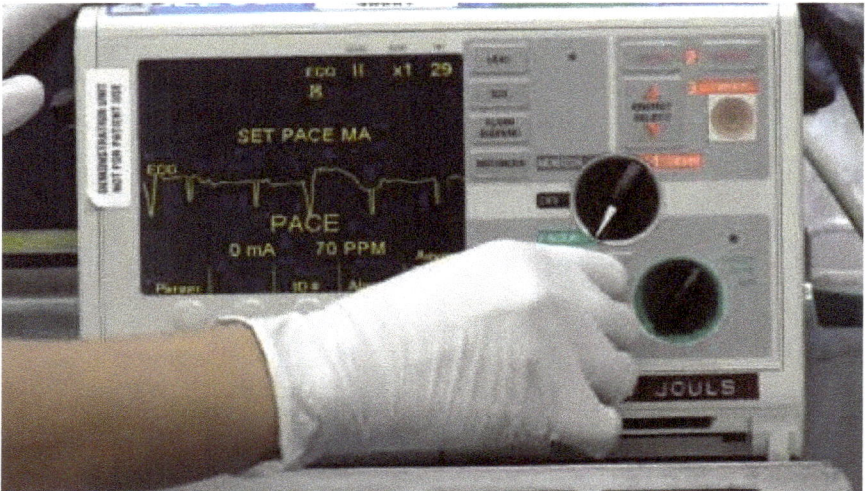

Fig.1.8.1. Pacing mode

Transcutaneous Pacing (TCP) is a temporary means of pacing a patient's heart during an emergency and stabilizing the patient until a more permanent means of pacing is achieved. It is accomplished by delivering pulses of electric current through the patient's chest, stimulating the heart to contract.

1. Unsynchronized Cardioversion

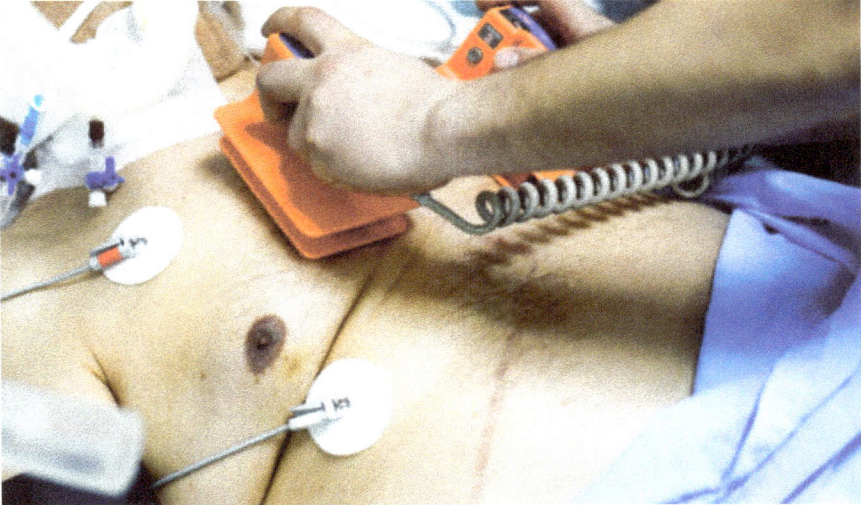

Overview

Defibrillation is a valuable and standard treatment for ventricular fibrillation (VF) and pulseless ventricular tachycardia in patients with cardiac arrest in the emergency department (Choi & Noh, 2021). The term defibrillation (shock success) is commonly described as the termination of VF for at least 5 seconds following the shock (Gliner & White, 1999; White, 1983). VF often recurs after successful shocks, but this recurrence should not be equated with shock failure (Van Alem et al., 2003). Furthermore, shock success using the typical definition of defibrillation should not be confused with resuscitation outcomes such as restoring a perfusing rhythm (ROSC), survival to hospital admission, or survival to hospital discharge (Cummins et al., 1991).

Objectives

- By the end of this section, you should be able to:
  - ◦ Recall the indication of defibrillation in the ED

○ Understand the importance of rapid defibrillation in VF and pulseless VT.

○ Summarize the steps involved in the termination of VF or pulseless VT with defibrillation.

○ Translate the technique of cardiac defibrillation in a patient experiencing sudden cardiac arrest secondary to ventricular dysrhythmia.

Indications

- Ventricular fibrillation (VF)
- Pulseless ventricular tachycardia (VT)
- Cardiac arrest due to or resulting from VF

Contraindications

- **Absolute**

  ○ Conscious patient

  ○ Presence of a pulse

  ○ Pulseless electrical activity (PEA)

  ○ Asystole

  ○ Multifocal atrial tachycardia

  ○ Defibrillation without knowing the rhythm

  ○ Second defibrillation before 2 min (or five cycles) of CPR,

  ○ An advanced directive, Physician Order for Life-Sustaining Treatment (POLST), indicating no cardiopulmonary resuscitation (CPR) or do not resuscitate (DNR)

- **Relative**

  ○ Potential electrical catastrophe (explosive environment [i.e., operating rooms])

  ○ Dysrhythmias due to enhanced automaticity such as in digitalis toxicity and catecholamine-induced arrhythmia (because the mechanism of tachycardia remains after the shock)

Factors that are no contraindications

- Chest trauma.
- Automatic implantable cardiac defibrillators (AICDs).
- The patient is on a wet or moist surface.
- Piercings on the chest.

Materials and Medications

- Electrocardiogram (ECG) monitor/defibrillator.
- Self-adhesive defibrillation pads or defibrillation paddles (paddles may be more successful than self-adhesive pads, but they have more complications and pose more danger to operators).
- Conductive gel for Defibrillation paddles (not ultrasound gel).
- ECG electrodes.
- Supplemental oxygen.
- Intubation equipment as needed

Procedure

- Defibrillation should be promptly performed in conjunction with or before administration of induction or sedative agents to facilitate intubation.
  - Assess the ABCs (airway, breathing, circulation).
- Open the airway with a head tilt/chin lift (or jaw thrust in a suspected traumatic patient).
- If the patient is apnoeic, provide breaths with a bag-valve-mask (BVM) and observe chest rise.
- Check for pulses. If absent, start CPR.
- CPR should be initiated before any shock while getting all equipment ready for at least 2 min to provide adequate circulation to the brain and heart.
  - Wipe off the patient's chest if moist or wet.
  - Remove transdermal patches, jewellery, and piercings if possible.
- Attach ECG electrodes to the patient.

- The self-adhesive defibrillation pads or defibrillation paddles can be used as ECG electrodes to access the rhythm.
- **Paddles:**
    - ○ With conductive gel applied to the metal surface, place one paddle on the patient's right chest, just below the clavicle, near the sternal border.
    - ○ The other should be on the left chest, midaxillary line above the fifth or sixth intercostal space.
    - ○ The long axis of the paddles should be perpendicular to the ribs to allow for better transduction of current through the chest.

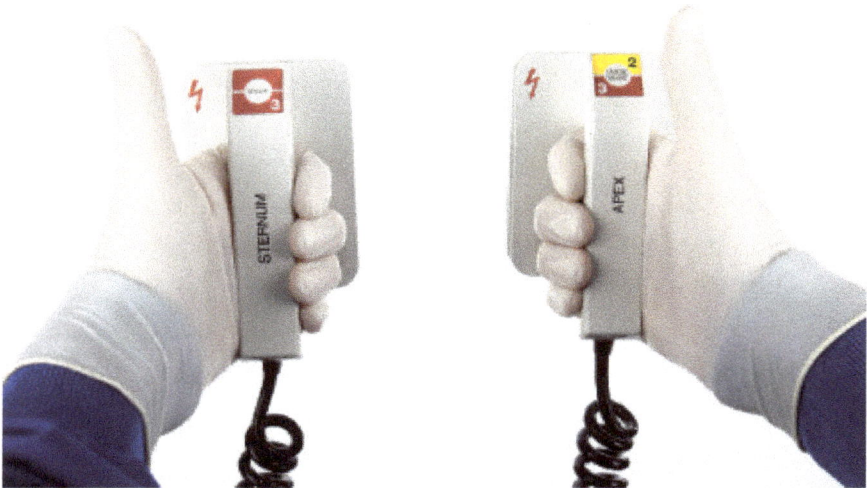

Fig.1.8.2. Defibrillator paddles

- **Pads:**
    - ○ Same placement as paddles, except that pad, can be placed in any orientation if they are in full contact with the chest. If a lot of breast tissue is present, push the tissue to one side or lift it away and place the paddles or pads underneath.

■ An error in pad or paddle placement can distort the rhythm into looking like a rhythm that does not require defibrillation.

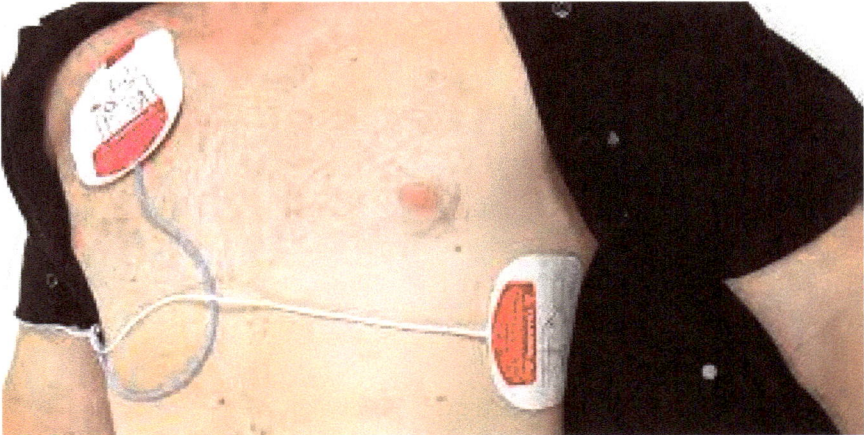

Fig.1.8.3. Defibrillator pads placement

- Place the ECG monitor/defibrillator into a mode to acquire a rhythm from the pads or paddles. Then, stop CPR and assess the rhythm and pulse for no longer than 10 s.
- If VF or pulseless VT is observed, switch the defibrillator to charge mode.
- Charge to 200 J. Continue CPR while the defibrillator is being charged.
- When the defibrillator indicates that it is charged, clearly order that everyone stop touching the patient and observe no physical contact before defibrillating the patient.
- If using the paddles, apply extra force to the chest through the paddles to deflate the lungs to allow for better defibrillation. The operator should observe a muscle twitch during defibrillation.
    ○ Restart CPR for 2 min or five cycles.
- Another operator may charge (but not fire) the defibrillator while CPR is being performed to expedite the time between pulse/rhythm check and the initiation of a shock.

- After 2 min or five cycles of CPR, assess the rhythm and pulse repeat steps above and give appropriate Advanced Cardiac Life Support (ACLS) medications.
- If the successful return of spontaneous circulation (ROSC) occurs, initiate the hypothermia protocol per hospital guidelines.

Complications

- Skin burns (most common and likely due to improper technique).
- Injury to cardiac tissue (myocardial necrosis secondary to burn): ST-segment elevation that lasts longer than 2 min usually indicates myocardial injury unrelated to the shock.
- Abnormal heart rhythms (usually benign like atrial, ventricular, and junctional premature beats).

2. Synchronized Electrical Cardioversion

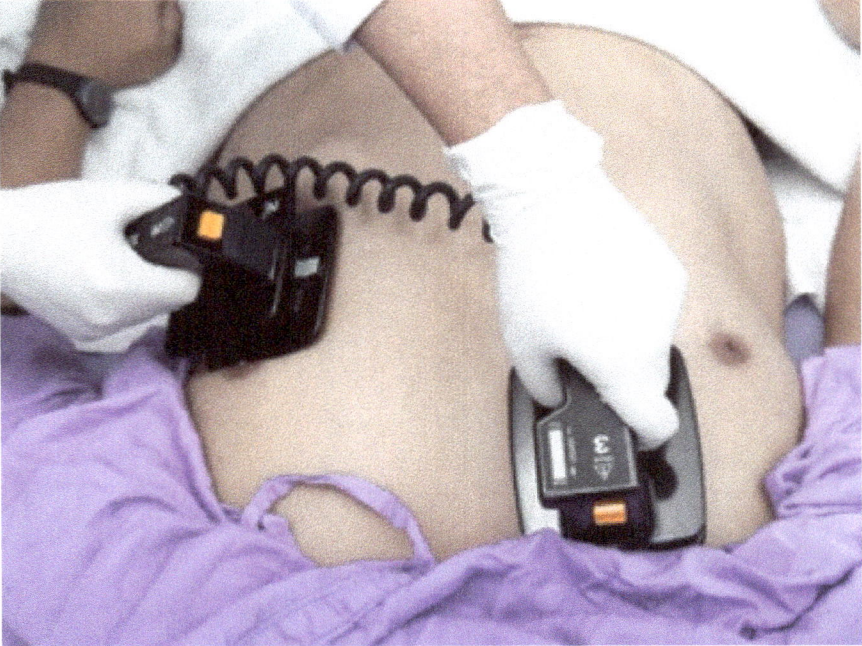

Overview

Synchronized cardioversion is shock delivery that is timed (synchronized) with the QRS complex. This synchronization avoids shock delivery during the relative refractory portion of the cardiac cycle when a shock could produce VF. Synchronized cardioversion is recommended to treat supraventricular tachycardia due to reentry, atrial fibrillation, atrial flutter, and atrial tachycardia. Synchronized cardioversion is also recommended to treat monomorphic VT with pulses. Cardioversion is not effective for the treatment of junctional tachycardia or multifocal atrial tachycardia (Link et al., 2020).

Objectives

- By the end of this section, you should be able to:
  - Recall the indication of cardioversion in the ED
  - Understand the importance of cardioversion in tachyarrhythmias.
  - Summarize the steps involved in the cardioversion of tachyarrhythmias in the ED.
  - Translate the technique of electrical cardioversion in a patient with tachydysrhythmias.

Indications

- Non-sinus-rhythm tachycardias with a pulse including:
  - Atrial fibrillation
  - Atrial flutter
  - Monomorphic ventricular tachycardia (VT)
  - Refractory or unstable supraventricular tachycardia (SVT)
- *Unstable signs and symptoms including acute coronary syndrome, decreased level of consciousness, chest pain, dyspnoea, pulmonary oedema, and hypotension.*

Contraindications

- **Absolute**
  - Ventricular fibrillation and pulseless or polymorphic (irregular) VT require unsynchronized electrical cardioversion (defibrillation), not synchronized cardioversion.
  - Known atrial thrombus.
  - Sinus tachycardia.
- **Relative**
  - Digitalis toxicity-related tachycardia
  - Atrial fibrillation of greater than 48 h duration without anticoagulation
  - Multifocal atrial tachycardia
  - Electrolyte abnormalities

○ Left atrial diameter greater than 4.5 cm

○ Patients with a low probability of maintaining sinus rhythm and readily return to atrial fibrillation

○ Patients with sick sinus syndrome or sinoatrial blockage who will require a pacemaker for maintenance of stable rhythm

Materials and Medications

- Airway management equipment (laryngoscopes, endotracheal tubes)
- Cardiac monitoring, pulse oximetry, end-tidal CO2 monitoring
- Cardioverter/defibrillator
- Sedation and analgesic medications.

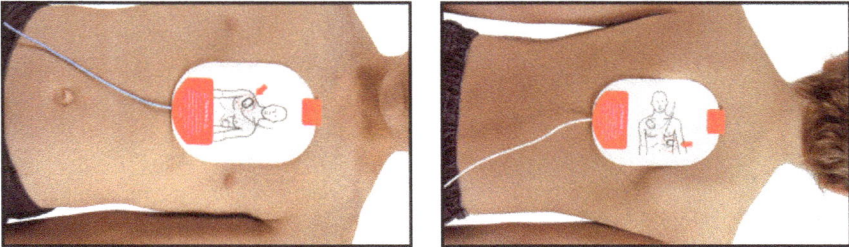

Fig.1.8.4. Paediatric pads placement for cardioversion
EM Safety Services

Procedure

- Obtain a 12-lead ECG and intravenous (IV) access.
- If possible, correct underlying electrolyte abnormalities that may cause or contribute to the patient's arrhythmia.
- Discuss risks, benefits, and alternatives (including pharmacological cardioversion) with the patient and obtain consent.
    ○ Prepare airway equipment and Advanced Cardiac Life Support (ACLS) code drugs.
    ○ Consider IV sedation (e.g., propofol, midazolam).
    ○ Provide IV analgesia (e.g., fentanyl, morphine).

- Place defibrillator adhesive pads (8- to 12-cm diameter in adults) or paddles on the patient.
- Paediatric-sized pads/paddles should be used if the patient is less than 10 kg.
- The first paddle/pad is placed to the right of the sternum at the second/third intercostal space.
- The second paddle/pad can be placed in one of two equally efficacious positions:
    - Anterolateral position—left fourth/fifth intercostal space in the midaxillary line.
    - Anteroposterior position—between the spine and the edge of the left scapula.
        - Turn the defibrillator/cardioverter into synchronized mode—marker above R-waves will be present.
        - Select the energy level to be delivered based on the underlying rhythm.
    - Announce that you will deliver the shock on the count of three and ensure that everyone is clear of the patient.
        - Deliver the shock by pressing the button marked "SHOCK."
    - If using paddles, apply firm pressure and keep paddles in place until shock is delivered.
        - Reassess the patient's pulse and cardiac rhythm.
        - Repeat with escalating energy in a stepwise fashion if cardioversion is unsuccessful.

Cardioversion dose

In 2010, the American Heart Association issued guidelines for initial energy requirements for monophasic and biphasic waveforms:

- *Regular VT (with pulses):* Adults: 100 J (monophasic or biphasic), 200 J for subsequent shocks

- *Atrial fibrillation:* 120–200 J (biphasic), 200 J (monophasic), 360 J for subsequent shocks
- *Atrial flutter and paroxysmal SVT:* 50–100 J (biphasic), 100 J for subsequent shocks
- *Paediatric dosage (regular and pulsed VT or SVT):* 5–1 J/kg, up to 2 J/kg for subsequent shocks.
- *Torsade de pointes:* defibrillation dose, not synchronised

Complications

- Superficial burns if there is inadequate gel.
- Induced arrhythmias (bradycardia in patients with previous inferior myocardial infarction, atrioventricular block, VT, ventricular fibrillation, asystole).
- Improperly synched cardioversion may rarely induce ventricular fibrillation.
    - Ectopy of the atria or ventricle in first 30 min after cardioversion
    - Atrial clot embolization in patients without adequate anticoagulation
- Apnoea, hypoxia, hypercarbia, or hypotension may occur from sedation/analgesia.
- Medical professionals who touch the patient during shock delivery may be shocked or burned.
- Rarely fire has occurred because of poor pad placement and a hyperoxygenated environment.

3. Transcutaneous Pacing

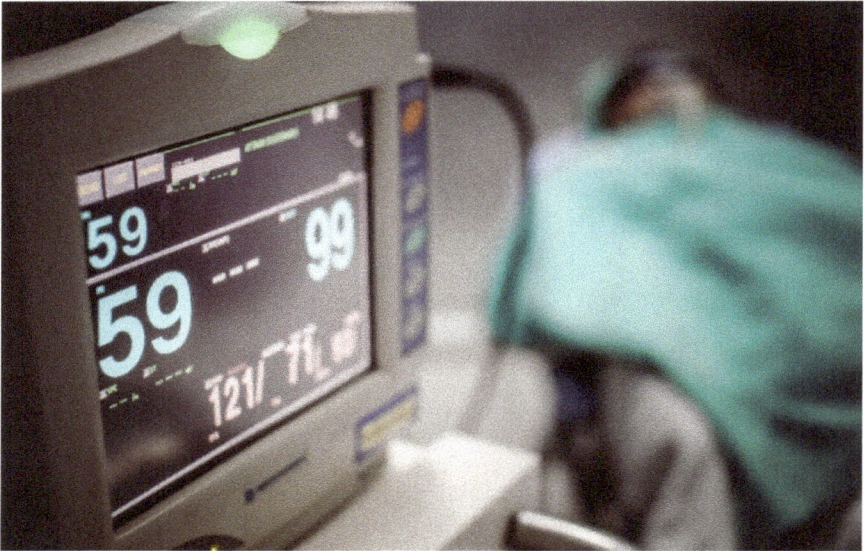

Overview

- Pacing is not effective for asystolic cardiac arrest and may delay or interrupt the delivery of chest compressions. Therefore, pacing for patients in asystole is not recommended. There are two types of artificial pacemakers: *temporary* and *permanent*.

  - Permanent (epicardial) pacemakers are implanted using a surgical procedure to treat permanent conduction problems.

  - Temporary pacemakers are used in emergencies for transient conduction disturbances or prophylactically for anticipated dysrhythmias.

    - Temporary pacemakers may be invasive (transvenous) or non-invasive (transthoracic).

    - Temporary non-invasive pacemakers are typically available to clinicians as part of a cardiac resuscitation system, complete with defibrillation, cardioversion, and monitoring capabilities.

Indications

- Hemodynamically unstable (i.e., hypotension, pulmonary oedema, chest pain, shortness of breath, or evidence of decreased cerebral perfusion) bradyarrhythmias refractory to medical therapies
- As a bridge to a transvenous or permanent pacemaker
- As an overdrive pacer in tachyarrhythmias
- Controversially, within the first 10 min of a witnessed asystolic cardiac arrest
- In children only with bradycardia associated with a known congenital cardiac defect or after cardiac surgery

Contraindications

- **Absolute**
  - None
- **Relative**
  - Bradyarrhythmia associated with hypothermia (ventricles are more prone to defibrillation-resistant fibrillation)
  - Prolonged cardiac arrest (>20 min)
  - Bradyarrhythmia in children (usually secondary to hypoxia or a respiratory issue)
  - The patient is unable to tolerate the procedure despite sedation and analgesia.

Materials and Medications

- Pacemaker device (modern units offer combined pacer and defibrillator functions)
- One set of standard electrocardiogram (ECG) electrodes
- One set of pacer pads
- Code cart and airway equipment (prophylactically)
- Sedation and analgesia (benzodiazepine and an opioid)

- Midazolam: 0.2–0.10 mg/kg IV push and may repeat with 25 % of initial dose after 3–5 min. Do not exceed 2.5 mg/ dose or a cumulative dose of 5 mg.
- Fentanyl: 1–2 mcg/kg IV slow push over 1–2 min, may repeat the dose in 30 min. (Fentanyl is the opioid of choice because it is less likely to exacerbate any hypotension.)

Procedure

- Time permitting, clean and dry the skin, and shave any excess hair off the chest.
  - Administer any appropriate sedation and analgesia.
- Attach the ECG electrodes to both the input port of the pacemaker unit and the patient.
- The white lead is placed just above the right clavicle, the black lead is just above the left clavicle, and the red lead is around the left midaxillary line.
- Attach the pacer pads either in the anteroposterior or anterolateral positions as pictured below (avoid placement over an implanted pacemaker or defibrillator.
- Turn the machine on and switch it to synchronous (or on-demand) mode.
- Asynchronous (or fixed) mode fires impulses with no regard to the intrinsic cardiac cycle, increasing the likelihood of an R on T phenomenon, which could result in ventricular tachycardia or fibrillation.
- Synchronous (or on-demand) mode will not fire an electrical impulse when a QRS complex is sensed; this is the preferred mode for transcutaneous pacing.
- Set the desired heart rate: typically, 60–80 beats/min to achieve adequate perfusion.
- Select a lead on the pacemaker unit and then press Start.
- Slowly increase the output current until electrical capture is denoted by a visible pacemaker spike, which will precede every QRS complex on the ECG monitor.

- Electrical capture is usually achieved between 50 and 100 mA.
- If a patient is unconscious or truly deteriorating quickly or in cardiac arrest, it may be prudent to set the initial currents at maximum to ensure rapid capture and then decrease the current to just above that at which electrical capture was achieved.
- After electrical capture is appreciated on the monitor, assess for mechanical capture by palpating a pulse at a rate that corresponds to the machine is set at. Improved blood pressure or the resolution of chest pain, shortness of breath, or altered mental status also suggests that the heart rate has improved, and perfusion has been restored.
- When pacing in overdrive for tachyarrhythmias, the pacer rate is set 20–60 beats/min faster than the detected tachycardic rate.
- Bear in mind that rhythm acceleration or the induction of ventricular fibrillation is a possibility with pacing, hence the recommendation of always having a code cart and airway equipment in the room.

Further reading

Update- Cardioversion: https://www.uptodate.com/contents/cardioversion-for-specific-arrhythmias

Medscape-Defibrillation & cardioversion: https://emedicine.medscape.com/article/80564-overview

Open Anaesthaesia- Transcutaneous pacing: https://www.openanesthesia.org/transcutaneous_pacing/

References

Choi, H. J., & Noh, H. (2021). Successful defibrillation using double sequence defibrillation: Case reports. Medicine, 100(10).

Cummins, R. O., Chamberlain, D. A., Abramson, N. S., Allen, M., Baskett, P. J., Becker, L., . . . Eisenberg, M. S. (1991). Recommended guidelines for uniform reporting of data from out-of-hospital cardiac arrest: the Utstein Style. A statement for health professionals from a task force of the American Heart Association, the European Resuscitation Council, the Heart and Stroke Foundation of Canada, and the Australian Resuscitation Council. Circulation, 84(2), 960-975.

Gliner, B. E., & White, R. D. (1999). Electrocardiographic evaluation of defibrillation shocks delivered to out-of-hospital sudden cardiac arrest patients. Resuscitation, 41(2), 133-144.

Goyal, A., Chhabra, L., Sciammarella, J. C., & Cooper, J. S. (2021). Defibrillation. In StatPearls. StatPearls Publishing. Copyright © 2021, StatPearls Publishing LLC.

Link, M., Atkins, D. L., Passman, R. S., . . . E., R. (2020). Part 6: Electrical Therapies-Automated External Defibrillators, Defibrillation, Cardioversion, and Pacing Circulation, 2010(122), S706–S719. https://doi.org/https://doi.org/10.1161/CIRCULATION-AHA.110.970954

Van Alem, A. P., Chapman, F. W., Lank, P., Hart, A. A., & Koster, R. W. (2003). A prospective, randomized, and blinded comparison of first shock success of monophasic and biphasic waveforms in out-of-hospital cardiac arrest. Resuscitation, 58(1), 17-24.

White, J. D. (1983). Transthoracic pacing in cardiac asystole. The American journal of emergency medicine, 1(3), 264-266.

| 9 |

Cricothyroidotomy

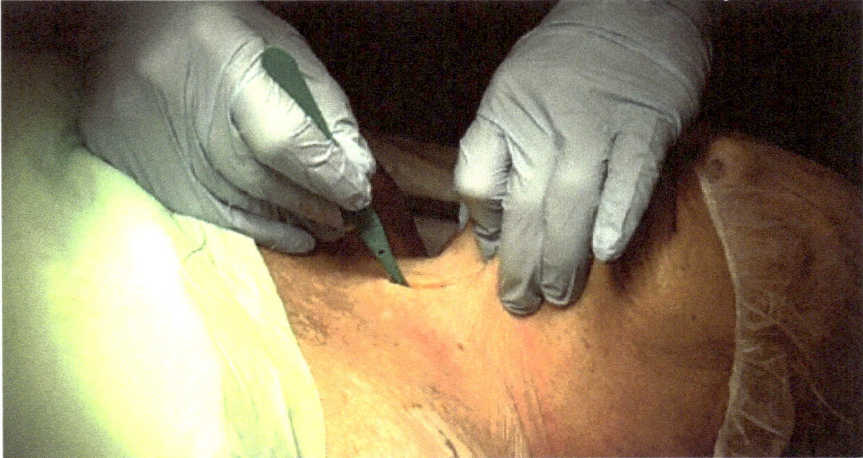

Overview

Cricothyroidotomy is an emergency procedure indicated in patients with severe respiratory distress who have failed orotracheal or nasotracheal intubation (Hsiao & Pacheco-Fowler, 2008). In other words, the procedure is used to obtain an airway when other, more routine methods are ineffective or contraindicated (Khan, 2019). The procedure requires the insertion of a tube after an incision in the cricothyroid membrane lying between the thyroid and cricoid cartilages to facilitate ventilation. Establishing an adequate airway in the face of medical emergencies is a skill that healthcare providers must master to minimise patient morbidity and prevent death (Khan, 2019). Because cricothyroidotomy is infrequently performed, emergency clinicians responsible for airway management must retain familiarity with the necessary equipment and relevant anatomy (Sakles, 2021).

Objectives

- By the end of this chapter, you should be able to:
  - Recognise the anatomical structures involved in a cricothyroidotomy.
  - Mention the indications and contraindications for a cricothyroidotomy.
  - Recognise the potential complications associated with cricothyroidotomy.

Indications

- **Can't Intubate, Can't Ventilate (CICV) scenario**
  - Trauma causing oral, pharyngeal, or nasal haemorrhage
  - Facial muscle spasms or laryngospasm
  - Uncontrollable emesis
  - Upper airway stenosis or congenital deformities
  - Clenched teeth
  - Tumour, cancer, or another disease process or trauma causing mass effect
- **Airway obstruction indications include the following:**
  - Oropharyngeal oedema (e.g., anaphylaxis)
  - Foreign body obstruction
- **The following are relative indications for cricothyroidotomy:**
  - Cervical spine immobilization secondary to injury
  - Maxillofacial injuries

Contraindications

- Airway protection is achievable using a less invasive strategy
- Tracheal transaction
- The presence of laryngeal pathology (e.g., tumour, fracture)
- Paediatric patients younger than 8 years
- Other relative contraindications to performing a cricothyroidotomy are:

○ Coagulopathy,

○ Massive neck swelling or Hematoma in the neck

○ Distortion of the anatomy.

○ Unfamiliarity with the technique

Equipment

- Yankauer suction
- Scalpel (preferably #20 blade)
- Gum elastic bougie
- Cuffed tracheostomy tube 6.0
- 10 cc syringe
- Securement device
- Ventilator and tubing

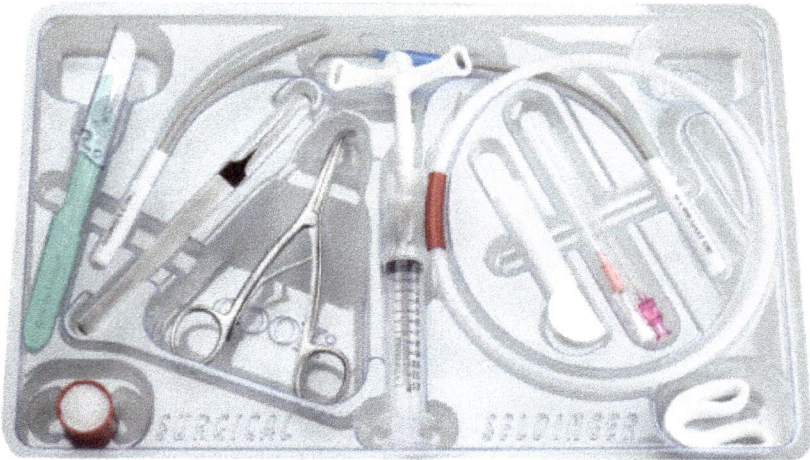

Fig.1.9.1. Can't intubate, can't ventilate emergency kit

Landmarks

- Thyroid Cartilage
- Cricothyroid Membrane/Ligament
- Cricoid Cartilage
- Trachea

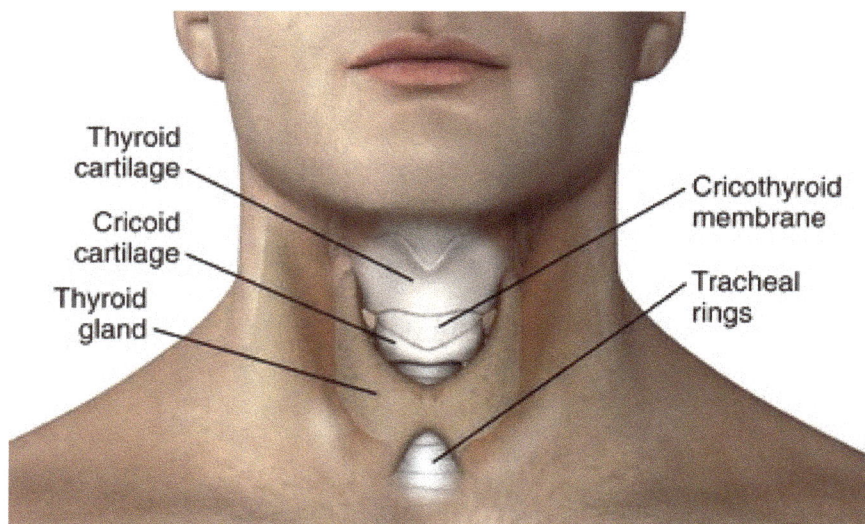

Fig.1.9.2. Cricothyroidotomy landmarks

The cricothyroid membrane is bordered superiorly by the thyroid carti-lage, inferiorly by the cricoid cartilage, and laterally by the bilateral cricothy-roideus muscles.

Pre-procedural care

- Before any intubation, especially a potential "difficult airway," a physician should go through a difficult airway algorithm, reduc-ing both the anxiety and difficulty of the final step in that path-way, the emergent cricothyrotomy.
- Identify critical neck anatomy and landmarks in case a cricothy-rotomy becomes necessary.
- Ensure that all equipment should be readily available at the bed-side (Kovacs & Sowers, 2018).
- Verbalise loudly to your team that you are in a ***can't intubate can't oxygenate*** scenario.

Procedure

- With your non-dominant hand, locate the cricothyroid membrane with your index finger while stabilizing the larynx between the thumb and middle finger.
- Create a 3-5 cm vertical incision through the skin overlying the cricothyroid membrane.
- Bluntly dissect with fingers through the subcutaneous tissue until the cricothyroid membrane is visible.

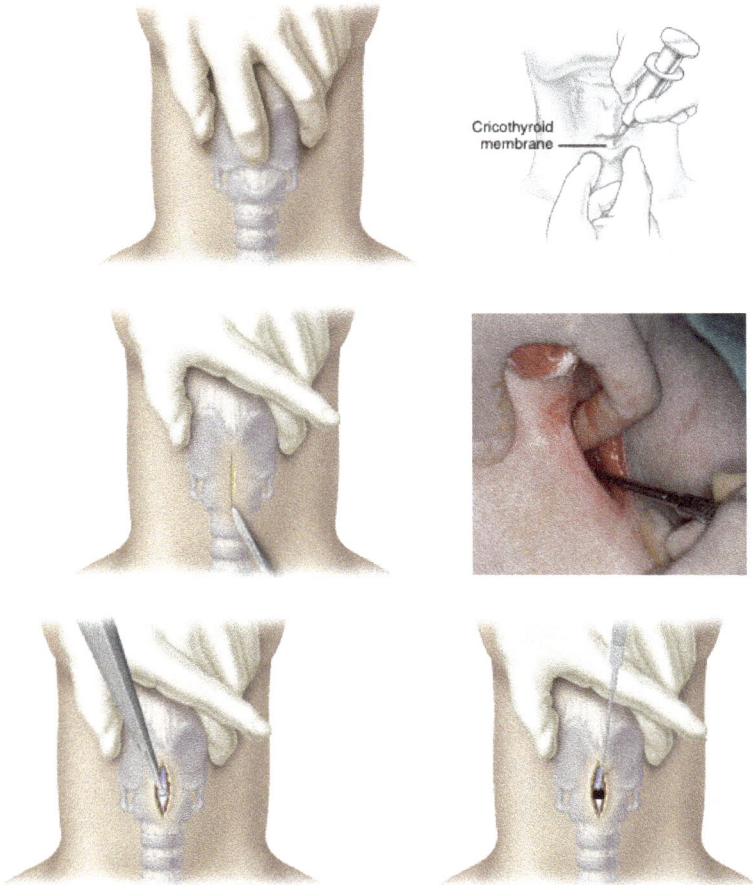

Fig.1.9.3. Step-by-step diagram of traditional surgical cricothyrotomy.
From Custalow CB: Color Atlas of Emergency Department Procedures. Philadelphia, Elsevier Saunders, 2005.

- Using the scalpel, puncture the cricothyroid membrane, slicing horizontally.
- Insert your finger through the incision.
- Slide a gum elastic bougie through the incision, using your finger to guide it inferiorly, into the trachea.
- Pass a 6.0 cuffed endotracheal tube over the bougie, until the balloon is no longer visible and inflate the cuff.
- Using a BVM, confirm placement with end-tidal capnography.
- Secure the ET tube in place with a securement device (Braude et al., 2009).

The standard technique described by Bramwell et al. (Bramwell et al., 1999):

- Immobilize the larynx and identify the cricothyroid membrane by palpation with the index finger of your non-dominant hand.
- This is achieved by identifying the inferior border of the thyroid cartilage and the superior border of the cricoid cartilage in the midline of the neck.
- While continuing to hold the larynx stable, create a vertical incision in the skin overlying the CTM in the midline of the neck, extending the incision approximately 3-5 cm in length.
- After creating your vertical skin incision, palpate the CTM and create a horizontal incision through the membrane.
- Be sure to direct your scalpel caudally to avoid the vocal cords and create the incision carefully, avoiding the posterior wall of the trachea.
- Keep the tip of your index finger in the incision through the CTM while you insert a tracheal hook into the hole, under the thyroid cartilage. Put upwards traction on the thyroid cartilage.
- Insert a trousseau dilator to extend the horizontal incision vertically.
- Insert the tracheostomy tube through the trousseau dilator and advance it caudally into the trachea.

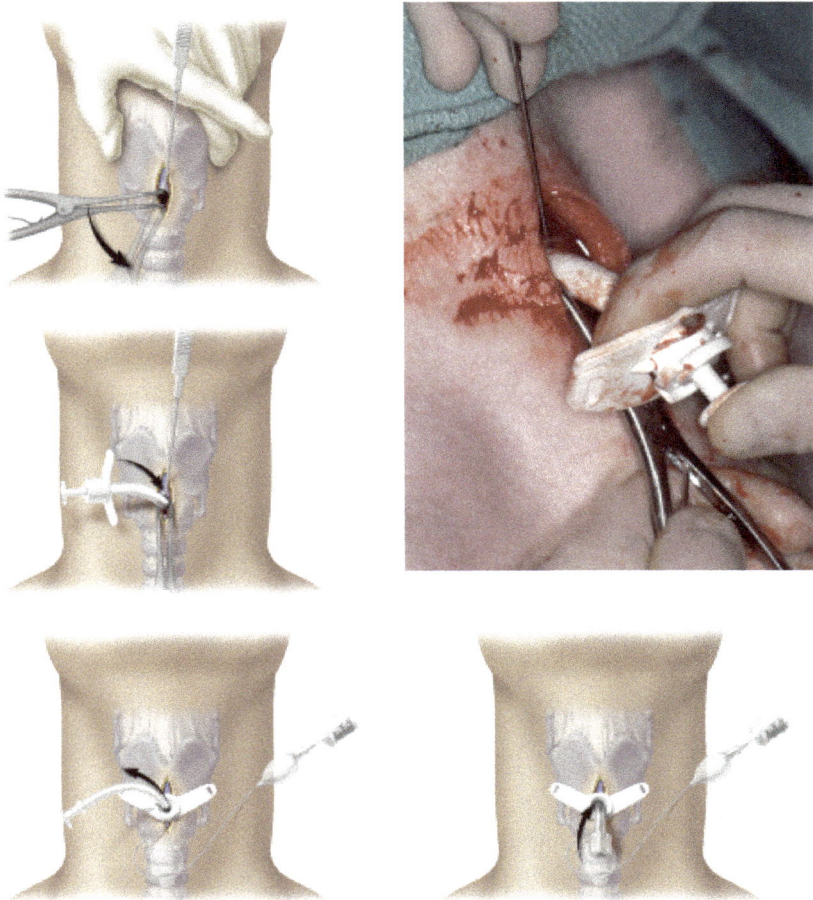

Fig.1.9.4. Step-by-step diagram of traditional surgical cricothyrotomy.
From Custalow CB: Color Atlas of Emergency Department Procedures. Philadelphia, Elsevier Saunders, 2005.

- Remove the trousseau dilator and tracheal hook.
- Remove the obturator of the tracheostomy tube.
- Insert the inner cannula of the tracheostomy tube.
- Inflate the balloon.
- Attach the tube to a BVM or ventilator.

Complications
- Bleeding

- ETT misplacement (a false passage, through the thyrohyoid membrane, unintentional tracheostomy)
- Hoarseness, dysphonia, or vocal cord paralysis
- Subglottic or laryngeal stenosis
- Damage to the thyroid cartilage, cricoid cartilage, or tracheal rings
- Perforated oesophagus
- Infection
- Aspiration

Further reading

BMJ article- Emergency cricothyroidotomy performed by inexperienced clinicians—surgical technique versus indicator-guided puncture technique: https://emj.bmj.com/content/30/8/646

References

Bramwell, K. J., Davis, D. P., Cardall, T. V., Yoshida, E., Vilke, G. M., & Rosen, P. (1999). Use of the Trousseau dilator in cricothyrotomy. J Emerg Med, 17(3), 433-436. https://doi.org/10.1016/s0736-4679(99)00012-8

Braude, D., Webb, H., Stafford, J., Stulce, P., Montanez, L., Kennedy, G., & Grimsley, D. (2009). The bougie-aided cricothyrotomy. Air Med J, 28(4), 191-194. https://doi.org/10.1016/j.amj.2009.02.001

Hsiao, J., & Pacheco-Fowler, V. (2008). Cricothyroidotomy. N Engl J Med, 358(e25). https://doi.org/10.1056/NEJMvcm0706755

Khan, H. (2019). Cricothyroidotomy. Medscape. Retrieved 2 Dec. 2021 from https://emedicine.medscape.com/article/1830008-overview

Kovacs, G., & Sowers, N. (2018). Airway Management in Trauma. Emerg Med Clin North Am, 36(1), 61-84. https://doi.org/10.1016/j.emc.2017.08.006

Sakles, J. (2021). Emergency cricothyrotomy (cricothyroidotomy). Uptodate. Retrieved 03 Dec. 2021 from https://www.uptodate.com/contents/emergency-cricothyrotomy-cricothyroidotomy

> ## *Percutaneous Transtracheal Jet Ventilation*

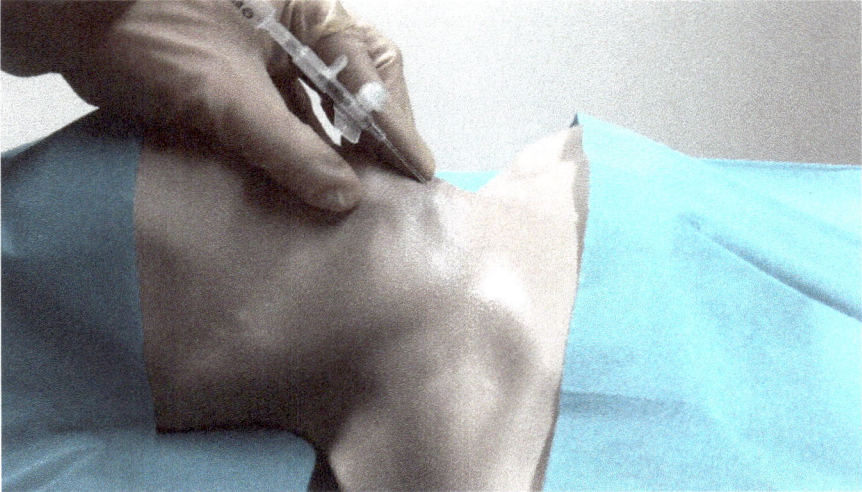

Overview

Before percutaneous transtracheal jet ventilation (PTJV) can start, a needle cricothyroidotomy must be performed. PTJV is broadly viewed as a lifesaving procedure that can provide sufficient, temporary oxygenation and ventilation with less training and complications than a surgical airway, a last resort for obtaining an airway in the algorithm. **Needle cricothyroidotomy** is an emergency airway procedure where an over-the-needle catheter is passed through the cricothyroid membrane. It provides a temporary secure airway to oxygenate and ventilate a patient in severe respiratory distress in whom less invasive techniques (e.g., bag-valve-mask ventilation, laryngeal mask ventilation, endotracheal intubation) have failed or are not likely to be successful (i.e., "can't intubate, can't ventilate") (Jorden et al., 1985; Kofke et al., 2011). **Surgical cricothyroidotomy** is an emergent airway procedure in which the incision is made in the cricothyroid membrane and passes a tracheostomy or endotracheal tube into the trachea. The standard, four-step, and Seldinger techniques are common methods of surgical cricothyroidotomy. Needle cricothyroidotomy can be achieved on patients of any age but is judged to be favoured to surgical cricothyroidotomy in infants and children up to 10 to 12 years of age because it is anatomically easier to perform with less potential injury to the larynx and surrounding structures (Chan et al., 1999; Sise et al., 1984).

Objectives

By the end of this chapter, you should be able to:

- Outline the indications for percutaneous transtracheal jet ventilation.
- Explain the contraindications of percutaneous transtracheal jet ventilation.
- Highlight the complications following a percutaneous transtracheal jet ventilation
- Describe the technique of performing percutaneous transtracheal jet ventilation.

Indications

- Failure to control the airway by other means
- As a temporary measure while preparing for definitive airway control
- Securing the airway in crash airways in infants and small children

Contraindications

- *Absolute*
  - Transection of the trachea below the cricothyroid membrane
- *Relative*
  - Inability to identify the cricothyroid landmarks
  - Anatomical distortion to the cricothyroid membrane
  - Supraglottic obstruction (preventing gas exhalation)

Equipment

- Sterile PPE (sterile gown & gloves, mask, face shield, hair net)
- 14-ga needle catheter (length ~2in)
- High-pressure non-collapsible oxygen tubing
- Oxygen source with the flow at 10-15L/min
- Plastic syringe, 3mL, Luer lock tip
- Inner adapter of 7.5 mm endotracheal tube

Pre-procedural care

- Positioning is like surgical cricothyrotomy, placing patient supine with head in a neutral position
- Set up materials listed above, attach 3-5mL syringe containing 1-2 cc of sterile NS to large-bore needle catheter.
- Prep the neck with chlorhexidine.
- Put on sterile gear.

Procedure

- Attach the tubing and the hand-operated regulator valve to wall oxygen and place the distal end of the tubing near the patient in preparation for ventilation.
  - Adjust the regulator to maximum pressure, 50 psi if possible.
  - Palpate the cricothyroid membrane just distal to the thyroid prominence.
- Sterilise the area with a suitable cleansing agent.
- Use the thumb and index finger of the non-dominant hand to stabilise the trachea for the procedure.
- Attach the TTJV catheter (or angiocatheter) to the syringe.
- Advance the catheter through the cricothyroid membrane at a 30–45° caudal direction while aspirating with the syringe.
- Return of air confirms entry into the trachea.
- If lidocaine is utilised, it can then be injected to prevent spasms during the procedure.

- Fully advance the angiocatheter and secure it while the needle and syringe are withdrawn.
- Remove the needle, secure it to the skin, and connect it to the regulator hose.
- Secure the distal end of the oxygen tubing (distal to the hand-operated valve) to the catheter.

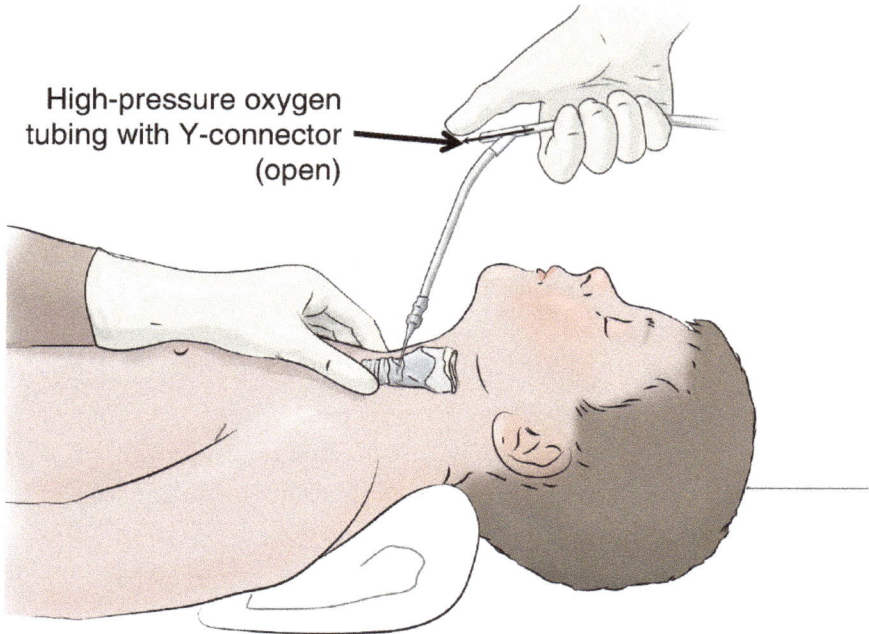

High-pressure oxygen tubing with Y-connector (open)

Fig.1.9.5. Percutaneous transtracheal jet ventilation
Credit - Morgan Schellenberg et al.

- If a BVM is used as the oxygen source:
  - Attach a 3-mL syringe to the angiocatheter.
  - Attach the BVM with the 7–0 endotracheal tube (ETT) connector to the end of the plungerless 3-mL syringe.
- Operate the valve 12–20 times a minute with long periods to allow gas exhalation and exchange.
- Preparations should be made for a definitive airway as soon as possible—preferably within 15 min.

Post-procedural care

- Kinking the catheter
- Nicking the skin prior to the procedure may prevent this
- Coughing in the conscious patient
- Usually not a problem is given most patient's unconscious
- Insert a few millilitres of lidocaine into the larynx
- Punctured the subclavian artery with a needle
- Withdraw the needle immediately
- Single SC artery puncture without laceration rarely causes harm

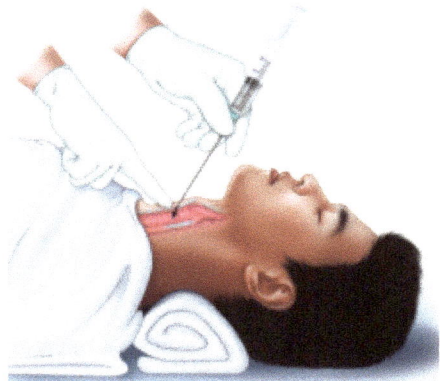

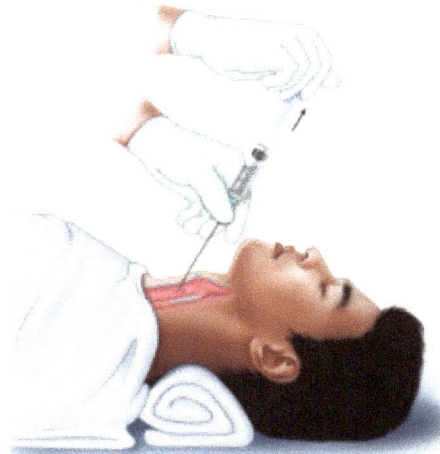

Complications

- Pneumothorax
- Pneumomediastinum
- Subcutaneous emphysema
- Catheter kink or misplacement
- Hypercarbia and respiratory acidosis
- Barotrauma
- Coughing in conscious patients
- Aspiration
- Persistent stoma

Fig.1.9.6. Percutaneous transtracheal jet ventilation
Credit - Clint Masterson

Further reading

Roberts & Hedges' Clinical Procedures in EM. 6th edition. pg 120-133

Life in the Fastlane- Cannula Cricothyroidotomy: http://lifeinthe-fastlane.com/ccc/cannula-cricothyroidotomy/

References

Chan, T. C., Vilke, G. M., Bramwell, K. J., Davis, D. P., Hamilton, R. S., & Rosen, P. (1999). Comparison of wire-guided cricothyrotomy versus standard surgical cricothyrotomy technique. J Emerg Med, 17(6), 957-962.

https://doi.org/10.1016/s0736-4679(99)00123-7

Jorden, R. C., Moore, E. E., Marx, J. A., & Honigman, B. (1985). A comparison of PTV and endotracheal ventilation in an acute trauma model. J Trauma, 25(10), 978-983. https://doi.org/10.1097/00005373-198510000-00009

Kofke, W. A., Horak, J., Stiefel, M., & Pascual, J. (2011). Viable oxygenation with cannula-over-needle cricothyrotomy for asphyxial airway occlusion. In Br J Anaesth (Vol. 107, pp. 642-643). https://doi.org/10.1093/bja/aer279

Sise, M. J., Shackford, S. R., Cruickshank, J. C., Murphy, G., & Fridlund, P. H. (1984). Cricothyroidotomy for long-term tracheal access. A prospective analysis of morbidity and mortality in 76 patients. Ann Surg, 200(1), 13-17. https://doi.org/10.1097/00000658-198407000-00002

| 10 |

End-Tidal Capnography

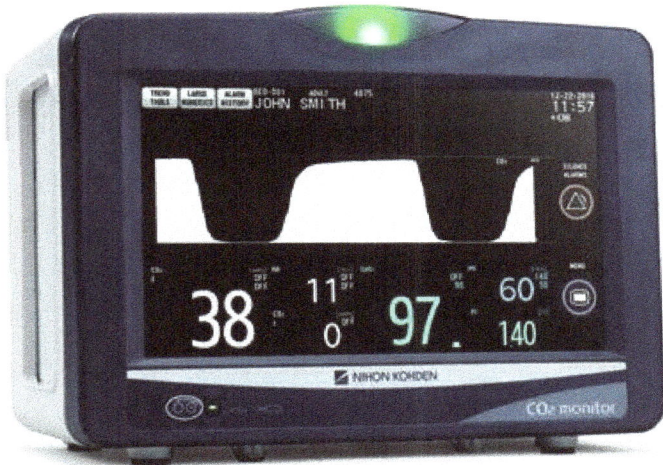

Overview

End-tidal capnography (end-tidal CO2, PETCO2, ETCO2) is a non-invasive method for continuously monitoring the partial pressure of carbon dioxide in exhaled breath (ETCO2) to evaluate a patient's ventilatory status (Page, 2013). This is depicted in a graphical form, with time on the X-axis and expired partial pressure of CO2 on the Y-axis: the result is a capnography trace or waveform (Kerslake & Kelly, 2017). The end-tidal CO2 (ETCO2) is the maximal partial pressure or concentration of CO2 in the respiratory gases at the end of an exhaled breath. Emergency physicians must always look for a non-invasive, reliable instrument to detect life-threatening conditions in patients. Capnography should be continuously monitored in all patients with an artificial airway. Failure to use capnography in patients dependent on an artificial airway contributed to more than 70% of the ICU-related airway deaths (Kerslake & Kelly, 2017).

Objectives

- By the end of this session, you should be able to:
  - Understand the basic components and phases of a capnography
  - Identify abnormal capnography waveforms as related to numerous airway-breathing-circulation problems.
  - Consider the clinical pertinence of capnography in the emergency department.
  - Make a diagnosis of specific medical conditions based on the ETCO2 graph
  - Influence the treatment decisions based on ETCO2 variations

Normal End-tidal capnography waveform

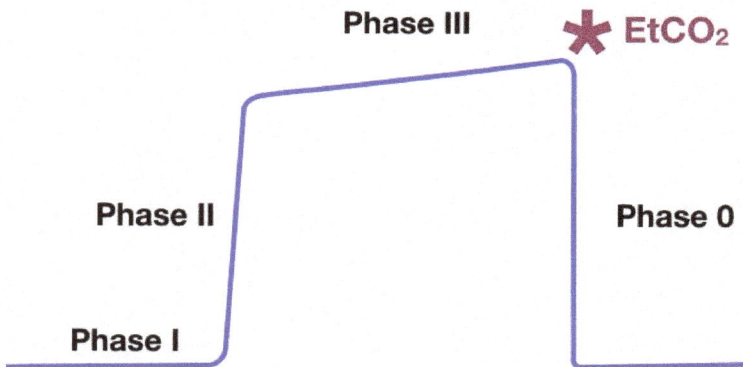

Fig.1.10.1. Normal End-tidal capnography waveform

1. **Phase I-Respiratory Baseline:** represents inspiration, and therefore no CO2 is detected. The end of phase I represents the beginning of expiration, but because the initial gases expired originate from unventilated dead space, the capnography trace remains at zero.

2. **Phase II- Expiratory Upstroke:** is a rapid uptick in the amount of CO_2 measured which represents the first gas that is being sampled from the alveoli, i.e., initial exhalation.

3. **Phase III-Expiratory Plateau:** It describes the amount of CO_2 in all the alveoli, on average. Reflects the alveolar expiratory flow (a small increase in $PECO_2$), which happens at the peak at the end of tidal expiration ($ETCO_2$). In this phase, $PECO_2$ is close to alveolar carbon dioxide tension ($PACO_2$). Note that if the alveoli all contained the same partial pressure of CO_2, phase III would be completely horizontal.

4. **Phase IV-Inspiratory Downstroke:** represents the beginning of the next breath, with the CO_2 content returning rapidly to zero.

Clinical uses of Capnography

- Confirmation of tracheal intubation
- Assessing tracheal tube and tracheostomy patency and position
- Monitoring adequacy of ventilatory support
- Use during percutaneous tracheostomy placement
- Monitoring patients with raised intracranial pressure
- Monitoring response to the treatment of bronchospasm
- Estimation of cardiac output

Arguably the most important role of capnography in cardiac arrest (with ongoing CPR) is to confirm that the airway is patent (Kerslake & Kelly, 2017).

- Capnography has several roles in cardiac arrest:
  - Confirmation that the airway is patent and present within the trachea
  - Monitoring ventilation rate during CPR and avoiding hyperventilation

- Assessing the adequacy of chest compressions during CPR
- Identifying return of spontaneous circulation (ROSC) during CPR
- Prognostication during CPR.

Limits of capnography

- End-tidal CO2 levels do not necessarily correspond to paCO2 levels obtained on arterial blood gas (Rieves & Bleess, 2021).
- Arterial – end-tidal PCO2 (a-ET PCO2) difference is, therefore, a good measure of dead space ventilation, except when the phase III plateau is steeply up-sloping, which can result in a zero or negative a-ET PCO2 difference.
- In patients with abnormal lung function, the gradient will stretch depending on the severity of the lung disease.
- EtCO2 in patients with lung disease, such as obstructive lung disease, is only useful for trending ventilatory status over time; not as a single number spot check that may or may not correlate with the pCO2 (Rieves & Bleess, 2021).
- Reduced cardiac output, poor pulmonary perfusion, and pulmonary embolism are common situations that result in an increased a-ET PCO2.
- These conditions will cause an underestimation of PaCO2 from EtCO2.

Causes of Abnormal ETCO2
Flat EtCO2 trace

- Ventilator disconnection
- Airway misplaced – extubation, oesophageal intubation
- Capnograph not connected to the circuit
- Respiratory/Cardiac arrest
- Apnoea test in "brain death" dead patient
- Capnography obstruction

Increased EtCO2 trace

- **CO2 Production**
  - Fever
  - Sodium bicarbonate
  - Tourniquet release
  - Venous CO2 embolism
  - Overfeeding
- **Pulmonary perfusion**
  - Increased cardiac output
  - Increased blood pressure
- **Alveolar ventilation**
  - Hypoventilation
  - Bronchial intubation
  - Partial airway obstruction
  - Rebreathing
- **Apparatus malfunctioning**
  - Exhausted CO2 absorber
  - Inadequate fresh gas flows
  - Leaks in ventilator tubing
  - Ventilator malfunctioning

Decreased EtCO2 trace

- **CO2 production**
  - Hypothermia
  - Pulmonary perfusion
  - Reduced cardiac output
  - Hypotension
  - Hypovolemia
  - Pulmonary embolism
  - Cardiac arrest

- **Alveolar ventilation**
  - Hyperventilation
  - Apnoea
  - Total airway obstruction
  - Extubation
- **Apparatus malfunctioning**
  - Circuit disconnection (note low airway pressures)
  - Leaks in the sampling tube
  - Ventilator malfunctioning

A sudden drop in etco2 to zero "dopes"	A sudden increase in etco2
• Displacement/ Disconnection • Obstruction/ Pneumothorax • Equipment failure, • Breath Stacking	• ROSC during cardiac arrest • Correction of ET tube obstruction
Sudden change in baseline (not to zero)	**Elevated inspiratory base-line**
• Calibration error • CO_2 absorber saturated: check capnograph with room air • Water drops in analyser or condensation in airway adapter	• CO_2 rebreathing (soda-lime exhaustion) • Contamination of CO_2 monitor (sudden elevation of baseline and top line) • Inspiratory valve malfunction (elevation of the baseline, prolongation of the downstroke, prolongation of phase III)

Common capnogram patterns

1. Normal

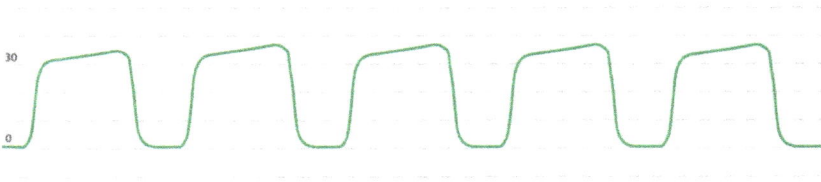

Fig.1.10.2. This is a normal capnogram that has all the phases that are easily appreciated. Note the gradual upslope and alveolar "Plateau"

2. Flatline

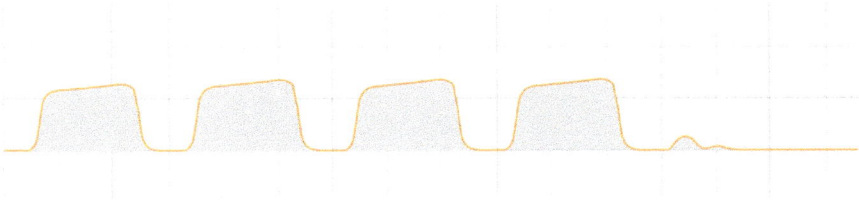

Fig.1.10.3. Initially, we notice some CO_2 returning through the tube. Subsequent breaths reveal how the end-tidal graph is dropping, the patient is becoming more hypoxic.

- **Causes of flat line:**
    - Oesophageal intubation
    - Ventilator disconnection
    - Airway obstruction (patient suddenly bit down on the tube)
    - ETT perforation (the end-tidal gas is escaping via the hole before it gets to the capnograph)
    - Capnograph disconnection or obstruction
    - Water droplet contamination of capnography module
    - Apnoea test in a brain-dead patient
    - Cardiac/respiratory arrest

3. Up-sloping plateau phase (increased alpha-angle)

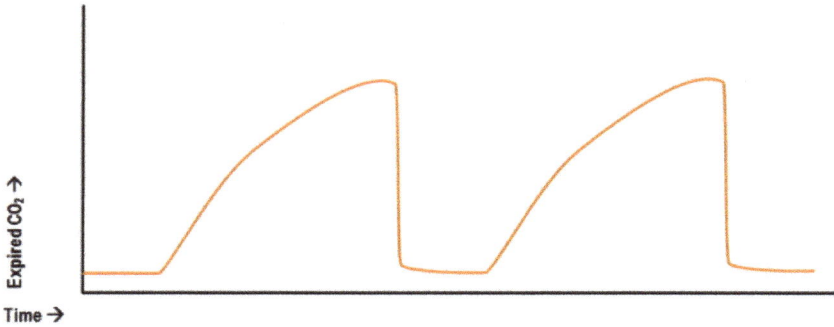

Fig.1.10.4. A Classical sawtooth slope of the asthmatic patient. As the airway obstruction in the bronchi worsens, the slope of the transitional phase becomes more gradual. Mild obstruction will produce an uptick in the slope of the top of the waveform. Severe obstruction will make the entire waveform resemble a shark fin.

- **Causes:**
  - Ventilation-perfusion mismatch
  - Lower airway obstruction: bronchospasm, asthma, COPD
  - Partial airway obstruction: pathological, secretions, tube kinking

4. Endobronchial intubation

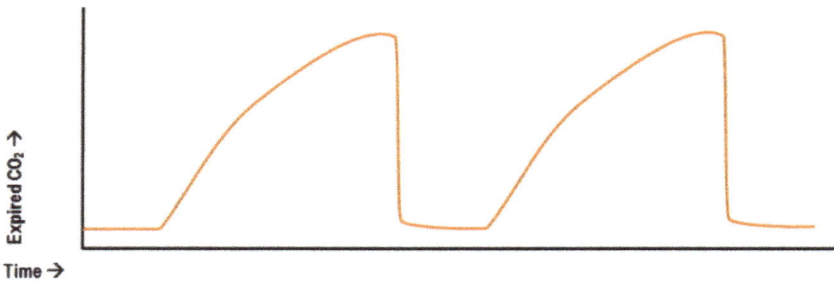

Fig.1.10.5. Bifid waveform indicates the differential ventilation of two lungs. The ETT is inserted mainly in the right main bronchus, the airflow through the right lung is the best, and right-sided gas forms the first (brisk and steep) part of the waveform. Then, appears a secondary transitional phase, which is the gas from the left lung escaping slowly up into the ETT.

5. High plateau and end-tidal CO2

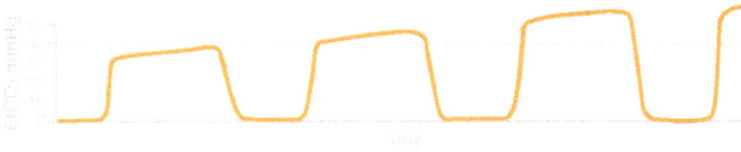

Fig.1.10.6. Hypoventilation In this capnogram, there is a gradual increase in the EtCO2. ETCO2 tracing never returns to zero baseline as the patient is rebreathing CO2. This may result from a faulty expiratory valve, or (in an anaesthetic machine) saturation of the CO2 system.

- **Possible Causes:**
  - Increased CO2 production (metabolic), e.g., malignant hyperpyrexia.
  - Respiratory depression for any reason
  - Narcotic overdose
  - CNS dysfunction
  - Heavy sedation

6. Low plateau and end-tidal CO2

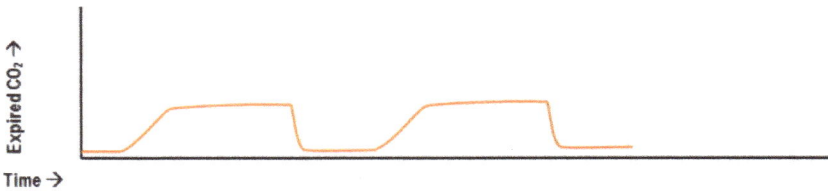

Fig.1.10.7. This is a future of hyperventilation such as in hypothermia where the total body CO2 production is significantly decreased, and the end-tidal CO2 is abnormally low. This can also be seen in a low-cardiac-output state generating a low end-tidal CO2 because there is not enough flow across the pulmonary circulation. Deep anaesthesia and muscle paralysis will result in a similar pattern.

- **Possible Causes:**
  - Cardiopulmonary arrest
  - Pulmonary embolism
  - Sudden hypotension, massive blood loss
  - Cardiopulmonary bypass

7. Progressively rising plateau and baseline

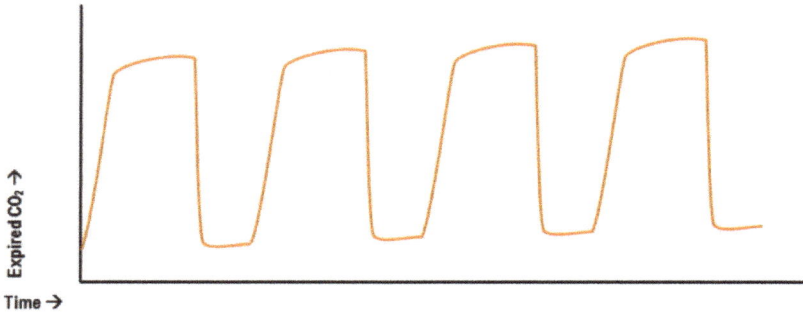

Fig.1.10.8. This feature usually appears if the CO2 absorbing lime bucket is saturated, the circuit becomes inundated with expired CO2 and the baseline gradually increases.

8. Reversal of alveolar slope in emphysema

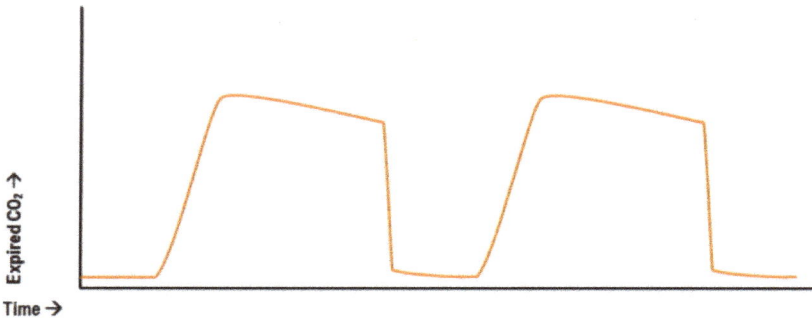

Fig.1.10.9. This is usually seen in emphysema where the alveolar slope is reversed. With a relatively poor gas exchange surface, the compliance of the lungs abnormally increases and the alveolar gas exchanges very rapidly. Therefore, the graphical representation of arterial CO2 is the early peak, not the end-tidal value. This is followed by a backward diffusion into the patient of the gas in the ventilator tubing to generate an equilibration between the higher CO2 inside the patient and the lower CO2 in the ventilator circuit, leading to a gradual drop of the total CO2 concentration in the capnograph-adjacent tubing.
Deranged physiology, 2019

9. Cardiogenic Oscillations

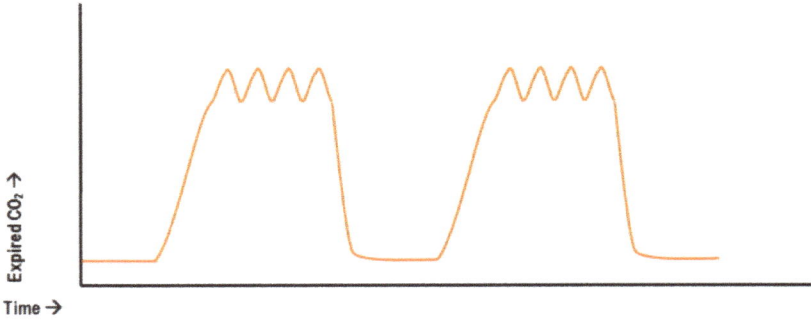

Fig.1.10.10. This is the graphical representation of an extra-large heart pulsation, transmitted to the lung parenchyma. Cardiogenic oscillations are caused by changes in thoracic volume secondary to expansion and contraction of the myocardium with each heartbeat. They are usually seen in patients with small tidal volumes and slow respiratory rates and are of little physiologic consequence.

10. Notched plateau phase

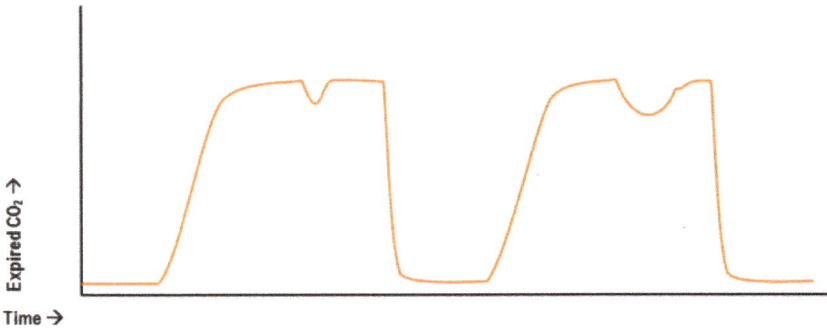

Fig.1.10.11. This capnography waveform demonstrates the "curare cleft" in the alveolar plateau. This is caused by the patient making spontaneous respiratory effort during mechanical ventilation due to neuromuscular blockade wearing off.

11. Pigtail Capnogram

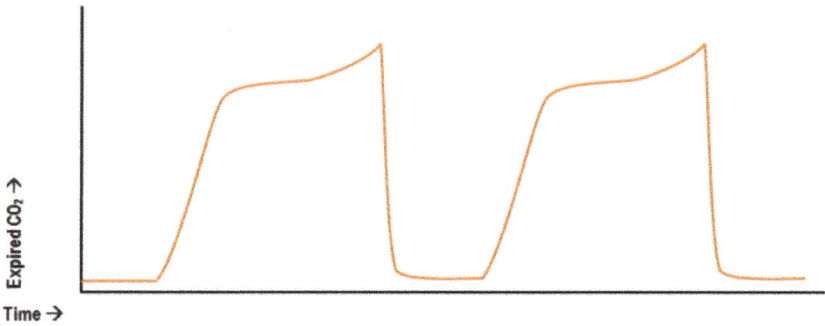

Fig.1.10.12. This is a "pigtail" capnogram seen in poor lung compliance, pregnancy, and obese patients. The sudden peak of pre-inspiratory expired CO2 is due to sudden airway closure. This happens when a poorly compliant lung breaks the last few millilitres of CO2-rich gas from the alveoli before the collapse of the lung parenchyma also occludes the small bronchi and places an end to the escape of gas.
Deranged physiology, 2019

Further Reading

EMCrit - Waveform capnography in the intubated patient by Josh Farkas: https://emcrit.org/ibcc/co2

Hamed Aminiahidashti et al., Applications of End-Tidal Carbon Dioxide (ETCO2) Monitoring in Emergency Department; a Narrative Review: https://www.ncbi.nlm.nih.gov/pmc/articles/PMC5827051/

References

Deranged physiology. (2019). Abnormal capnography waveforms and their interpretation. Deranged Physiology. Retrieved 06 Dec. 2021 from https://derangedphysiology.com/main/cicm-primary-exam/required-reading/respiratory-system/Chapter%205593/abnormal-capnography-waveforms-and-their-interpretation

Kerslake, I., & Kelly, F. (2017). Uses of capnography in the critical care unit. BJA Education, 17(5), 178-183. https://doi.org/10.1093/bjaed/mkw062

Page, B. (2013). "Riding the Waves"- The Role of Capnography in EMS. Retrieved 06 Dec. 2021 from http://centegra.org/wp-content/uploads/2013/06/Riding-the-Waves-ETCo2.pdf

Rieves, A., & Bleess, B. (2021). Be All End-Tidal: The Expanding Role Of Capnography In Prehospital Care. EMS Med. Retrieved 09 Dec. 2021 from http://www.naemsp-blog.com/emsmed/2017/3/22/be-all-end-tidal-the-expanding-role-of-capnography-in-prehospital-care

| 11 |

Escharotomy

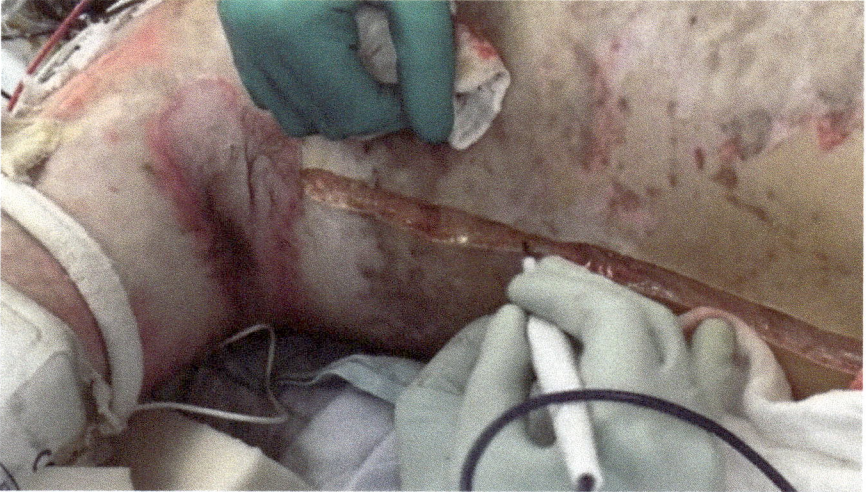

Overview

Burns typically present acutely and may be caused by heat, chemical, electrical, or radiation. Burns are classified as superficial (first degree), partial thickness (second degree) burns and full-thickness (third-degree) burns. Circumferential, full-thickness burns on limbs or trunk can create a splinting or tourniquet effect which compromises limb circulation and may reduce respiratory muscle movement, resulting in limited respiratory function (Zhang et al., 2021). An escharotomy is the surgical section of the nonviable eschar, the tough, inelastic mass of burnt tissue that results from full-thickness circumferential and near-circumferential skin burns (Pal, 2021). If left untreated, it can cause distal ischaemia, compartment syndrome, respiratory failure, tissue necrosis, or death (Zhang et al., 2021).

Objectives

- By the end of this chapter, you should be able to:
    - Outline the indications for an escharotomy.
    - Describe the technique used for escharotomy.
    - Recognise the complications of escharotomy.

Indications

The escharotomy is generally indicated within the first 48 hours of injury, due to initial injury from the primary source, and secondarily due to resuscitation and development of tissue oedema (Orgill & Piccolo, 2009):

- Full circumferential thickness burns
- Partial-thickness burns result in circulatory or respiratory compromise.

Contraindications

- Burns that will heal without surgical reconstruction (superficial burns)
- When there is no compromise to respiration or circulation.

Equipment

- Marking pen
- Sterile preparation, such as chlorhexidine or non-alcoholic povidone-iodine
- Sterile drapes
- Local anaesthetic +/- sedation
- Diathermy cauterization device
- Alginate dressing
- Scalpel +/- cutting diathermy

Pre-procedural care

- Escharotomy does not mandate multiple tools and can be performed at the bedside.

- A general anaesthetic is not usually needed, although sedation can be required.
- A local anaesthetic is needed to infiltrate unburnt skin, into which the escharotomy will extend.
- A scalpel or cutting diathermy can be used to make the incision, and a diathermy cauterization device should be used to manage the bleeding (White & Renz, 2008; Wong & Spence, 2000).

Procedure

- Clean the surgical site with povidone-iodine solution
- Drape with sterile drapes.
- Use diathermy to incise the eschar up to the subcutaneous fat.
- Consider fasciotomy with the escharotomy in case of severely burned limbs (if compartment pressures are greater than 30 mm Hg).
- Continue with the incision down through to the level of the sub-cutaneous fat until you feel an immediate release in tissue pressure with a perceptible popping sensation.
- Carry the incisions approximately 1 cm proximal and distal to the extent of the burn.

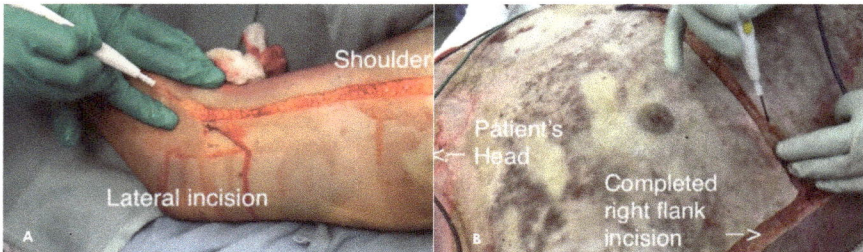

Fig.1.11.1. (A) Lateral forearm incision and (B) transverse thoracic escharotomy incision

- The incisions should extend across joints to permit for decompression of neurovascular structures.
- Careful with the neurovascular bundle
- For the escharotomy of the chest, neck, limbs, and digits, check the diagram below.

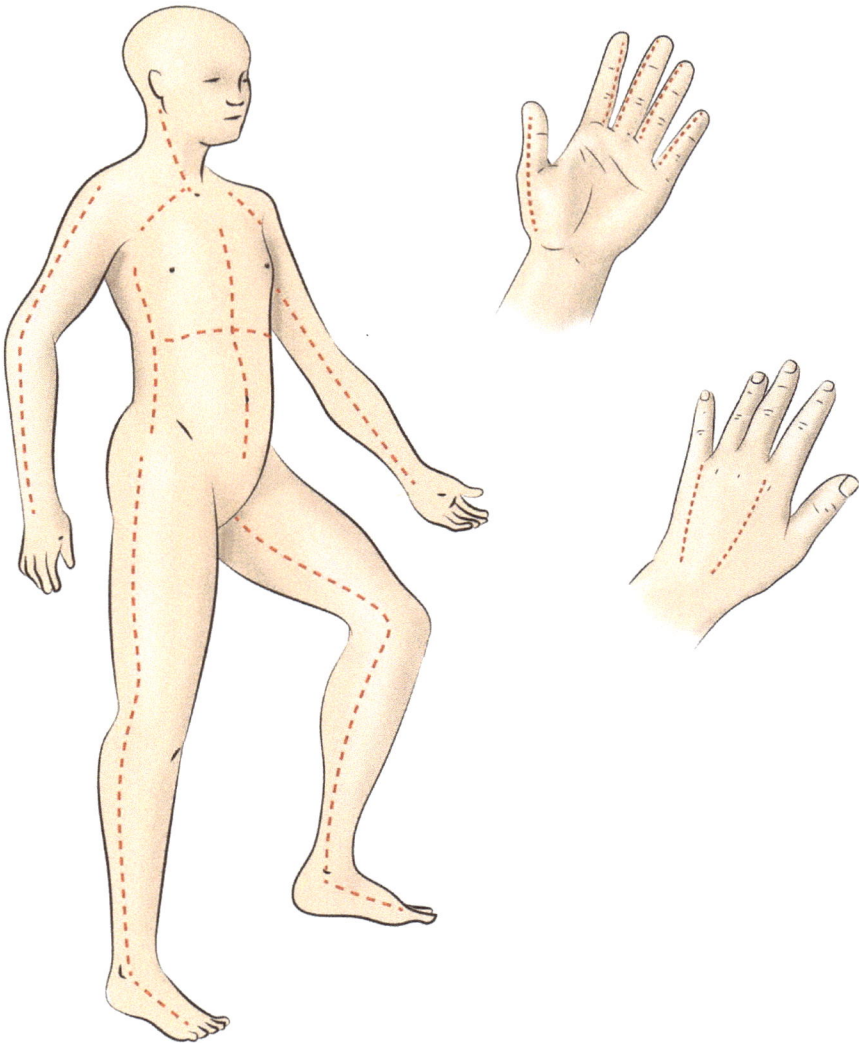

Fig.1.11.2. Diagrammatic representation of escharotomy incisions
(Yin et al., 2018)

Post-procedural care

- Use the diathermy to control bleeding from escharotomy incisions.
- Apply topical antimicrobial and dressings to prevent infection.

- Check the capillary filling pressures or compartment pressures or use a handheld doppler to assess the adequacy of the escharotomy.

Complications

- **Complications of inadequate decompression:**
  - Muscle necrosis
  - Nerve injury
  - Gangrene resulting in an amputation of the limb or digits
  - Respiratory compromise due to inadequate ventilation as a result of the compressive effect of the chest and upper torso burns
  - Abdominal compartment syndrome with visceral hypoperfusion as a result of the abdominal wall and upper torso burns
- **Systemic complications of inadequate decompression:**
  - Myoglobinuria,
  - Renal failure,
  - Hyperkalaemia,
  - Metabolic acidosis
- **Complications of an escharotomy are as follows:**
  - Excessive blood loss
  - Inadvertent fasciotomy
  - Incision/injury to the underlying healthy tissue including neurovascular structures, especially in the extremities and digits
  - Bacteraemia and septic shock
  - Infection of the open escharotomy wounds

Further reading

MSD Manual - How To Do Burn Escharotomy: https://www.msdmanuals.com/en-gb/professional/injuries-poisoning/how-to-do-

skin,-soft-tissue,-and-minor-surgical-procedures/
how-to-do-burn-escharotomy

References

Orgill, D. P., & Piccolo, N. (2009). Escharotomy and decompressive therapies in burns. J Burn Care Res, 30(5), 759-768. https://doi.org/10.1097/BCR.0b013e3181b47cd3

Pal, N. (2021). Emergency Escharotomy. Medscape. Retrieved 23 Dec. 2021 from https://emedicine.medscape.com/article/80583-overview

White, C. E., & Renz, E. M. (2008). Advances in surgical care: management of severe burn injury. Crit Care Med, 36(7 Suppl), S318-324. https://doi.org/10.1097/CCM.0b013e31817e2d64

Wong, L., & Spence, R. J. (2000). Escharotomy and fasciotomy of the burned upper extremity. Hand Clin, 16(2), 165-174, vii.

Yin, C., Demetriades, D., & Garner, W. (2018). Bedside Escharotomies for Burns. In D. Demetriades, K. Inaba, & P. D. Lumb (Eds.), Atlas of Critical Care Procedures (pp. 251-254). Springer International Publishing. https://doi.org/10.1007/978-3-319-78367-3_28

Zhang, L., Labib, A., & Hughes, P. G. (2021). Escharotomy. In StatPearls. StatPearls Publishing. Copyright © 2021, StatPearls Publishing LLCPal, N. (2021). Emergency Escharotomy. Medscape. Retrieved 23 Dec. 2021 from https://emedicine.medscape.com/article/80583-overview

| 12 |

Fasciotomy

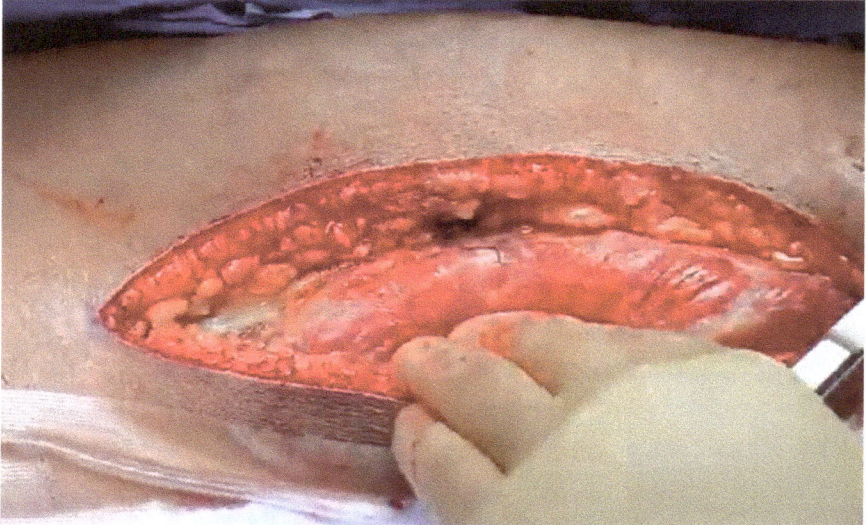

Overview

Fasciotomy is a clinical procedure that decompresses acute compartment syndrome (Wood, 2017). Compartment syndrome is caused by the combination of raised interstitial tissue pressure and the non-compliant nature of the fascia and osseous structures that make up a fascial compartment. Acute compartment syndrome often occurs in the leg and the forearm in the setting of acute trauma. Therefore, a high index of suspicion is essential for the early detection of compartment syndrome from the whole interdisciplinary team and the low threshold for intervention needed by the responsible healthcare professional (Ormiston & Marappa-Ganeshan, 2021). A fasciotomy consists of fascial incisions and remains the only effective way to treat acute compartment syndrome.

Objectives

- By the end of this chapter, you should be able to:
  - Recognise the indications for fasciotomy.
  - Describe the technique of fasciotomy.
  - Review the potential complications and clinical significance of fasciotomies.

Indications

- Classical features of compartment syndrome:
- Pain that is out of proportion to clinical findings
- Pain with passive stretch of involved muscles
- Pain with palpation of involved compartment
- Pressure increase within the compartment as measured
- A compartment pressure of 30 mm Hg is commonly an indication for fasciotomy
- *No universal agreement exists on indications for emergency fasciotomy.*

Contraindications

- There is no absolute contraindication to performing a fasciotomy.
- Delayed presentation: if the clinician suspects compartment syndrome of having been present for more than 12 hours, there is a potential risk of reperfusion injury.
- Fasciotomy 3-4 days after onset of compartment syndrome can lead to infection and kidney failure in a setting of devascularised and necrotic muscle (Arató et al., 2009).

Equipment

- Skin preparation with an antiseptic solution
- Skin scalpel
- Inside scalpel
- Forceps

- A simple hand-held retractor (Langenbeck)
- Diathermy
- Dressing

Procedure

Davey, Rorabeck and Fowler Technique: Single-incision Fasciotomy of the Leg

- The skin incision starts at the lateral malleolus and spreads proximally along the fibula for the entire length of the compartment (Wood, 2017).
- Expose the fascial layer– beware of injury to the superficial peroneal nerve at this stage.
- Create a longitudinal incision in the anterior and lateral fascial compartments.
- Recognize the soleus in the superficial posterior compartment begin to develop the plane between the distal third of the soleus and the lateral compartment.
- Remove the soleus and the deeper flexor hallucis longus from the posterior fibula. Be aware the peroneal neurovascular bundle will be immediately medial to the fibula.
- Retract the peroneal vessels posteriorly to expose the fascial attachment of the tibialis posterior to the fibula, make a longitudinal incision.
- Apply appropriate wound dressing.

Mubarak and Harges Technique: Double Incision Fasciotomy of the Leg

- **Anterolateral Incision**
  - ○ Create a 20 cm anterior skin incision centred between the crest of the tibia and the fibula.

- Identify the anterior intramuscular septum, make a longitudinal incision on either side into the anterior and lateral compartments (Wood, 2017).

- **Posteromedial Incision**
  - Create a second skin incision beginning 2 cm proximal and 2 cm superior to the medial malleolus of the tibia, extending proximally in line with the tibia longitudinally.
  - Carefully use blunt dissection to identify the fascial layer, the long saphenous vein, and the saphenous nerve; retract these anteriorly (Wood, 2017).
  - Make an incision along the length of the posterior fascial compartment.
  - Make another fascial incision over the flexor digitorum longus muscle immediately posterior and medial to the tibia to release the posterior compartment.

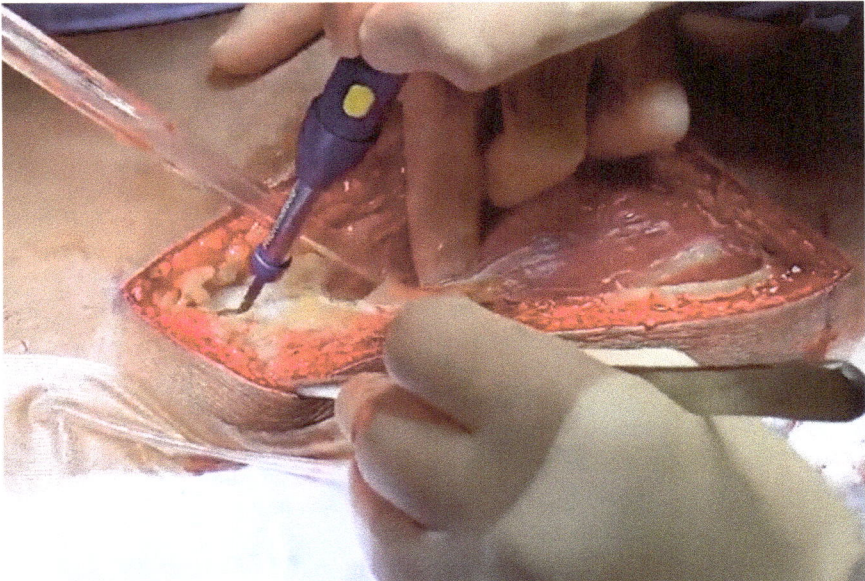

Fig.1.12.1. Fasciotomy - Incision of the fascia

Forearm Fasciotomy

- **Volar Incision**
  - Make a large skin incision starting just radial to the flexor carpi ulnaris and extending proximally to the medial epicondyle.
  - Extend the incision distally to the wrist crease, cross the wrist crease diagonally towards the hypothenar eminence, and into the palm to facilitate a carpal tunnel release.
  - Make a longitudinal incision into the superficial fascial compartment.
  - Retract the flexor carpi ulnaris, the ulnar neurovascular bundle medially.
  - Retract the flexor digitorum superficialis medially.
  - This exposes the deep fascial compartment; make a fascial incision onto the flexor digitorum profundus (Wood, 2017).
  - Extend both fascial incisions to the transverse carpal ligament.
- **Dorsal Incision**
  - Make a skin 10cm incision between the extensor digitorum communis and extensor carpi radialis brevis starting 2cm distal to the lateral epicondyle.
  - This incision will allow you to release the fascia over the mobile wad immediately.
  - Develop the subcutaneous plane posteriorly to expose the extensor retinaculum and release the fascia to decompress the posterior compartment (Wood, 2017).

Post-procedural care
- Delayed wound closure
- Elevate the affected extremity for 24-48 hours after the procedure.
- Check for complications

- Urgent referral to orthopaedic or plastic surgery

Complications

- Muscle necrosis
- Rhabdomyolysis
- Acute renal failure
- Excessive bleeding
- Infection
- Scarring
- Chronic pain
- Tissue damage that causes loss of nerve or muscle function
- Future corrective surgeries, which may include amputation

Further reading

Semantic Scholar - Lower Extremity Fasciotomy: Indications and Technique: https://www.semanticscholar.org/paper/Lower-Extremity-Fasciotomy%3A-Indications-and-Bowyer/cd4ad3fd11d2b7f9bd626960eb49fd39bf1ce4dd

References

Arató, E., Kürthy, M., Sínay, L., Kasza, G., Menyhei, G., Masoud, S., . . . Jancsó, G. (2009). Pathology and diagnostic options of lower limb compartment syndrome. *Clin Hemorheol Microcirc, 41*(1), 1-8. https://doi.org/10.3233/ch-2009-1145

Ormiston, R. V., & Marappa-Ganeshan, R. (2021). Fasciotomy. In *StatPearls*. StatPearls Publishing. Copyright © 2021, StatPearls Publishing LLC.

Wood, J. (2017). *Fasciotomy*. Medscape. Retrieved 23 Dec. 2021 from https://emedicine.medscape.com/article/1894895-overview

| 13 |

Large Joint Clinical Examination

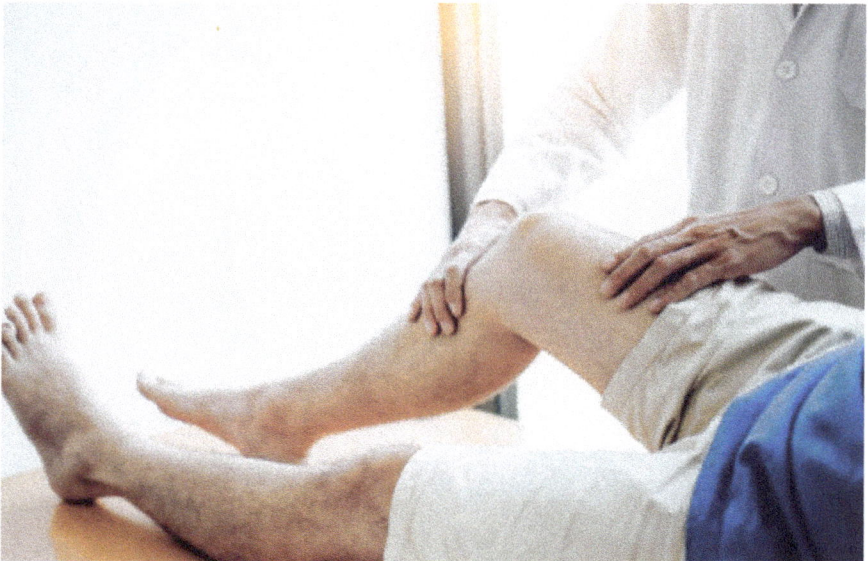

Overview

The emergency department continually encounters patients with knee conditions. This ranges from simple swelling, trauma, infection to a significant traumatic injury. The ability to correctly examine the knee is an essential tool for an emergency physician to address diagnosis and treatment correctly and must never be superseded by the imaging studies requested for the patient (Rossi et al., 2011). Accurate diagnosis mandates a good understanding of knee anatomy, typical pain patterns in knee injuries, and components of frequently encountered causes of knee pain, as well as specific physical examination skills (Calmbach & Hutchens, 2003). History taking should contain elements of the patient's pain, mechanical symptoms (locking, popping, giving way), joint effusion (timing, amount, recurrence), and mechanism of injury. Physical examination should include careful inspection, palpation, assessment of joint effusion, range-of-motion testing, evaluation of ligaments for injury or laxity, and assessment of the menisci (Calmbach & Hutchens, 2003). According to the Ottawa knee rules (Hwang, 2020).

Objectives

- By the end of this chapter, you should be able to:
    - Understand steps needed for a reasonable knee examination
    - Conduct adequate examination to acquire the extent of the problem
    - Rule out what structures are involved
    - Determine when imaging studies may or may not be helpful.
    - Reassess after treatment for any improvement or deterioration.

Red flags

- Below symptoms may indicate that something more sinister may be going on:
    - Bilateral pins and needles or numbness in the lower limb (LL).
    - Problems with bowel and bladder function where the patient is unable to feel themselves going to the toilet.
    - Paraesthesia in the groin region.

- Loss of pulses in the LL (Vascular compromise).
- Obvious deformity.

Inspection

- **Skin**
  - Check the skin for any discolouration, wounds, previous scars, or gross deformity.
- **Soft Tissues**
  - Inspect for any swelling, asymmetry, or any muscle atrophy
- **Bony**
  - Length - compared to the contralateral side
  - Position - genu varum or valgus; flexion contractures
  - Look for any gross deformity or malalignment
- **Gait**
  - Varus thrust: Suggests possible LCL or PLC insufficiency or injury
  - Antalgic: Shortened stance phase on the affected side
  - Patella tracking
  - Flexed knee gait: due to tight Achilles' tendon or hamstrings

Palpation

- **Bony**
  - Joint line: feel for any tenderness medially or laterally
  - Patella: feel for any facet pain
  - Tibial tubercle
- **Soft-tissue structures**
  - Pes anserine bursae
  - Patellar & Quadriceps tendon
  - Iliotibial band
  - Collateral ligaments

○ Popliteal fossa: feel for any pain with Baker's cyst or popliteal aneurysm

- **Swelling**
  ○ Pre-patellar bursitis
  ○ Intra-articular effusion: patella balloting, milking
  ○ Traumatic hemarthrosis: suggestive of any intra-articular fracture or ligament rupture

Neurovascular

- **Motor**
  ○ Knee flexion - sciatic nerve
  ○ Knee extension - femoral nerve
  ○ Foot plantarflexion - tibial nerve
  ○ Foot dorsiflexion - deep peroneal nerve
- **Sensory**
  ○ Medial thigh - obturator nerve
  ○ Anterior thigh - femoral nerve
  ○ Posterolateral leg - sciatic nerve
  ○ Dorsal foot - peroneal nerve
  ○ Plantar foot - tibial nerve
- **Pulses**
  ○ Popliteal
  ○ Dorsal pedis
  ○ Posterior tibial
- **Reflexes**
  ○ Patellar (L4)
    - Hypoactive/absent is concerning for L4 radiculopathy
    - Hyperactive may indicate UMN injury

1. Patellofemoral Assessment

- An evaluation for effusion should be conducted with the patient supine and the injured knee in extension.
- The suprapatellar pouch should be milked to determine whether an effusion is present.
- Patellofemoral tracking is assessed by observing the patella for smooth motion while the patient contracts the quadriceps muscle. The presence of crepitus should be noted during palpation of the patella.

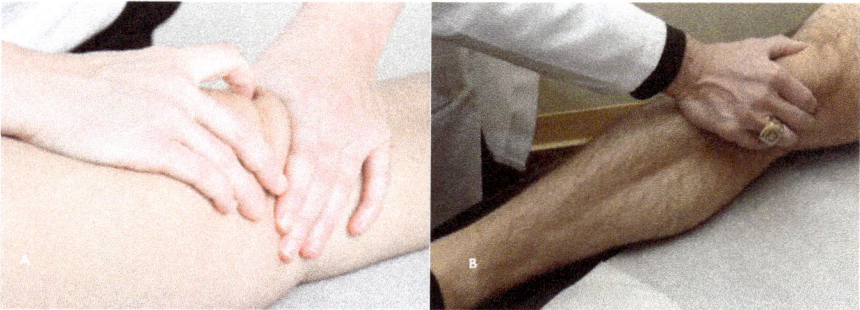

Fig.1.13.1. (A) Assessment of the patella and (B) lateral patella apprehension test

A. Patellar Apprehension Test

- With fingers placed at the medial aspect of the patella, the physician attempts to sublux the patella laterally. If this manoeuvre reproduces the patient's pain or a giving-way sensation patellar subluxation is the likely cause of the patient's symptoms.
- Both the superior and inferior patellar facets should be palpated, with the patella subluxed first medially and then laterally

2. Anterior Cruciate Ligament

A. Anterior drawer

- **Description**
  - The Anterior Drawer test examines for any tearing or laxity of the ACL ligament.
- **Manoeuvre**
  - Have the patient lying on their back with their knee bent as close to 90° as possible, with the foot resting on the table. Place both hands behind the tibia and pull the tibia forward, using a force between 5-10Kg.
  - The test can also be performed with the foot externally rotated (turned out) to 15°.
- **Positive Findings**
  - Increased anterior movement of the tibia on the injured side compared to the non-injured side is a positive test.
  - Up to 3 mm of forward movement of the tibia is considered normal.
  - The Grading: Grade 1 = 5 mm, Grade 2 = 5 to 10 mm, Grade 3 > 10 mm.

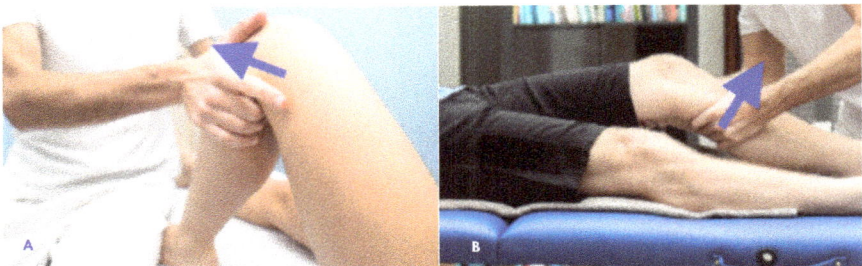

Fig.1.13.2. Knee examination - (A) Anterior drawer test and (B) Lachman test

B. The Lachman test

- It is another means of assessing the integrity of the anterior cruciate ligament.
- The test is performed with the patient in a supine position and the injured knee flexed to 30 degrees.
- The physician stabilizes the distal femur with one hand, grasps the proximal tibia in the other hand, and then attempts to sublux the tibia anteriorly.
- The lack of a clear endpoint indicates a positive Lachman test.

Knee X-Ray indications: Ottawa Knee rules (Acute)

- *Age ≥ 55 years*
- *Isolated patella tenderness*
- *Tenderness of head of the fibula*
- *Inability to flex knee 90°*
- *Inability to bear weight (4 steps) immediately after injury and in the emergency department*

3. Posterior cruciate ligament

A. Posterior drawer

- **Description:**
  - The posterior drawer test is used to examine the Posterior Cruciate Ligament (PCL).
- **Manoeuvre**
  - Have the patient lying on their back with their knee bent as close to 90° as possible with their foot resting on the table.

- Place both hands behind the tibia and push backwards on the proximal shin/tibia looking for instability backwards.
- Use a force between 15-20 lbs.

- **Positive Findings**
  - Upon application of a posterior force to the upper shin, an increase in backwards motion in comparison to the other side is indicative of a positive test.

4. Medial & Lateral collateral ligaments

A. Valgus stress test

- **Description**
  - The valgus stress test checks for medial joint laxity, which usually represents an injury to the medial collateral ligament (MCL).
- **Manoeuvre**
  - Have the patient lie on their back. Position one hand at the joint line on the outer part of the knee.
  - Have the other hand fixed on the ankle of the affected side.
  - Flex the knee between 20° and 30° and apply a medial or valgus force to the knee.
- **Positive Findings**
  - A positive test demonstrates increased medial joint laxity compared to the unaffected side.
  - Grading system: Grade 1= 5mm, Grade 2= 5 to 10mm, Grade 3= >10 mm.
  - To test the MCL, as well as the posterior medial capsule, the test can be repeated at 0° with the knee in full extension.

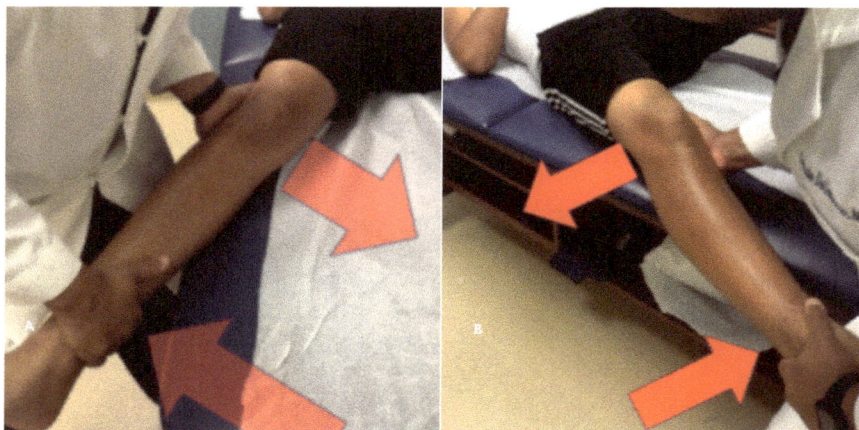

Fig.1.13.3. Knee examination - (A) The valgus stress test and (B) The varus stress test

B. Varus stress test

- **Description**
    - The varus stress test checks for joint laxity on the outside of the knee, which usually represents an injury to the lateral collateral ligament (LCL).
- **Manoeuvre**
    - With the patient lying on their back, position one hand at the joint line on the outer part of the knee.
    - Fix the other hand on the ankle of the affected side.
    - Flex the knee between 20° and 30° and apply a lateral or varus force to the knee.
    - This can be done either by reaching over the top of the knee or by approaching the patient from the inside aspect of the knee with the leg off to the side.
    - The test can also be repeated at 0° with the knee in full extension.
- **Positive Findings**
    - A positive test demonstrates increased lateral joint laxity compared to the unaffected side.

○ Grading system: Grade 1= 5mm, Grade 2= 5 to 10mm, Grade 3= >10 mm.

○ Place the other hand over the knee, with the thumb and fingers on the joint line.

○ Gently rotate the tibia with the heel internally rotated with a mild valgus force (for the lateral compartment) and externally rotated with a mild varus force (for the medial compartment).

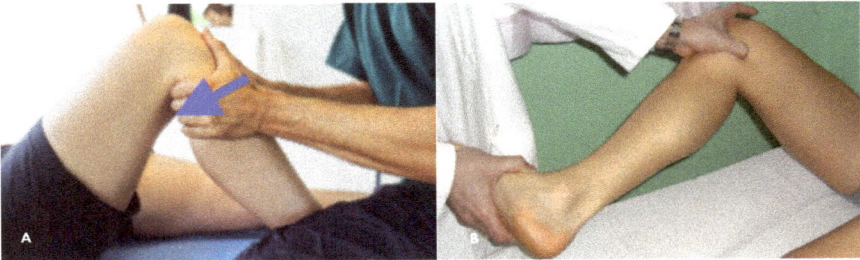

Fig.1.13.4. Knee examination - (A) Posterior drawer test and (B) McMurray test

5. Menisci

A. McMurray's test

- **Description**
  ○ This test checks for meniscal tears and other internal derangements in the knee.
- **Manoeuvre**
  ○ With the patient supine, and their hip and knee bent to 90°, grasp the heel in one hand.
- **Positive Findings**
  ○ Painful clicking along the joint line or any pain over the joint line that reproduces the patient's symptoms is a positive test.

B. Thessaly's test

- **Description**
  - ○ This functionally tests meniscus tears in the standing position.
  - ○ Since bending and twisting movements while weight bearing often reproduce pain from meniscus tears, this test recreates the exacerbating movements.

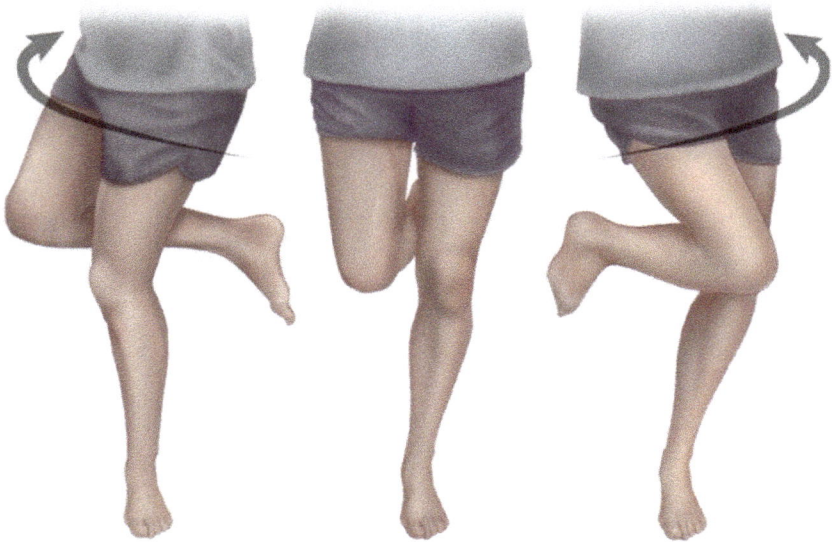

©UWorld

Fig.1.13.5. Knee examination - Thessaly's test

- **Manoeuvre**
  - ○ Have the patient stand on one foot with the foot flat on the floor.
  - ○ Hold the patient's hand for support and have them initially bend on the standing knee to 5° of flexion. Ask the patient to twist at the knee, making sure they are internally and externally rotating at the knee rather than at the pelvis or back.
  - ○ Check for any reproduction of pain symptoms.

○ Next, have the patient bend the knee deeper to 20°degrees and again actively twists on the knee.

- **Positive Findings**
  ○ The twisting movement will reproduce the pain of a meniscal injury.
  ○ The pain is typically localised to the joint line, and patients typically have more pain with the knee bent at 20° rather than 5°.

Further reading

Stanford Medicine- Introduction to the Knee Exam: https://stanfordmedicine25.stanford.edu/the25/knee.html

References

Calmbach, W. L., & Hutchens, M. (2003). Evaluation of patients presenting with knee pain: Part I. History, physical examination, radiographs, and laboratory tests. Am Fam Physician, 68(5), 907-912.

Hwang, C. (2020). Calculated decisions: Ottawa Knee Rule. Emerg Med Pract, 22(Suppl 8), Cd11-cd12.

Rossi, R., Dettoni, F., Bruzzone, M., Cottino, U., D'Elicio, D. G., & Bonasia, D. E. (2011). Clinical examination of the knee: know your tools for diagnosis of knee injuries. Sports medicine, arthroscopy, rehabilitation, therapy & technology : SMARTT, 3, 25-25. https://doi.org/10.1186/1758-2555-3-25

2. Shoulder Clinical Examination

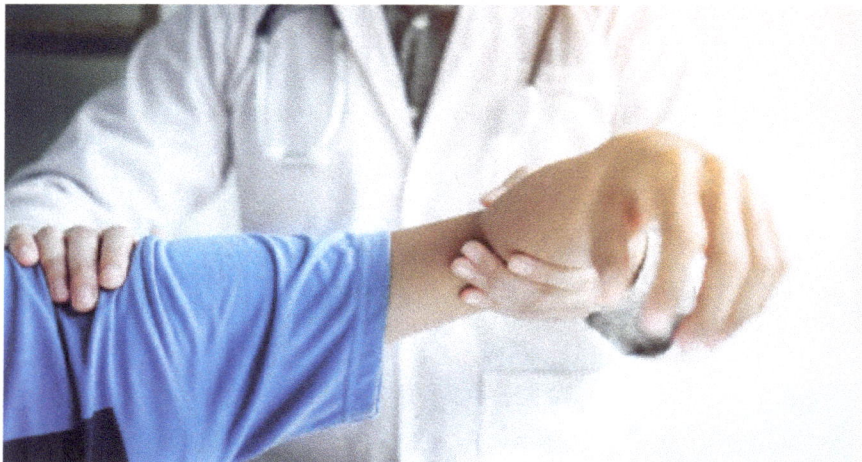

Overview

Shoulder pain is one of the most common complaints in the emergency department (ED) setting. The aetiology is usually traumatic due to accident and fall or sports injury but, it can also originate from a non-traumatic cause such as degenerative disease or osteoarthritis. ED physician is expected to identify relevant clinical signs using basic examination skills by keeping in mind the four components of musculoskeletal examinations- look, feel, move, and special tests to identify any shoulder lesion. This book provides a clear step-by-step approach to examining the shoulder in the emergency department.

Objectives

- By the end of this chapter, you should be able to:
  - Understand steps needed for a reasonable shoulder examination
  - Conduct adequate examination to acquire the extent of the problem
  - Rule out what structures are involved

- Determine when imaging studies may or may not be helpful.
- Reassess after treatment for any improvement or deterioration.

Patient History

- Be attentive to the patient's past medical history as this may rule out red flags and direct the shoulder examination
- History of presenting complaint: how long have you been having these complaints, how did it happen, any history of trauma?
- The distribution and severity of the pain: Is the pain preventing the patient from doing his activities or aggravated with certain positions or movements
- Self-medication and other therapies the patient has tested
- Any previous shoulder complaints in the past: course, treatment and result of the treatment
- Association between the complaints and profession or sport and training

Inspection

- **Start by comparing both shoulders**
  - Atrophy or Hypertrophy
  - Symmetry
  - Skin
  - Swelling
  - Scars
  - Scapular winging

Palpation

- **Bony prominences:**
  - Cervical spinous processes
  - Sternoclavicular joint
  - Clavicle
  - Acromioclavicular joint

  ◦ Acromion
  ◦ Coracoid process
  ◦ Scapular spine
- **Muscles and soft tissues:**
  ◦ Deltoid
  ◦ Rotator cuff tendon insertion / greater tuberosity
  ◦ Long head of the biceps tendon in the groove
  ◦ Paraspinal muscles
  ◦ Periscapular region

Range of motion
- **Cervical spine**
  ◦ Flexion
  ◦ Extension
  ◦ Lateral flexion
  ◦ Rotation
- **Shoulder**
  ◦ Compare both shoulders for active and passive motion
  ◦ Forward elevation: Normal is 180°
  ◦ Abduction: normal is 90 with the scapula stabilized
- *External rotation at 90 degrees abduction*
- *External rotation at the side, 80 degrees considered normal*
- *Internal rotation to vertebral height: T4-T8 considered normal*
- *Internal rotation at 90 degrees abduction*

Neurovascular exam
- **Sensation:** check all dermatomes from C4 to T1:
  ◦ C4 – Top of Shoulders
  ◦ C5 – Lateral Deltoid
  ◦ C6 – Tip of Thumb
  ◦ C7 – Distal Middle Finger
  ◦ C8 – Distal 5th Finger
  ◦ T1 – Medial Forearm

- **Motor:** check all myotomes
    - C4 – Shoulder Elevation/Shrug
    - C5 – Shoulder Abduction
    - C6 – Elbow Flexion, Wrist Extension
    - C7 – Elbow Extension, Wrist Flexion
    - C8 – Thumb Abduction/Extension
    - T1 – Finger Abduction
- **Vascular**
    - Brachial artery pulse
    - Radial artery pulse
    - Ulnar artery pulse

Special tests

1. Frozen shoulder: external rotation

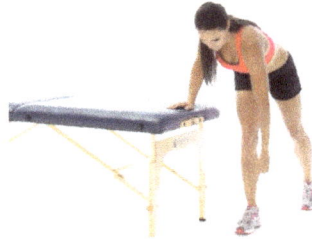

Fig.1.13.6. Codman's pendulum test

- To improve range of motion, special exercises such as Codman's Pendulum can be performed to help relax the muscles around the shoulder, reduce pain, and increase motion.

A. CODMAN'S PENDULUM

- Have the patient stand in a relaxed position and tell them to swing their weak arm in a circular motion while keeping their shoulder nice and relaxed.
- Be sure they swing their arm in both the clockwise and counterclockwise directions.

2. Rotator cuff strength testing

A. Empty can test

- **Description:**
    - The empty can test is used to evaluate the strength and integrity of the supraspinatus muscle and tendon.
- **Manoeuvre:**
    - Have the patient stand with their shoulder abducted to 90° and horizontally adducted forward 30° with the thumbs pointing down towards the floor, as if they are pouring out a can.
    - Ask the patient to maintain this position.
    - Proceed to apply downward resistance to the patient's forearm.
    - A variation of this test can be done at 30° abduction instead of 90°, where the supraspinatus should function in relative isolation.
- **Positive findings:**
    - Decreased strength or pain on resisted testing.

B. Full can test

- **Description:**
    - This test assesses the function of the Supraspinatus muscle and tendon of the shoulder complex.
- **Manoeuvre:**
    - The patient is in a seated or standing position,
    - Having their arm in 90° of elevation in the scapular plane with maximum external rotation of the glenohumeral joint. The patient's thumb should be pointing up.

- ○ The physician stabilizes the shoulder while applying a downward force to the arm whilst the patient attempts to resist this movement (Timmons et al., 2017).
- **Positive findings:**
  - ○ This test is deemed positive if the patient experiences pain or weakness with resistance to the shoulder complex.

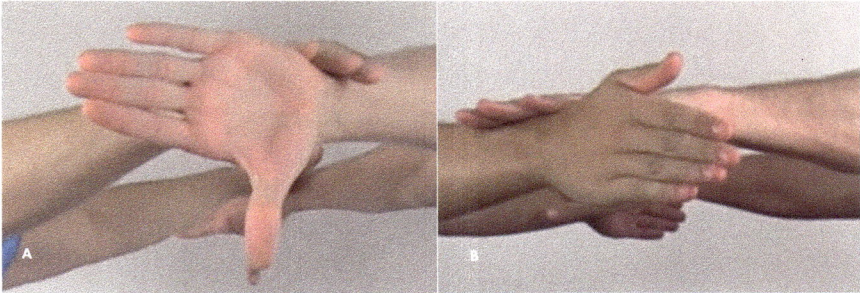

Fig.1.13.7. Shoulder examination - (A) Empty can test and (B) Full can test

C. External rotation

- **Description:**
  - ○ The external rotation test examines the strength of the infraspinatus and teres minor.
- **Manoeuvre:**
  - ○ With the patient's arms at their side, externally rotated 45° and elbow flexed to 90°, the examiner applies an internal rotation moment to assess the strength of the external rotators.
- **Positive Findings:**
  - ○ Decreased strength or pain on resisted testing.
  - ○ A significant weakness of the infraspinatus may be indicative of suprascapular nerve palsy, where the infraspinatus become denervated.
  - ○ This can be due to trauma, ganglion cyst or illness.

D. Lift-off test

- **Description:**
  - ○ The lift off test evaluates the muscular strength of the sub-scapularis.
- **Manoeuvre:**
  - ○ With the patient seated or standing, have them internally rotate their arm behind their back.
  - ○ Then ask the patient to lift the back of their hand off their lower back.
  - ○ If they are unable to complete this task, apply resistance to the palm to assess the strength of the subscapularis.
- **Positive findings:**
  - ○ Inability to lift the dorsum of hand off the back.

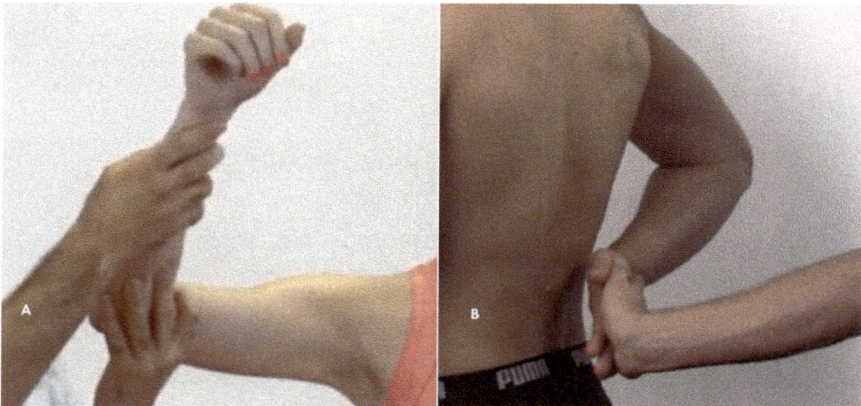

Fig.1.13.8. Shoulder examination - (A) External rotation test and (B) Lift off test

3. Impingement/rotator cuff special tests

A. Neer's impingement

- **Description:**
  - ○ The Neer's impingement test assesses the presence of impingement of the rotator cuff, primarily the supraspinatus,

as it passes under the subacromial arch during forward flexion.

- **Manoeuvre:**
  - ○ Stabilise the scapula with one hand while applying passive forced flexion of the arm.
- **Positive findings:**
  - ○ Pain in the anterior shoulder or reproduction of the patient's symptoms.

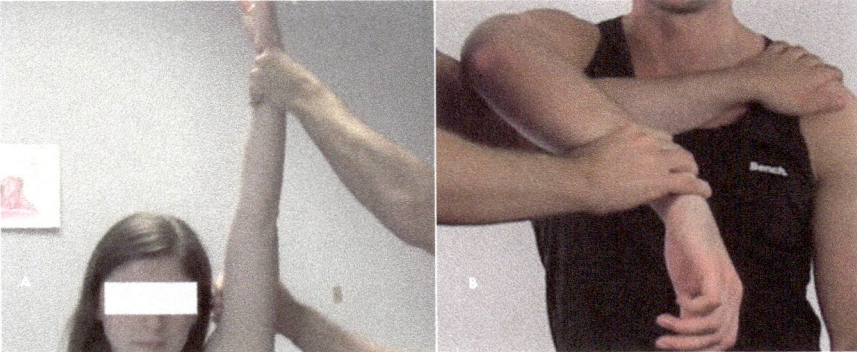

Fig.1.13.9. Shoulder examination - (A) Neer's impingement test and (B) Hawkins Kennedy impingement test

B. Hawkins Kennedy impingement test

- **Description:**
  - ○ The Hawkin's test is used to evaluate impingement of rotator cuff and subacromial bursa.
- **Manoeuvre:**
  - ○ The patient is seated or standing and with their arm forward flexed to 90°and their elbow bent to 90°.
  - ○ Stabilise the top of the shoulder while internally rotating the arm at the forearm.
- **Positive Findings:**
  - ○ Pain in the anterior shoulder or reproduction of the patient's symptoms with the test.

4. Instability special tests

A. Load and shift test

- **Description:**
  - The Load and Shift test examines integrity of shoulder stability in the anterior and posterior directions.
- **Manoeuvre:**
  - Have the patient seated or supine with their arm relaxed and resting at their side.
  - Grasp the head of the humerus with thumb and fingers and apply an anterior and posterior glide from the resting position.
- **Positive Findings:**
  - Excessive gliding of the humeral head is a positive test.

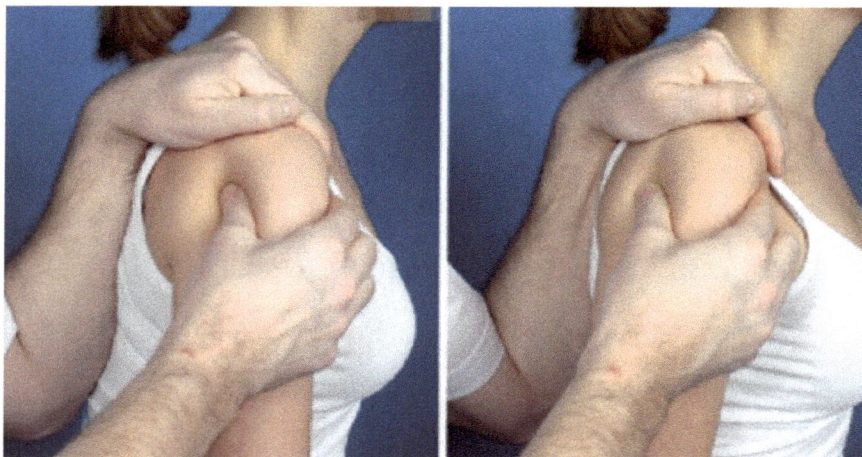

Fig.1.13.10. Load & Shift test

B. Apprehension- relocation test

- **Description:**
  - **The apprehension test** assesses for anterior instability of the shoulder.

- ○ **The relocation test,** described by Jobe (Jobe et al., 1989), is used in conjunction with the apprehension test to distinguish between anterior instability and primary impingement of the shoulder.
- **Manoeuvre:**
  - ○ To perform the apprehension test, have the patient supine, with their arm abducted and elbow flexed to 90°. Gently externally rotate the arm.
  - ○ Once the patient becomes apprehensive or complains of pain, proceed with the relocation and surprise test by applying a posterior force to the humeral head.
- **Positive Findings:**
  - ○ For the apprehension test, the patient may complain of pain or be apprehensive that their arm may dislocate as it is externally rotated.
  - ○ The relocation test is positive if the symptoms of apprehension reduce, or if the clinician can externally rotate the shoulder further without any increase in pain or apprehension.
  - ○ If the symptoms persist following the posterior directed force, the pain is associated with primary impingement and not anterior shoulder instability.

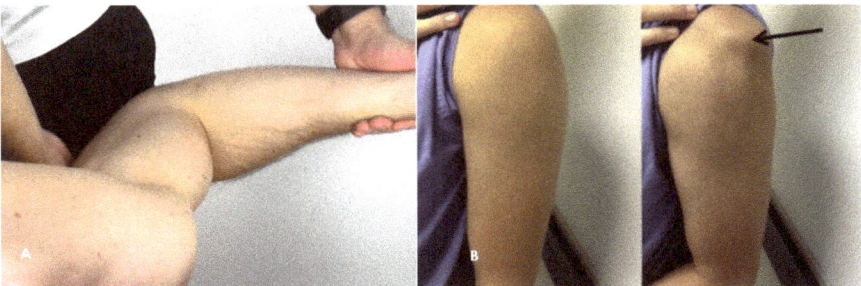

Fig.1.13.11. Shoulder examination - (A) Apprehension test and (B) Sulcus sign. (1) Patient at rest. (2) Patient after voluntary anterior and inferior subluxation. Note anterior skin dimpling below the acromion (black arrow).

C. Sulcus sign

- **Description:**
  - ○ The sulcus sign tests for inferior instability caused by laxity of the inferior glenohumeral ligament complex.
- **Manoeuvre:**
  - ○ Have the patient seated with their arm resting at their side. Grasp the patient's upper arm and apply a distal force to it.
- **Positive Findings:**
  - ○ Increased inferior movement of the humeral head or the visible development of a sulcus at the glenohumeral joint are positive findings.
  - ○ A positive test can often suggest that the patient has multi-directional instability, especially if there are other signs of joint instability.

5. Labral special tests

A. O'Brien's test

- **Description:**
  - ○ This test examines the integrity of the glenoid labrum and the acromioclavicular joint (O'Brien et al., 1998).
- **Manoeuvre:**
  - ○ With the patient seated or standing, instruct the patient to raise their arm into 90° of forward flexion with their elbow extended, and then adduct their arm 10-15°.
  - ○ Have the patient internally rotate their arm and point their thumb down to the ground.
  - ○ Apply a downward force to the arm.
  - ○ Then instruct the patient to externally rotate their arm and point their thumb towards the ceiling. Again, apply a downward force.

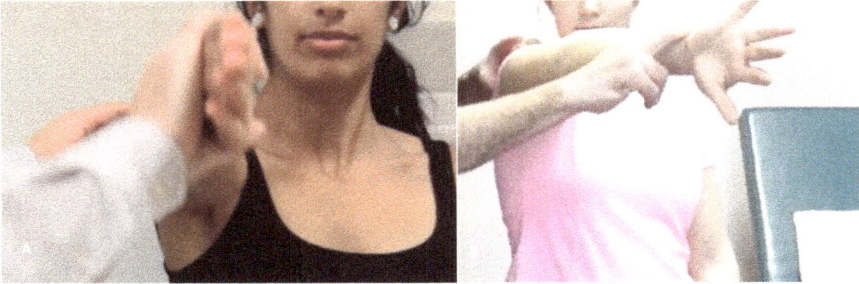

Fig.1.13.12. Shoulder examination - A&B: O'Brien's test

- **Positive Findings:**
  - Positive findings for labral pathology occur when the first test reproduces pain, while the second test decreases or eliminates pain.
  - The pain associated with labral tears is deep in the shoulder.
  - Pain situated over the acromioclavicular joint is associated with acromioclavicular joint pathology such as osteoarthritis or a shoulder separation, rather than labral pathology.
  - Pain in the AC joint is usually equal with the palm down or the palm up.

Further reading

Apprehension (Crank) Test for Anterior Shoulder Dislocation- Shoulder Instability: https://www.youtube.com/watch?v=_JA-qvX-cUdQ

Physiotutors. Full Can Test- Shoulder Impingement: https://www.youtube.com/watch?v=NuBOHdm20cc

References

Jobe, F. W., Kvitne, R. S., & Giangarra, C. E. (1989). Shoulder pain in the overhand or throwing athlete. The relationship of anterior instability and rotator cuff impingement. Orthop Rev, 18(9), 963-975.

O'Brien, S. J., Pagnani, M. J., Fealy, S., McGlynn, S. R., & Wilson, J. B. (1998). The active compression test: a new and effective test for diagnosing labral tears and acromioclavicular joint abnormality. Am J Sports Med, 26(5), 610-613. https://doi.org/10.1177/03635465980260050201

Timmons, M. K., Yesilyaprak, S. S., Ericksen, J., & Michener, L. A. (2017). Full can test: Mechanisms of a positive test in patients with shoulder pain. Clin Biomech (Bristol, Avon), 42, 9-13. https://doi.org/10.1016/j.clinbiomech.2016.12.011

3. Ankle Clinical Examination

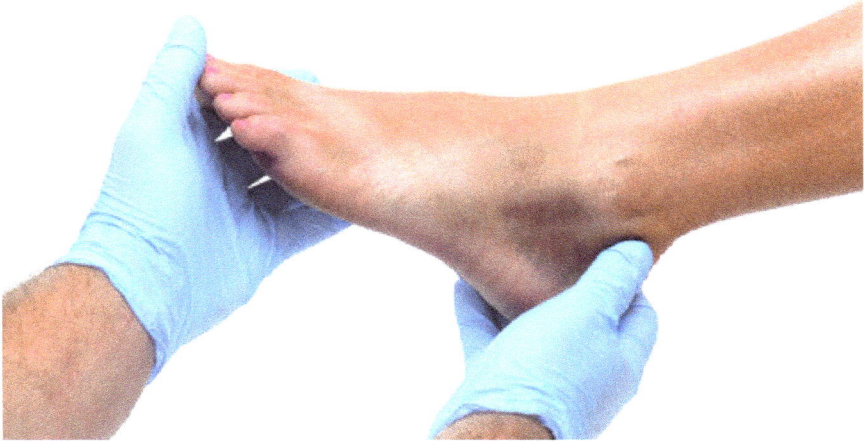

Overview

Patients commonly present with foot and ankle problems in the emergency department (ED). The ankle and the foot anatomy are complex with many joints; therefore, many ED physicians find it challenging to assess these patients (Papaliodis et al., 2014). The Aetiology of foot and ankle problems varies from pain, swelling, deformity, stiffness, instability and/or abnormal gait to major trauma. Therefore, the physical exam of the ankle is of paramount significance for the clinical evaluation of a patient presenting to our ED. This book will familiarize you with some basic manoeuvres and physical signs required to assess the presence and the severity of structural lesions involving the ankle.

Objectives

- By the end of this chapter, you should be able to:
    - Understand steps needed for a reasonable ankle examination
    - Conduct adequate examination to acquire the extent of the problem

○ Rule out what structures are involved

○ Determine when imaging studies may or may not be help-ful.

○ Reassess after treatment for any improvement or deterio-ration.

Red flags

• Below symptoms may indicate that something more sinister may be going on:

○ Obvious deformity

○ Incontinence

○ Paraesthesia in the groin region

○ Bilateral pins and needles or numbness in the lower limb (LL)

○ Bowel and bladder dysfunction

○ Positive Babinski sign

○ Loss of pulses in the LL

Inspection

• Compare both ankles without shoes or socks:

○ Swelling or joint effusion

○ muscle atrophy

○ Erythema

○ Deformity

○ Ecchymosis(recent Trauma)

○ Overlying skin changes

○ Scars suggesting old Trauma

Palpation

○ Palpate any swellings or lumps

○ Areas of tenderness should be localised by checking bony prominences and tendon insertions

○ Check for the pulses and the skin temperature

Range of Motion

- Ankle, subtalar, mid-tarsal, and toe joints should be examined systematically
- Muscle power and tendons may be checked by testing inversion, eversion, etc against resistance
- **Range of movement:** from a neutral point at right angles to the leg, the range of plantar and dorsiflexion should normally be 55 and 15 degrees
- **Lateral ligament stress test** - grasp the heel and forcibly invert the foot while feeling for the opening of the lateral side of the ankle between the tibia and talus
- **Inferior tibiofibular ligament test** - dorsiflexion of the foot induces pain when the tibia is displaced laterally

Special tests

1. Talar tilt test

- **Description:**
  - ○ The Talar Tilt Test is a ligamentous stress test that examines the integrity of the lateral ankle ligaments, particularly the calcaneofibular ligament.
- **Manoeuvre:**
  - ○ Have the patient in the seated position, with their knee bent and foot in a neutral or slightly dorsiflexed position. Stabilise the distal tibia with one hand while applying an inversion force to the foot.
- **Positive Findings:**
  - ○ Positive findings include any pain in the ankle or increased joint laxity.
  - ○ Depending on the positioning of the ankle, pain may be experienced over either the calcaneofibular ligament or the anterior talofibular ligament.

2. Anterior drawer

- **Description:**
  - The anterior drawer test is used to examine the integrity of the anterior talofibular ligament, which is frequently injured during an inversion ankle sprain.

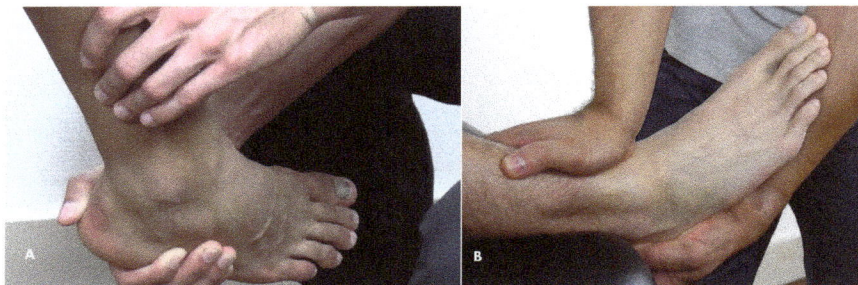

Fig.1.13.13. (A) Ankle Talar tilt test and (B) Ankle anterior drawer test

- **Manoeuvre:**
  - Have the patient seated with their knee bent and their ankle in a neutral position at 0° or 90° to the leg.
  - Stabilize the distal tibia with one hand, while grasping the heel with the other hand.
  - Apply an anterior force to the heel.
  - This test should be performed bilaterally to compare for differences in anterior translation.
- **Positive Findings:**
  - Pain or increased joint laxity in the injured ankle indicates disruption of the anterior talofibular ligament.
  - A dimple may also be visually seen by the clinician while performing this test.

3. External rotation or Kleiger's test

- **Description:**
    - ○ The test is used to help identify syndesmotic injuries.
- **Manoeuvre:**
    - ○ Have the patient seated with their knee bent on the exam table.
    - ○ Stabilise the distal tibia while externally rotating the foot.
    - ○ External rotation of the talus applies pressure to the lateral malleolus, causing a widening of the tibiofibular joint.
- **Positive findings:**
    - ○ Increased external rotation of the foot when compared bilaterally, or any pain in the anterolateral ankle joint is a positive finding.

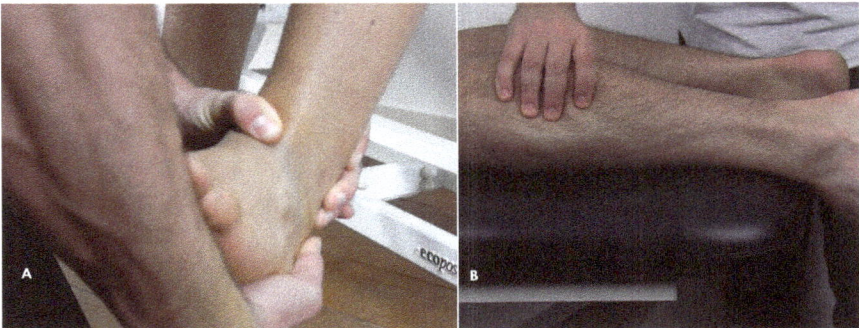

Fig.1.13.14. (A) Ankle Kleiger's test and (B) Thompson's test

4. Thompson's test

- **Description:**
    - ○ This test is utilised to evaluate the integrity of the heel cord.

- **Manoeuvre:**
  - Have the patient lying prone on a table with their foot extended off the edge. Squeeze the calf muscle at position slightly distal to the place of widest girth. Examine the movement at the foot.
- **Positive Findings:**
  - A positive test occurs when the calf is squeezed, and no plantar movement occurs at the foot. This indicates Achilles' tendon rupture.

5. Compression test

- **Description:**
  - This test examines the integrity of the distal tibiofibular joint. It can also assess for fractures of the tibia and fibula.
- **Manoeuvre:**
  - Have the patient sitting supine with their foot on the table. Grasp the mid-calf and squeeze the tibia and fibula together. Gradually move distally towards the ankle while continuing to apply the same amount of pressure.
- **Positive findings:**
  - Any pain in the lower leg may be indicative of a fracture or syndesmotic sprain.

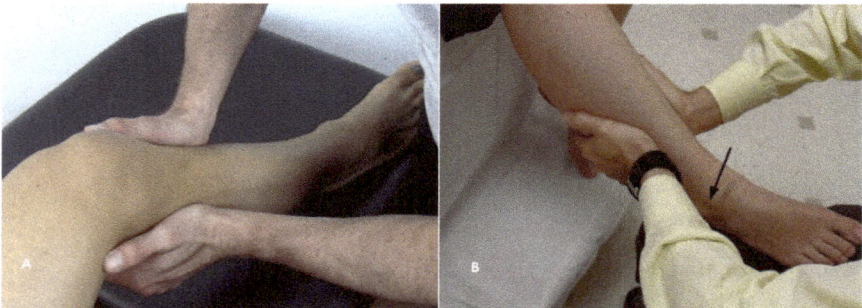

Fig.1.13.15. A&B: Ankle compression test

The Ottawa ankle rules

The Ottawa ankle rules are a clinical decision-making approach for deciding the radiographic imaging indications for ankle and midfoot injuries. The rules have 97.5% sensitivity and decrease by 35% the need for radiographs (Dowling et al., 2009).

- *An ankle x-ray is required only if there is any of the following is satisfied (Bachmann et al., 2003):*
    - point tenderness at the posterior edge (of distal 6 cm) or tip lateral malleolus
    - point tenderness at the posterior edge (of distal 6 cm) or tip medial malleolus
    - inability to weight bear (four steps) immediately after the injury and in the emergency department
- *A foot x-ray is required if any of the following (Bachmann et al., 2003) is satisfied:*
    - point tenderness at the base of the fifth metatarsal
    - point tenderness at the navicular
    - inability to weight bear (four steps) immediately after the injury and in the emergency department
    - The Ottawa ankle rules should apply with caution in children <6 years old (Runyon, 2009).

Further reading
Physiopaedia - Foot and Ankle Examination: https://www.physio-pedia.com/Foot_and_Ankle_Examination

Stanford medicine - Foot and Ankle Exam: https://stanfordmedicine25.stanford.edu/the25/Ankleandfootexam.html

References

Bachmann, L. M., Kolb, E., Koller, M. T., Steurer, J., & ter Riet, G. (2003). Accuracy of Ottawa ankle rules to exclude fractures of the ankle and mid-foot: systematic review. Bmj, 326(7386), 417. https://doi.org/10.1136/bmj.326.7386.417

Dowling, S., Spooner, C. H., Liang, Y., Dryden, D. M., Friesen, C., Klassen, T. P., & Wright, R. B. (2009). Accuracy of Ottawa Ankle Rules to exclude fractures of the ankle and midfoot in children: a meta-analysis. Acad Emerg Med, 16(4), 277-287. https://doi.org/10.1111/j.1553-2712.2008.00333.x

Papaliodis, D. N., Vanushkina, M. A., Richardson, N. G., & DiPreta, J. A. (2014). The foot and ankle examination. Med Clin North Am, 98(2), 181-204. https://doi.org/10.1016/j.mcna.2013.10.001

Runyon, M. S. (2009). Can we safely apply the Ottawa Ankle Rules to children? In Acad Emerg Med (Vol. 16, pp. 352-354). https://doi.org/10.1111/j.1553-2712.2009.00370.x

4. Hip Clinical Examination

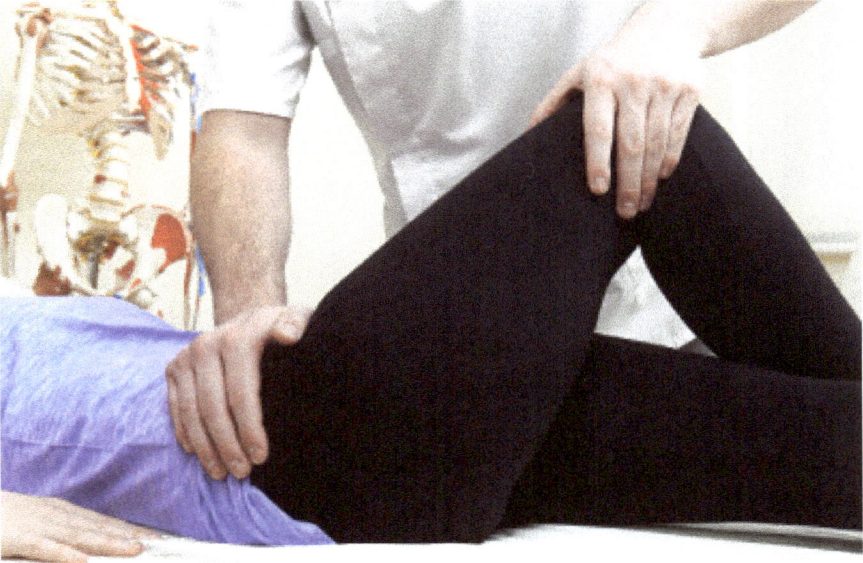

Overview

The Hip joint is one of the most important joints of our body; it plays a crucial role in locomotion. It is the second-largest weight-bearing joint in the body, after the knee joint. The spherical head of the femur forms the ball, which fits into the acetabulum, and ligaments connect the ball to the socket, thereby providing incredible strength and stability to the joint. Patients with hip complaints frequently present in the emergency department, and an emergency physician is expected to identify the relevant clinical signs using your examination skills. The examination of the hip joint will stick on the four components of the musculoskeletal examinations -look, feel, move and special tests. An assessment of a painful hip is relatively straightforward and dependable at detecting the existence of a hip joint problem. Hip joint conditions may go undetected, leading to secondary illnesses (Byrd, 2007). With a correct approach and systematic examination techniques, most hip joint conditions can be detected, and a proper treatment strategy can then be initiated based on an accurate diagnosis. This new guide provides a straightforward step-by-step approach to examining the hip in the emergency department.

Objectives

- By the end of this chapter, you should be able to:
  - Understand steps needed for a reasonable hip examination
  - Conduct adequate examination to acquire the extent of the problem
  - Rule out what structures are involved
  - Determine when imaging studies may or may not be helpful.
  - Reassess after treatment for any improvement or deterioration.

Red flags

- Any swelling
- Any deformity
- An inability to bear weight
- Sudden onset of pain
- A history of trauma
- Any lumps or bumps felt in the groin
- Any noticeable groin pulsations
- Constipation or vomiting
- Testicular swelling
- Haematuria
- Fever
- Lower limb neurological symptoms - weakness, numbness, or tingling
- Night pain, sweats, unintentional weight loss, appetite loss
- History of malignancy or steroid use
- High-risk sexual activity

Inspection

- Inspect the **anterior aspect** of the hip joints and lower limbs, noting any abnormalities:
  - Scars
  - Bruising
  - Swelling
  - Quadriceps wasting
  - Leg length discrepancy
  - Pelvic tilt
- Inspect the **lateral aspect** of the hip joints for any **flexion abnormalities**: fixed flexion deformity at the hip joint may indicate the presence of contractures secondary to previous trauma, inflammatory conditions or neurological disease.
- Inspect the **posterior aspect** of the hip joints and lower limbs, noting any abnormalities:
  - Scars
  - Muscle wasting

Palpation

- Temperature: may suggest an infection or inflammation
- Swelling: effusion, synovial thickening, extracapsular
- Tenderness: fell the lumbar spine, pelvis, greater trochanter, inguinal ligament, femoral triangle (hip joint), and the knee
- Vascular system: distal pulses, capillary refill
- Sensation (Neurological Examination) – Peripheral nerve skin sensation and power

Neurological assessment

- **Manual Muscle Testing:** the strength of the muscle groups surrounding the hip joint, namely the hip extensors, flexors, abductors, adductors, internal and external rotators should be graded and documented.
- Straight Leg Raise

- Dermatome Testing
- Skin sensation test

Gait

- At the end of the examination, ask the patient to walk, then turn and walk back whilst observing their gait paying attention to:
  - **Gait cycle:** note any anomalies of the gait cycle (e.g., abnormalities in toe-off or heel strike).
  - **Range of movement:** reduced in osteoarthritis, inflammatory arthritis
  - **Limping:** suggestive of joint pain or weakness.
  - **Leg length:** any discrepancy may suggest a joint pathology.
  - **Turning:** slow turns may be due to limitations in joint range of movement or instability.

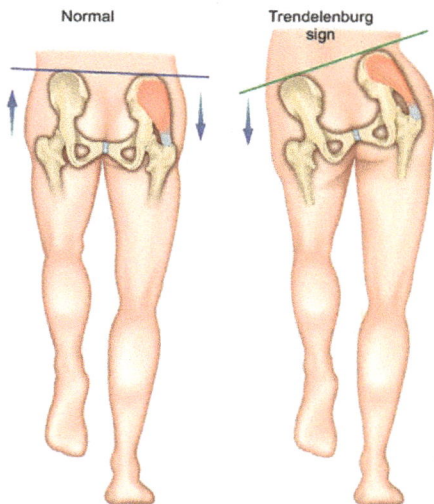

Fig.1.13.16. Normal vs Trendelenburg gaits

- **Trendelenburg's gait:** an abnormal gait provoked by the unilateral weakness of the hip abductor muscles following a superior gluteal nerve injury or L5 radiculopathy.

- **Waddling gait:** an abnormal gait induced by the bilateral weakness of the hip abductor muscles, commonly associated with myopathies (e.g., muscular dystrophy).
- **Assess the patient's footwear:** unequal sole wearing is suggestive of an abnormal gait.

Leg length assessment

- ED physician must be able to differentiate the true leg length discrepancy from an apparent discrepancy caused by other abnormalities (e.g., a leg appears shorter secondary to lateral pelvic tilt).
  - *Apparent leg length measurement: measure and compare the distance between the **umbilicus** and the **tip of the medial malleolus** of each limb.*
  - *True leg length measurement: measure from the **anterior superior iliac spine** to the **tip of the medial malleolus** of each limb.*

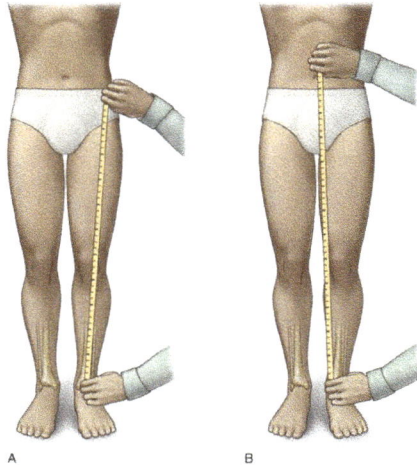

Fig.1.13.17. (A) True leg length vs (B) Apparent leg length

Straight Leg Raise test

- **Description:**
    - The Straight Leg Raise (SLR) test, described by Lasegue and is therefore referred to as *"Lasegue's test"*, is a commonly used test to identify impairment in disc pathology or nerve root irritation. It is useful in detecting disc herniation and neural compression (Pesonen et al., 2021), excessive nerve root tension (Kamath & Kamath, 2017) or compression (Das & Nadi, 2021). SLR test puts tensile stresses at the sciatic nerve and of traction at the lumbosacral nerve roots primarily from L4 ton S2.
- **Manoeuvre**
    - Each leg is tested individually with the unaffected leg being tested first.
    - Position the patient supine without a pillow under his/her head,
    - The clinician stands at the tested side with the distal hand around the patient's heel and proximal hand on the patient's distal thigh (anterior) to keep knee extension. Elevate the patient's leg by the posterior ankle while keeping the knee in a fully extended position.
    - Continue to lift the leg by flexing at the hip until the patient complains of pain or tightness in the back or back of the leg (Kamath & Kamath, 2017).
- **Positive findings**
    - If symptoms are primarily back pain, the primary cause is most likely a disc herniation applying pressure on the anterior theca of the spinal cord, or the pathology causing the pressure is more central.

○ If pain is primarily in the leg, it is more likely that the pathology causing the pressure on neurological tissue(s) is more lateral.

○ Disc herniations or pathology causing pressure between the two extremes are more likely to cause pain in both areas.

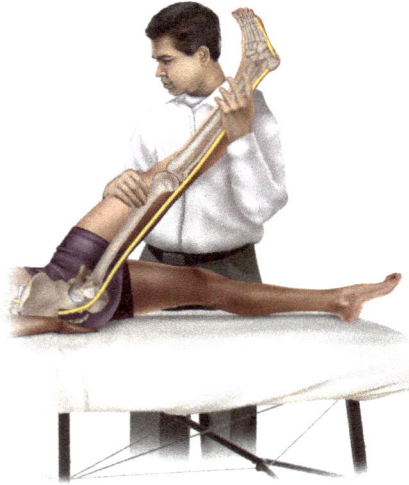

Fig.1.13.18. Straight leg raise test
Credit - Learn Muscles

Thomas Test

- **Description**
  - ○ Thomas' test is useful for hip flexion contractures.
  - ○ It assesses for anterior or lateral capsular restrictions or hip flexor tightness.
- **Manoeuvre**
  - ○ The patient is asked to lie supine.
  - ○ The clinician checks for lordosis which is a predictor of a tight hip flexor.

- Flex one hip bringing the knee to the chest and ask the patient to hold the knee to help stabilise the pelvis and flatten out the lumbar region.
- **Positive findings**
    - If the leg that is being tested (the leg on the table) does not have a hip flexion contraction it will remain on the testing table.
    - If a contracture is present, the leg will raise off the table.
- The test can also be achieved with the starting position of both knees fully flexed to the chest and slowly lowering the leg being tested to see if the leg makes it to the table:

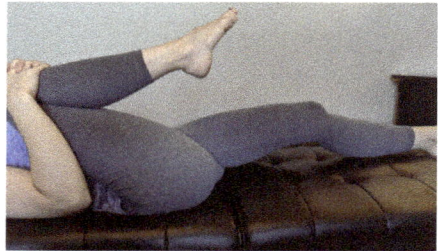

Fig.1.13.19. Positive Thomas test
Credit - Compropmed

    - Any lack of full hip extension with knee flexion less than 45° indicates iliopsoas tightness.
    - If a full extension is achieved in this position, this indicates rectus femoris tightness.
    - If any hip external rotation is observed, it may indicate iliotibial band tightness.

Trendelenburg's test

- Position patient
- If the patient is comfortable standing alone, stand behind the patient.
- Alternatively stand in front of the patient, with patient forearms placed on yours for support.
- Single-leg stance
- Ask the patient to raise each foot in turn off the ground.
- When the patient raises their right foot, the left hip abductors are being tested.

- When the patient lifts their left foot, the right hip abductors are being tested.
- Observe
- Position your hands on the patient's iliac crests.
- Watch carefully if the hip on the unsupported side lifts or droops.
- If the patient is using your arms for support, feel them pressing down on one of your arms if their hip abductors are unable to support their weight.
- Normally, abductors are strong enough to keep the pelvis level during a single leg stance, but it is normal to see a slight elevation of the pelvis on the unsupported site due to the abductor muscles contracting.
- **Positive sign**
    ○ A positive Trendelenburg's sign is pathological and involves sagging of the pelvis on the unsupported side due to the abductor muscles failing to stabilise the hip towards the weight-bearing femur.

Trendelenburg's gait

- Trendelenburg's gait implies the excessive up-down motion of the pelvis whilst walking arising because of compensatory mechanisms due to the drooping pelvis.
- Unilateral positive: Trendelenburg's sign produces a lurching gait.
- Bilaterally positive: Trendelenburg's sign produces a waddling gait.

FABER test or Patrick's test

- **Description**
    ○ To assess for the sacroiliac joint or hip joint being the source of the patient's pain.

- **Manoeuvre**
  - ○ Position the patient Supine.
  - ○ The patient's tested leg is positioned in a "figure-4" position, where the knee is flexed, and the ankle is placed on the opposite knee.
  - ○ The hip is put in Flexion, Abduction, and External Rotation (FABER).
  - ○ The clinician applies a posteriorly directed force against the medial knee of the bent leg towards the tabletop.
- **Positive findings**
  - ○ A positive test occurs when groin pain or buttock pain is produced.
  - ○ Due to forces going through the hip joint as well, the patient may experience pain if pathology is in the hip as well.

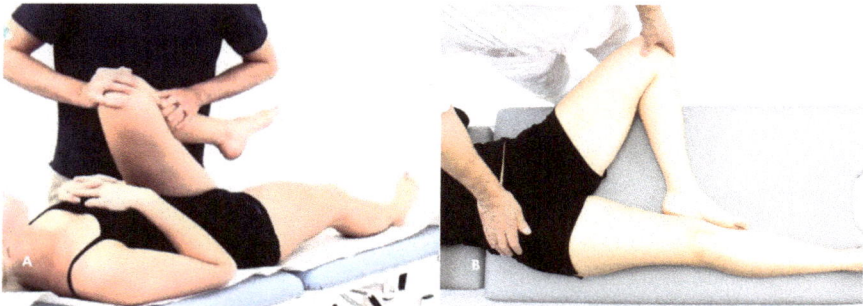

Fig.1.13.20. (A) FABER's test and (B) FADDIR's test

FADDIR test

- **Description**
  - ○ **FADIR test (Flexion, Adduction, Internal Rotation test)**is performed to evaluate for hip femoro-acetabular impingement.
- **Manoeuvre**
  - ○ The patient remains supine.

- The examined leg is passively flexed in knee and hip joints at 90 degrees.
- The physician then adducts and internally rotates the hip.
- The other leg is straight during the examination.

- **Positive findings**
  - The test is positive if, during the manoeuvre, the patient develops anterior groin or anterolateral hip pain. Positive test may indicate femoro-acetabular impingement

Ober Test

- **Description**
  - The Ober's test evaluates a tight, contracted, or inflamed Tensor Fasciae Latae (TFL) and Iliotibial band (ITB)
- **Manoeuvre**
  - The patient is in a side-lying position with the affected side up.
  - Flex the bottom knee and hip to flatten the lumbar curve.
  - Stand behind the patient and firmly stabilise the pelvis/ greater trochanter to prevent movement in any direction.
  - Then grasp the distal end of the patient's affected leg with your other hand and flex the leg to a right angle at the knee
  - Extend and abduct the hip joint then slowly lower the leg toward the table -adduct hip- until motion is restricted. Make sure that the hip does not internally rotate and flex during the test and the pelvis must be stabilised.
  - While letting the thigh drop in flexion and internal rotation would 'give in' to the tight TFL and not accurately test the length (Das & Nadi, 2021).
- **Positive findings**
  - Negative test: If the iliotibial band (ITB) is normal, the leg will adduct with the thigh slightly falling below the horizontal and the patient will not feel any pain.

○ Positive test: If the ITB is tight, the leg would stay in the abducted position and the patient would experience lateral knee pain.

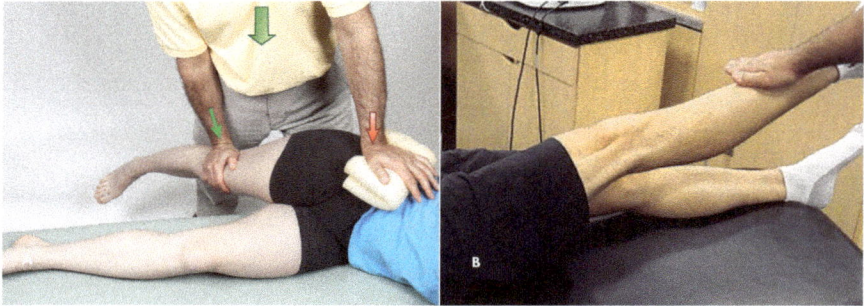

Fig.1.13.21. (A) Ober's test and (B) Stinchfield's test

Stinchfield's Test

- **Description**
  - ○ Stinchfield's test assesses for intraarticular hip pathology.
- **Manoeuvre**
  - ○ The patient lies supine,
  - ○ Ask the patient to flex her hip to 20-30 degrees with the knee fully extended and apply a resistive force.
- **Positive finding**
  - ○ Pain in the anterior groin with this manoeuvre indicates a positive test.

Ely's test

- **Description**
  - ○ Ely's test or Duncan-Ely test is used to assess rectus femoris spasticity or tightness (Marks et al., 2003).
- **Manoeuvre**
  - ○ The patient lies prone in a relaxed state.

- The physician is standing next to the patient, at the side of the leg that will be tested.
- One hand should be on the lower back, the other holding the leg at the heel.
- Passively flex the knee in a rapid fashion.
- The heel should touch the buttocks.
- Test both sides for comparison.

- **Positive finding**
  - The test is positive when the heel cannot touch the buttocks, the hip of the tested side rises up from the table, the patient feels pain or tingling in the back or legs.

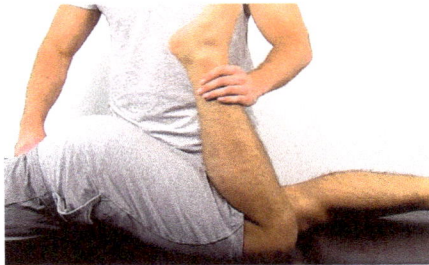

Fig.1.13.22. Ely's test

Further reading

Physiotutors- Thomas Test- Iliopsoas Tightness: https://www.youtube.com/watch?v=NMDd-4NspHs

Physiotutors -Straight Leg Raise or Lasègue's Test for Lumbar Radiculopathy: https://www.youtube.com/watch?v=LdAD9GNv8FI

Physiotutors - Patrick's / Faber / Figure Four Test: https://www.youtube.com/watch?v=89Qiht82zmg

Physiotutors – FADDIR's Test: https://www.youtube.com/watch?v=xyJUIhsL4lg

Clinical physio-Obers Test for Hip | Clinical Physio Premium: https://www.youtube.com/watch?v=ydO-_gc1yWo

The physio channel: How to do the Ely's Test for Rectus Femoris and Femoral Nerve pain: https://www.youtube.com/watch?v=rZqMHA9qh0U

References

Byrd, J. W. T. (2007). Evaluation of the hip: history and physical examination. *North American journal of sports physical therapy : NAJSPT*, *2*(4), 231-240.

Das, M. J., & Nadi, M. (2021). Lasegue Sign. In *StatPearls*. StatPearls Publishing. Copyright © 2021, StatPearls Publishing LLC.

Kamath, S. U., & Kamath, S. S. (2017). Lasègue's Sign. *J Clin Diagn Res*, *11*(5), Rg01-rg02. https://doi.org/10.7860/jcdr/2017/24899.9794

Marks, M. C., Alexander, J., Sutherland, D. H., & Chambers, H. G. (2003). Clinical utility of the Duncan-Ely test for rectus femoris dysfunction during the swing phase of gait. *Dev Med Child Neurol*, *45*(11), 763-768. https://doi.org/10.1017/s0012162203001415

Pesonen, J., Shacklock, M., Rantanen, P., Mäki, J., Karttunen, L., Kankaanpää, M., . . . Rade, M. (2021). Extending the straight leg raise test for improved clinical evaluation of sciatica: reliability of hip internal rotation or ankle dorsiflexion. *BMC Musculoskelet Disord*, *22*(1), 303. https://doi.org/10.1186/s12891-021-04159-y

| 14 |

Large Joint Aspiration

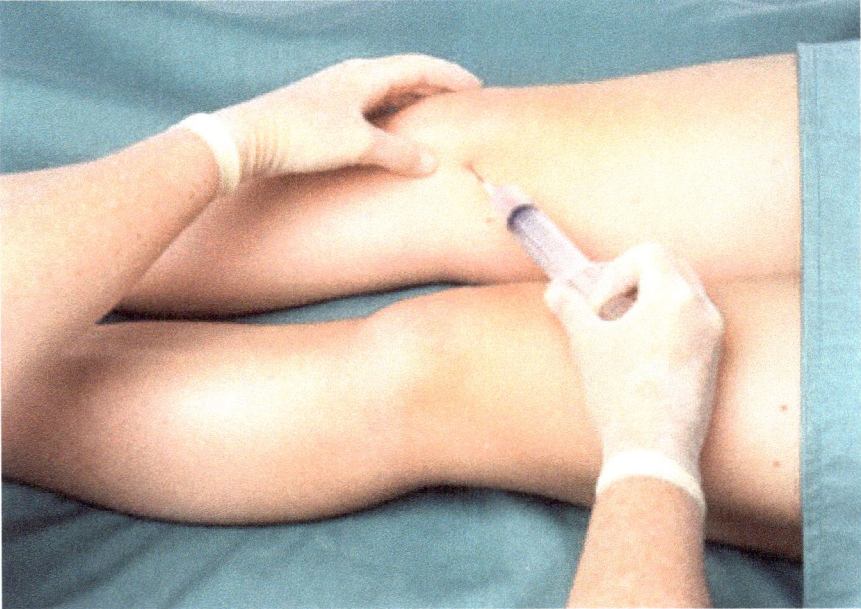

Overview

There are two principal indications for which a needle is inserted into a joint: diagnostic indication to aspirate joint fluid (arthrocentesis) or therapeutic indication to relieve joint pressure or inject medications. Often glucocorticoids, local anaesthetics (or a combination of the two) are injected into joints. Sometimes saline is used to diagnose a joint injury. The extensor surface of the joint is preferred as it lowers the risk of the tendon, ligament, and vascular injuries. When assessing synovial fluid, the rule-of-twos may be used to differentiate among normal, inflammatory, and septic fluid. Normal synovial fluid has fewer than 200 WBCs/mm³. Noninflammatory synovial fluid has 200–2000 WBCs/

mm³ and inflammatory synovial fluid has greater than 2000 WBCs/ mm³ (but <50,000 WBCs/mm³. Septic synovial fluid has greater than 75,000 WBCs/mm³. Only septic synovial fluid will have a positive Gram stain and culture. This section will highlight in detail diverse techniques commonly used in joint arthrocentesis in the emergency department.

Objectives
- By the end of this section, you should be able to:
    - Highlight the indications and contraindications of joint aspiration in the emergency department
    - Describe the techniques commonly used to aspirate different joints.
    - List possible complications associated with this procedure

Indications
- Diagnosis of septic joint
- Diagnosis of traumatic effusion
- Diagnosis of inflammatory effusion
- Diagnosis of crystal-induced arthritis
- Therapeutic relief of pain from effusion

Contraindications
- Severe coagulopathy
- Skin infection over the needle insertion site
- Joint prosthesis
- Patients with bacteraemia or sepsis (except to diagnose a septic joint)

Procedure
- Informed consent may be required.
- Position the patient appropriately.
- The joint should be placed in slight flexion.
- Palpate the joint and identify anatomical landmarks.

○ **For knee arthrocentesis**, the needle should be inserted at the midpoint of either the medial or the lateral side of the patella.

○ **For acromioclavicular (AC) joint arthrocentesis**, the needle should be inserted at the superior surface of the AC joint.

○ **For glenohumeral joint arthrocentesis,** there are two approaches:

- In the anterior approach, the needle is inserted into the groove lateral to the coracoid process.

- In the posterior approach (preferred), the needle is inserted below the posterior border of the acromion process and lateral to the border of the scapula.

- Prepare the skin and drape in a sterile fashion.

- Using lidocaine (drawn up in a 5-mL syringe), anaesthetise the skin with the 25-gauge needle.

- Secure the 18- to 22-gauge needle on the 5- to 50-Ml syringe (depending on the size of the joint) and insert it into the skin.

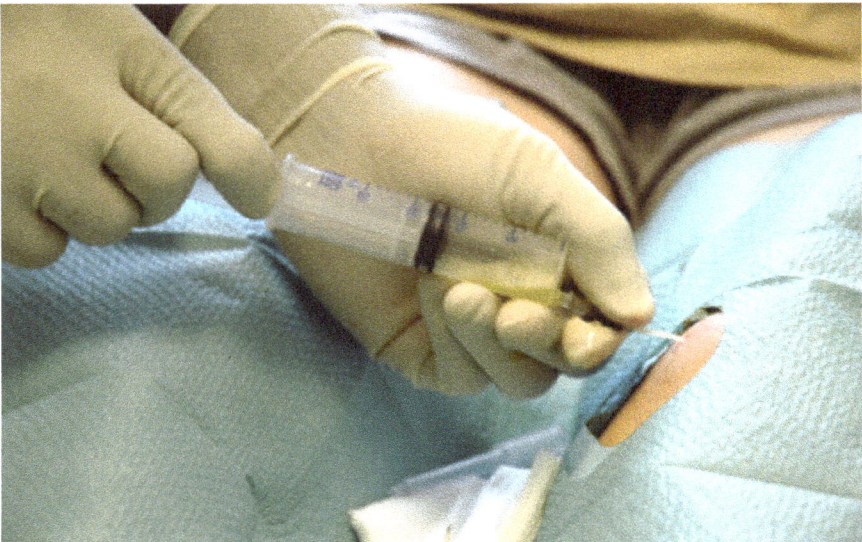

Fig.1.14.1. Knee arthrocentesis

- Advance the needle slowly into the joint space while aspirating until joint fluid can easily be withdrawn.
- While inserting the needle into the joint space, avoid scraping the needle against the bone.
- If fluid cannot be aspirated easily, the catheter can be repositioned further in the joint space or turned by 45° sequentially as needed.
- Once the joint fluid is aspirated, pull out the needle and hold pressure with gauze.
- Bleeding should be minimal.
- Place a band-aid or other dressing over the site.
- Send the synovial fluid to the laboratory.
- Generally, laboratory analyses may include:
  - Crystals,
  - Protein,
  - Glucose,
  - Cell count and differential,
  - Culture and sensitivity, and gram stain.

Complications
- Introduction of infection
- Bleeding
- Dry tap

Post-procedure care
- Ice, elevation, and analgesia (NSAIDs) to relieve pain.
- If considerable effusion, use an elastic bandage after the procedure to minimise swelling and pain.
- If intra-articular anaesthetic has been injected, prohibit joint mobility for at least 4 to 8 hours.
- If an intra-articular corticosteroid has been given, 24 to 48 hours of immobilisation may be required.
- If any redness, pain, and/or swelling > 12 hours after the procedure, the joint should be examined for possible infection.

| 15 |

Lateral Canthotomy & Cantholysis

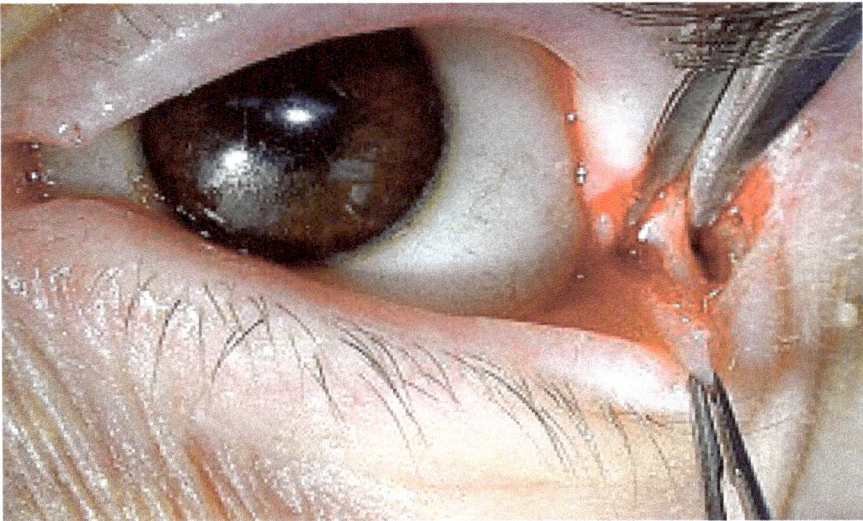

Overview

The orbital compartment is a fixed space with a restricted capacity for expansion. **Orbital compartment syndrome** is an ophthalmologic emergency manifesting with rapid, progressive vision loss, raised intraocular pressure, reduced extraocular motility, and pain in a patient with recent eye/orbital trauma or surgery (Brady, 2020). Blunt facial trauma may induce retrobulbar hematoma or extreme oedema into the retrobulbar space leading to an upsurge in pressure resulting in ischaemia to the retina and optic nerve. **If not managed promptly, this may lead to a** permanent visual loss (Pham et al., 2020). Lateral canthotomy and cantholysis (LCC) is a straightforward procedure to decompress a compartment syndrome of the orbit (McInnes & Howes, 2002). **This procedure** remains the **management of choice** and involves surgically exposing the **lateral canthal tendon** and its **inferior crus** to relieve intraorbital pressure (Pham et al., 2020). Irreversible vision loss can transpire if retina ischaemia time is greater than 90-120 minutes. LCC has the potential to save the vision and can be efficiently performed by the emergency physician (McInnes & Howes, 2002).

Objectives

- By the end of this module, you should be able to:
    - Identify the indications of lateral canthotomy and cantholysis (LCC)
    - Recall the contraindications of LCC
    - Describe the procedure of LCC
    - List potential complications following LCC

Indications

- Facial trauma and suspected orbital compartment syndrome. associated with:
    - Retrobulbar Bleed
    - Proptosis
    - Tender, hard eyeballs
    - Decreased Visual Acuity
    - Tender, hard eyeballs
    - Raise in intra-ocular pressure (**40 mmHg** and above of pressure requires decompression)

Contraindications

A potential globe rupture is a relative contraindication (Gushchin, 2020).

- Consider globe rupture if:

- ○ Enophthalmos
- ○ Conjunctival Tear
- ○ Hyphema
- ○ Irregular Shaped Pupil
- ○ Subconjunctival Haemorrhage

Equipment

- Chloraprep applicator
- Lidocaine 1% with needle and syringe
- Straight artery forceps
- Chlorhexidine
- Needle and syringe for lidocaine injection
- Tenotomy scissors
- Straight mosquito hemostat
- Forceps

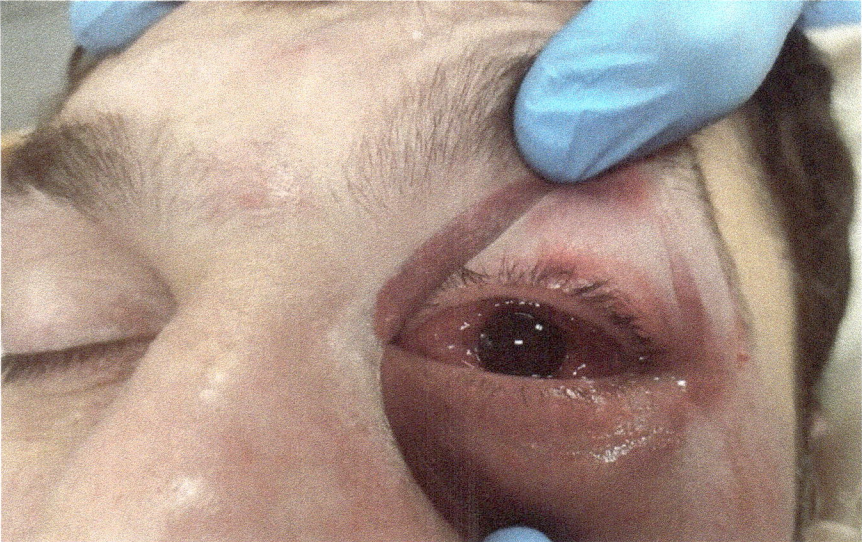

Fig.1.15.1. Orbital compartment syndrome

Relevant Anatomy for Lateral Canthotomy

- The medial and lateral canthal ligaments contain the eye within the orbit and eyelids.

- The lateral canthal tendon has two branches: a superior and an inferior.
- Cutting one, or both loosens the eyelids and allows the globe to expand out of the orbit and thus relieve pressure on the eye (Brady, 2020).

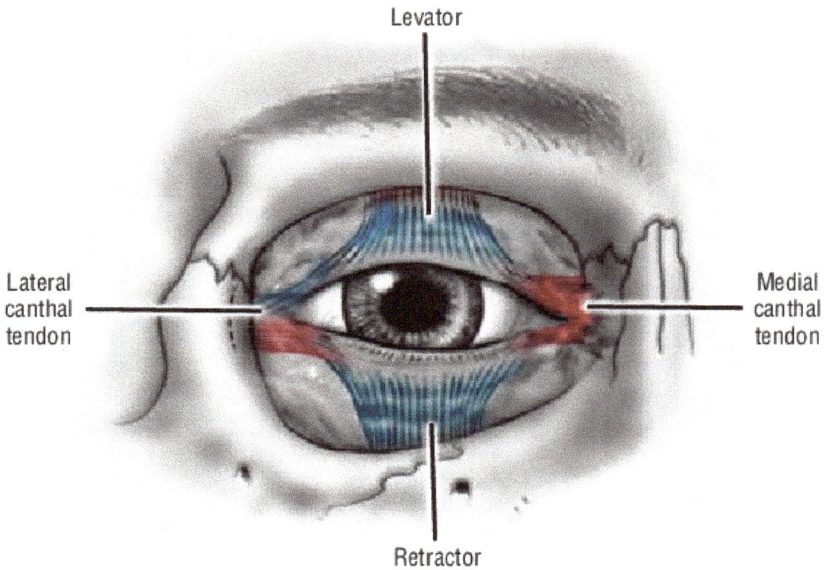

Fig.1.15.2. Anatomical Consideration of the eye
Semantic Scholar

Landmarks and Procedure

- The patient should be positioned supine with the head of the bed elevated 10-15° (Gushchin, 2020)
- Inform the patient about the procedure and obtain consent.
- Consider sedation
- Cleanse the area around the eye
- Infiltrate 1-2ml of 1% lignocaine with adrenaline into the lateral canthus. Do not injure the globe
- Devascularise the lateral canthus using a little clamp to clamp the tissues for about 15-30 seconds.

- Incise into the lateral canthus, staying away from the globe.
- Then cut the canthal tendons. These run superiorly and inferiorly and feel like guitar strings
- If bleeding, control with direct pressure. The eye pressure should reduce almost immediately.

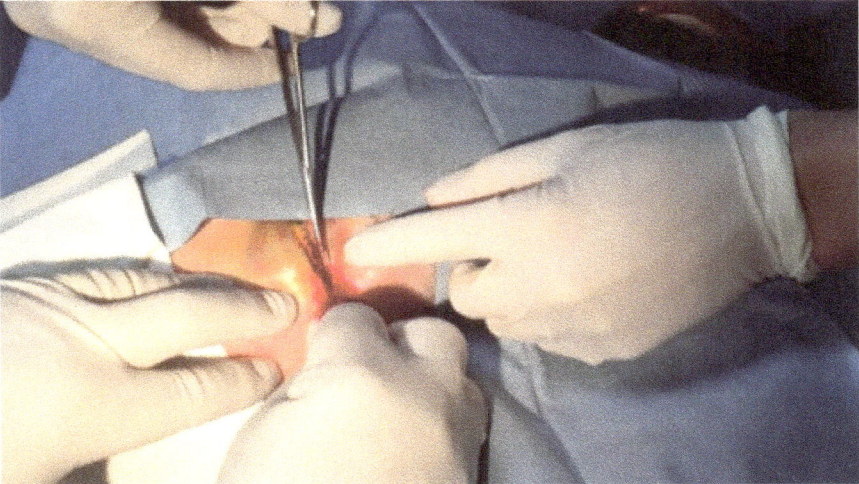

Fig.1.15.3. Lateral cathotomy- Incision into the lateral canthus
Resus Australia

Complications

- Iatrogenic injury to the globe or lateral rectus
- Ptosis due to damage to the levator aponeurosis (Weber et al., 2009)
- Injury to the lacrimal gland and lacrimal artery
- Bleeding
- Extensive cantholysis may result in ectropion (Vassallo et al., 2002)

Further reading

EM Curious-The Lateral Canthotomy: http://www.emcurious.com/blog-1/2014/9/25/the-lateral-canthotomy

References

Brady, C. (2020). How to do lateral canthotomy. MSD Manual. Retrieved 22 Dec. 2021 from https://www.msdmanuals.com/en-gb/professional/eye-disorders/how-to-do-eye-procedures/how-to-do-lateral-canthotomy

Gushchin, A. G. (2020). Lateral Canthotomy and Cantholysis. Medscape. Retrieved 23 Dec. 2021 from https://emedicine.medscape.com/article/82812-overview

McInnes, G., & Howes, D. W. (2002). Lateral canthotomy and cantholysis: a simple, vision-saving procedure. Cjem, 4(1), 49-52. https://doi.org/10.1017/s1481803500006060

Pham, B., Lin, B., & Pham, R. (2020). How to perform a lateral canthotomy. Eyeguru. Retrieved 22 Dec. 2021 from https://eyeguru.org/blog/lateral-canthotomy/

Vassallo, S., Hartstein, M., Howard, D., & Stetz, J. (2002). Traumatic retrobulbar hemorrhage: emergent decompression by lateral canthotomy and cantholysis. J Emerg Med, 22(3), 251-256. https://doi.org/10.1016/s0736-4679(01)00477-2

Weber, D., Shaw, S., & Winslow, J. (2009). Traumatic eye swelling. Subconjunctival and orbital emphysema with orbital floor fracture. Ann Emerg Med, 54(4), 635, 642.

| 16 |

Lumbar Puncture

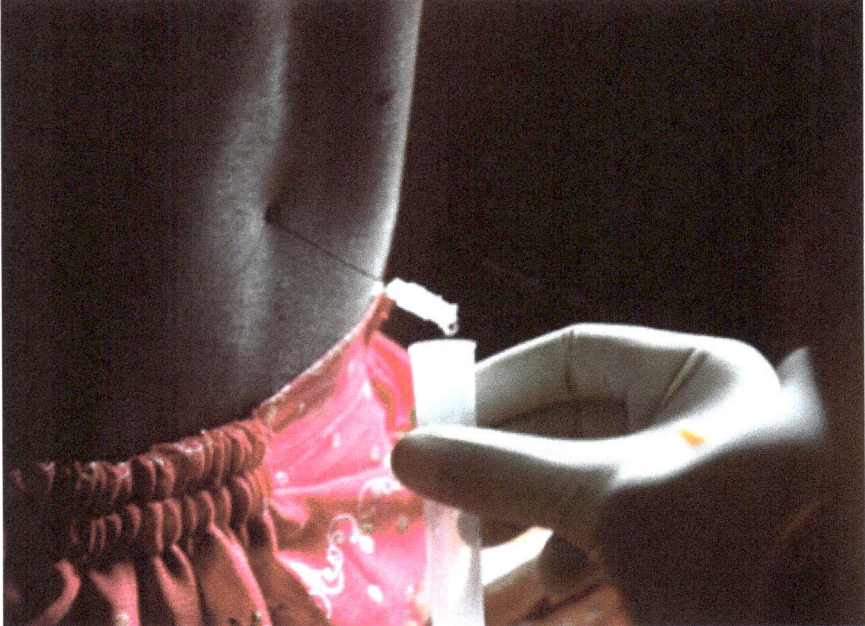

Overview

Lumbar puncture (LP) is a procedure that is often performed in the emergency department to obtain information about cerebrospinal fluid (CSF) (Cooper, 2011; Farley & McLafferty, 2008). LP with an examination of CSF is an essential diagnostic tool for various infectious and non-infectious neurologic conditions (e.g., bacterial meningitis or subarachnoid haemorrhage). LP is also sometimes used for therapeutic purposes (e.g., treatment of pseudotumor cerebri). CSF fluid analysis can also assist in the diagnosis of numerous other diseases (e.g., demyelinating diseases and carcinomatous meningitis). LP should be performed only after a neurologic examination but should never delay potentially life-saving interventions, such as administering antibiotics and steroids to patients with suspected bacterial meningitis (Shlamovitz, 2020).

Objectives

- By the end of this chapter, you should be able to:
  - Describe the indications and contraindications for lumbar puncture.
  - Explain the technique involved in a lumbar puncture.
  - Review the common complications of lumbar puncture.

Indications

- **Diagnostic**
  - Evaluation for the possibility of a central nervous system (CNS) infection: Viral, Bacterial, and Fungal Meningitis and Encephalitis
  - Evaluation for inflammatory processes: Multiple Sclerosis, Guillain-Barré syndrome
  - Evaluation for spontaneous subarachnoid haemorrhage (SAH)
  - Suspicion of CNS diseases: oncological and metabolic processes
- **Therapeutic**
  - Therapeutic reduction of cerebrospinal fluid (CSF) pressure
  - Procedures requiring lower body analgesia or anaesthesia
  - Intrathecal antibiotic administration for some types of meningitis
  - Chemotherapy and methotrexate for some forms of leukaemia and lymphomas

Contraindications

- **Absolute:**
  - ○ The presence of infected skin over the needle entry site
  - ○ The presence of unequal pressures between the supratentorial and infratentorial compartments.
- The latter is usually inferred from the following characteristic findings on computed tomography (CT) of the brain:
  - ○ Midline shift
  - ○ Loss of suprachiasmatic and basilar cisterns
  - ○ Posterior fossa mass
  - ○ Loss of the superior cerebellar cistern
  - ○ Loss of the quadrigeminal plate cistern
- **Relative:**
  - ○ Increased intracranial pressure (ICP)
  - ○ Coagulopathy
  - ○ Brain abscess
- **Indications for performing brain CT scanning before lumbar puncture** in patients with suspected meningitis include the following (Hasbun et al., 2001):
  - ○ Age > 60 years
  - ○ Immunocompromised patient
  - ○ Patients with known CNS lesions
  - ○ Seizure within 1 week of presentation
  - ○ Abnormal level of consciousness
  - ○ Focal findings on neurologic examination
  - ○ Evidence of papilledema seen on physical examination, with clinical suspicion of an elevated ICP

Consent

According to the GMC, the consent can be (GMC, 2019):

- *Informed consent*: the patient should be provided with all the information about what the procedure involves, including the benefits and risks, whether there are reasonable alternative treatments, and what will happen if the procedure fails.

- *Verbal consent*: The patient says they're happy to have the procedure done
- *Implied consent*: Assuming that the patient has voluntarily positioned him/herself to allow the procedure.
- *Voluntary:* the decision to either consent or not to consent to the procedure must be made by the patient and must not be influenced by pressure from medical staff, friends, or family.

All adults are presumed to have sufficient capacity to decide on their own medical treatment unless there's significant evidence to suggest otherwise GMC, 2019).

- ***Capacity:*** the patient must be capable of giving consent, which means they understand the information given to them and can use it to make an informed decision.
- In case of emergency or if a person ***does not have the capacity*** to decide about their treatment and they have not appointed a lasting power of attorney (LPA), emergency physicians should go ahead with the procedure if they believe it's in the person's best interests.
- If children are able to consent, they usually consent themselves. But someone with parental responsibility may need to give consent for a child up to the age of 16 to have treatment.

Equipment
- Spinal needle(s) with stylet
- Three-way stopcock (optional: drainage catheter)
- Manometer (optional: extension tube for higher opening pressures)

- Specimen tubes (may vary, but in general labelled 1–4, important to obtain from 1, 2, 3, 4 owing to cell count obtained from tubes 1 and 3)
- Local anaesthetic (lidocaine 1 or 2 %), 5- to 10-mL syringe and needle (25-gauge) for local anaesthesia
- Sterile drapes and gauze
- Mask, sterile gown, sterile gloves
- Antiseptic solution for skin preparation (Chloroprep or iodine)

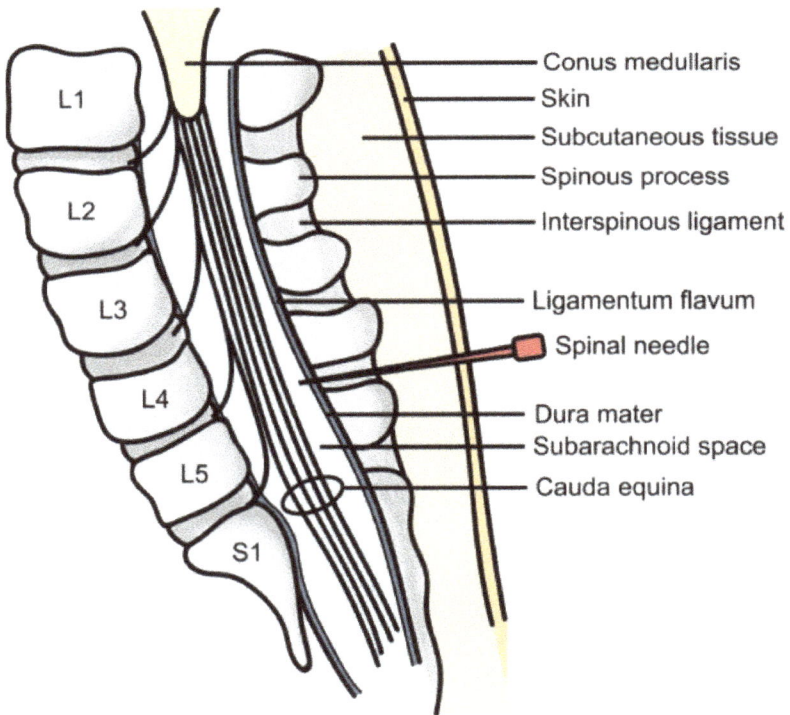

Fig.1.16.1. Lumbar puncture anatomical landmarks

Landmarks

- It is defined by palpation.
- Draw a visual line between the superior aspects of the iliac crests that intersects the midline at the L4 interspace.

- The L3–4 and L4–5 spaces are favoured because these points are below the termination of the spinal cord.
- Palpate the posterosuperior iliac crests with the midpoint of a visual line that connects the two crests representing the L4 spinous process.
- Palpate the space between the L3–4 or the L4–5 spinous processes and mark where the needle will be placed.
- **Ultrasound guidance (optional):**
  - Helpful in obese patients, patients with previous surgical scarring, or anyone in whom palpation of the spinous processes is not easily done.
  - Sonographic measurement of the dura mater strongly correlates with needle depth needed to obtain CSF.

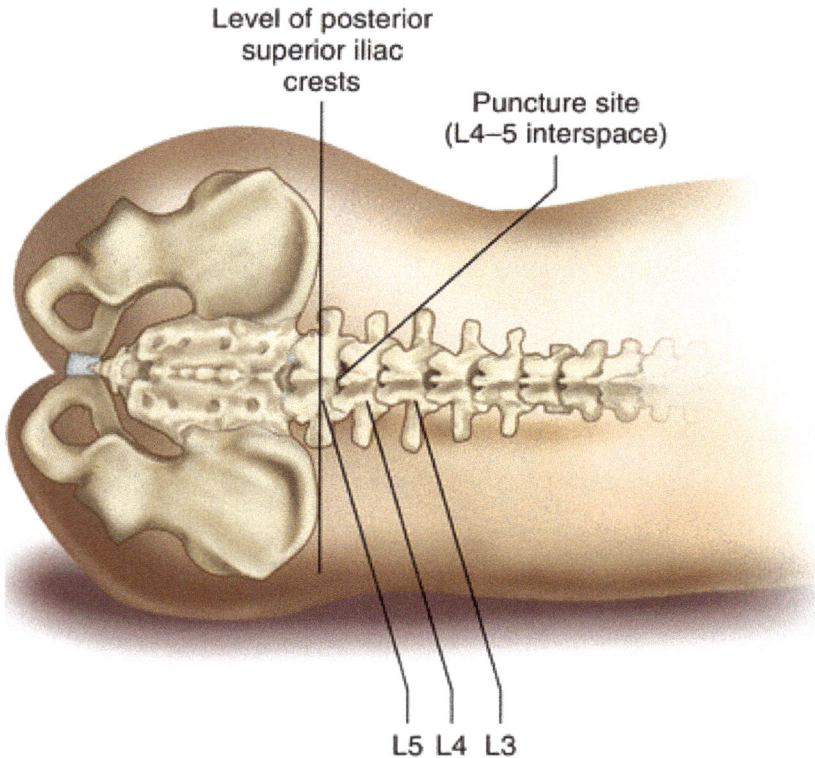

Level of posterior superior iliac crests

Puncture site (L4–5 interspace)

L5 L4 L3

Fig.1.15.2. Lumbar puncture Landmarks

Procedure

Positioning

- Determined by practitioner preference or patient capability.
- Options: lateral recumbent position, upright sitting position.
- The lateral recumbent position is preferred to obtain accurate opening pressure and to reduce the risk of post puncture headache.

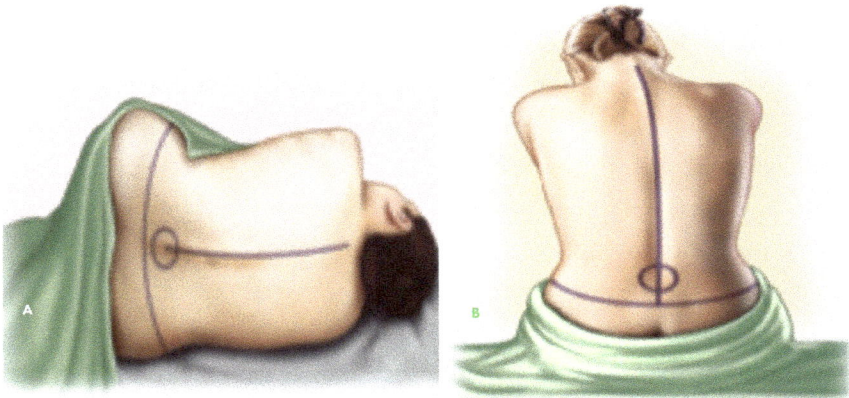

Fig.1.15.3. Lumbar puncture - (A) Left lateral decubitus position abd (B) Sitting position with general areas of insertion of the needle

- Both positions require the patient to arch the lower back toward the practitioner to open up the intervertebral spaces (obtain the "foetal position" or arch "like a cat").
- Shoulders and hips should remain aligned during the process.

Sterile Preparation

- After positioning and palpating the appropriate landmarks
- Dress in the suitable protective gear: mask, gown, and sterile gloves.
- Sterilely prepare the patient.
- Completely expose the patient's back.

- Clean the patient's back with an antiseptic solution
- Apply sterile drapes with the puncture site exposed.
- Inject local anaesthesia into the deep tissues
- Systemic sedatives and analgesics may also be used.

Needle insertion

- Insert the needle, cephalad with the bevel up, in the midline between the L3–4 or the L4–5 spinous process, and the stylet should be firmly in place.
- Initially parallel to the bed, but once into the subcutaneous tissue, the needle should be angled toward the umbilicus (slightly cephalad, 15°) with the bevel facing upward.
- If properly positioned, the needle passes through the skin; subcutaneous tissue; supraspinous ligament; interspinous ligament between the spinous processes; ligamentum flavum; epidural space including the internal vertebral venous plexus, dura, and arachnoid; into the subarachnoid space and between the nerve roots of the cauda equina.
- In most cases, a "pop" will be felt when the needle penetrates the ligamentum flavum, entering the subarachnoid space; then intermittent withdrawal should be done in 2-mm intervals to assess for CSF flow.
- If the bone is encountered during insertion, partially withdraw the needle without exiting the skin and readjust to a different angle more cephalad.
- If the tap is traumatic, CSF may be blood-tinged but should clear as more is collected.
- If it does not clear, it may indicate intracranial haemorrhage or subarachnoid blood.

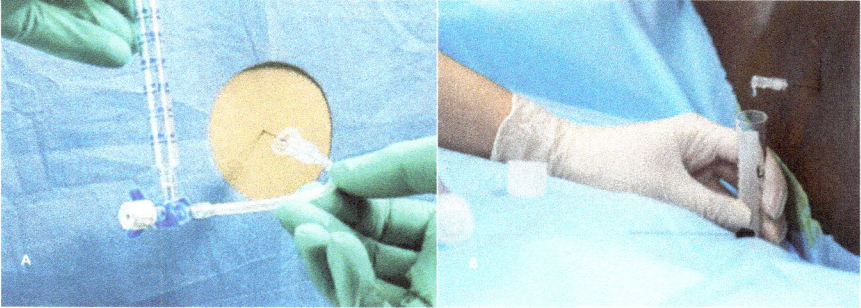

Fig.1.16.4. Lumbar puncture- (A) opening pressure measurement and (B) CSF collection

- Also, in traumatic patients, clotting will be seen in the tubes; clotting does not occur in SAH owing to defibrinated blood being present in the CSF.
- Blood-tinged CSF can also be seen in herpes simplex virus (HSV) encephalitis.
- A dry tap is usually due to incorrect positioning and misdirection of the needle, often due to a superior direction of the needle with obstruction by the lamina or spinous process of the superior or inferior vertebra. If the needle is too lateral, an inferior or superior articular process may be hit.
- If the flow slows down, rotate the needle 90° because a nerve root may be obstructing the opening.

Opening pressure measurement

- Must be performed in the lateral recumbent position.
- Although there are some conversion formulas from the sitting position, these are not standard of care.
- Once the needle is in the subarachnoid space and CSF is flowing from the needle, the three-way stopcock should be attached to the needle and the manometer should be attached to the stopcock to take a measurement.
- Use the flexible tube to connect the manometer to the hub of the needle.

- Note the height of fluid in the manometer after it stops rising (normal opening pressure, <20 cm Hg); it may be possible to see pulsations from cardiac or respiratory motion.
- Elevated CSF pressure is seen with meningeal inflammation, hydrocephalus, pseudotumor cerebri, SAH, and CHF.
- Decreased CSF pressure is seen in leakage of CSF and severe dehydration.

Collecting CSF fluid

- Collect at least 1–2 mL of CSF fluid in each tube, going from 1 to 4 and never aspirate because this can cause haemorrhage.
- After collecting the fluid, replace the stylet and remove the needle, clean the skin, and place a bandage over the puncture site.

General Recommendations
- *Tube 1:* glucose, protein, protein electrophoresis
- *Tube 2:* Gram stain, bacterial and viral cultures
- *Tube 3:* cell count and differential
- When ruling out SAH, cell count should be performed in tubes 1 and 3 or 1 and 4 to differentiate between SAH and traumatic tap.
- *Tube 4:* Any special tests: myelin basic proteins, lactate, pyruvate, and smear on cell concentrates all depend on suspicion.

Complications
- Implantation of epidermoid tumours: from introducing skin plug into the subarachnoid space and can be avoided by using stylet when advancing.
- Post lumbar puncture headache: most common, occurring in 36.5 % of patients within 48 h
- CSF leak: causes a headache when CSF leak through puncture site exceeds the rate of production

- Bleeding: most common in patients with bleeding diathesis; may result in spinal cord compression
- Epidural hematoma
- Infection: local cellulitis, abscess (local or epidural), or meningitis
- Herniation syndromes: high risk can be identified by computed tomography but may not completely identify all patients with increased ICP
- Backache: local or referred pain
- Cardiorespiratory compromise

Further reading

Uptodate - Lumbar puncture: https://www.uptodate.com/contents/lumbar-puncture-technique-indications-contraindications-and-complications-in-adults

References

Cooper, N. (2011). Lumbar puncture. Acute Med, 10(4), 188-193.

Farley, A., & McLafferty, E. (2008). Lumbar puncture. Nurs Stand, 22(22), 46-48. https://doi.org/10.7748/ns2008.02.22.22.46.c6358

GMC. (2019). Consent for treatment. General Medical Council UK. https://www.nhs.uk/conditions/consent-to-treatment/

Hasbun, R., Abrahams, J., Jekel, J., & Quagliarello, V. J. (2001). Computed tomography of the head before lumbar puncture in adults with suspected meningitis. N Engl J Med, 345(24), 1727-1733. https://doi.org/10.1056/NEJMoa010399

Shlamovitz, G. Z. (2020). Lumbar Puncture. Medscape. Retrieved 30 Nov. 2021 from https://emedicine.medscape.com/article/80773-overview

| 17 |

Non-Invasive Ventilation

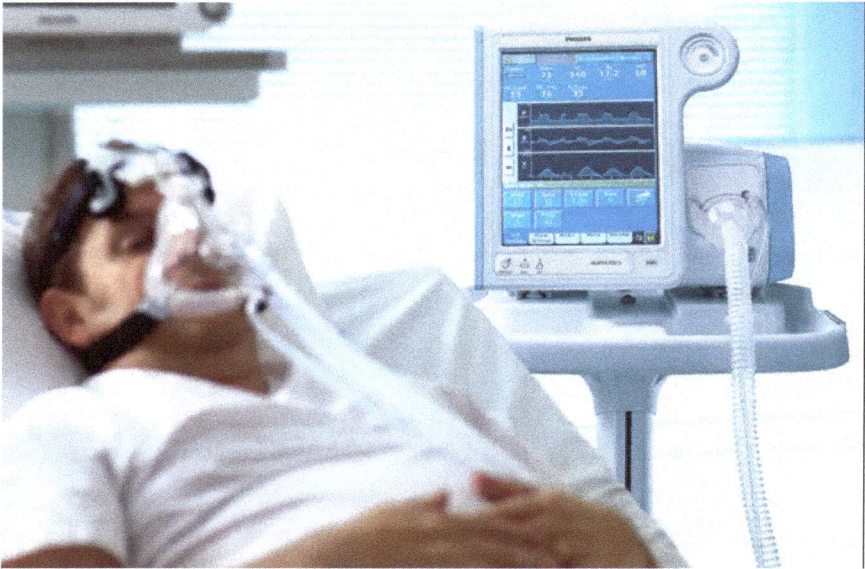

Overview

Around 3 million people live with COPD in the UK, which is the fifth leading cause of death. Type 2 respiratory failure happens in late disease-causing significant morbidity and mortality (Imperial College Healthcare NHS Trust, 2018). Non-invasive ventilation (NIV) provides ventilatory support through the patient's upper airway applying a mask or similar device. NIV is distinguished from the invasive technique which bypasses the upper airway with a tracheal tube, laryngeal mask, or tracheostomy (BMJ, 2002). Non-invasive ventilation (NIV) is currently the most effective treatment for these patients, reducing mortality by 50%. Unfortunately, NIV is stressful and frightening (Imperial College Healthcare NHS Trust, 2018). Modern NIV devices have several modes. The primary therapy delivered by NIV is called bi-level positive airway pressure because it uses two pressure levels (Wheatley, 2021).

- **Inspiratory positive airway pressure (IPAP)** – this increases the tidal volume per minute (the amount of air that moves in or out of the lungs with each respiratory cycle) and alveolar ventilation, as well as enabling carbon dioxide (CO_2) removal.
- **Expiratory positive airway pressure (EPAP)** – this opens the alveolar to allow for more gas exchange by increasing the surface area; it prevents dynamic airway collapse, decreases auto-positive end-expiratory pressure and increases the functional residual capacity of the lungs.

Objectives
- By the end of this chapter, you should be able to:
  - Understand the difference between non-invasive from invasive ventilation.
  - Highlight the indications and contraindications for NIV.
  - Learn the potential complications associated with NIV.

Common NIV modes and CPAP
Modern NIV devices have several modes (Wheatley, 2021):

- **Spontaneous timed:** Bi-level positive airway pressure ventilation (IPAP & EPAP) that spontaneously triggers a breath, with a timed back-up breath if an apnoea period occurs; the value determined by the difference between IPAP & EPAP (pressure support) is used to create sufficient tidal volume to aid the removal of carbon dioxide.
- **Spontaneous: Bi-level positive airway pressure** that is patient triggered without a timed backup breath

- **Continuous Positive Airway Pressure (CPAP):** A continuous flow of air pressure (also called positive end-expiratory pressure or EPAP)
- **Volume-targeted modes** (Average volume-assured pressure support): the delivery of a pre-set average assured volume, normally based on ideal patient weight (8-10ml/Kg), that is delivered between a range of IPAP upper and lower settings and a fixed EPAP setting.

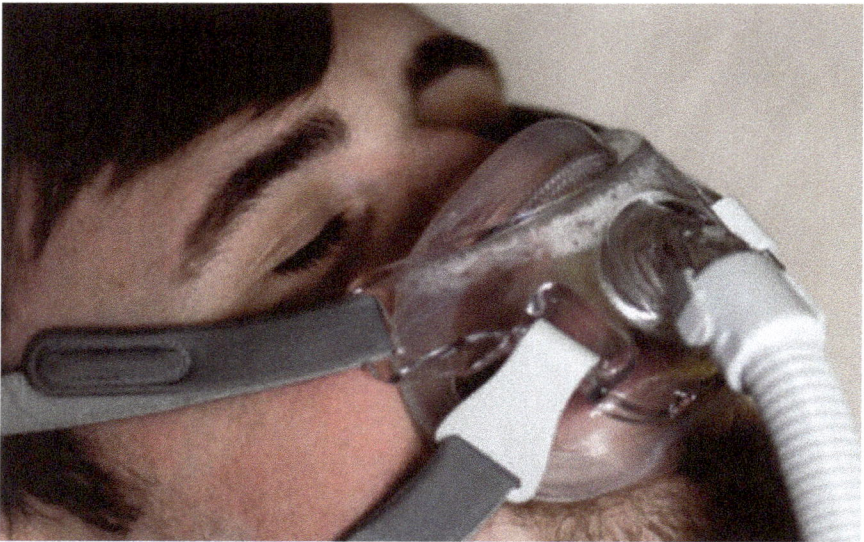

Fig.1.17.1. Non-invasive positive-pressure ventilation

- **Average volume-assured pressure support auto-EPAP**: the delivery of a pre-set average assured volume, normally based on ideal patient weight (8-10ml/Kg), that is delivered between a range of IPAP upper and lower settings with the added variable auto-EPAP range (which has upper and lower settings).
- **Pressure control:** Ventilator-timed breaths with IPAP and EPAP, with a set inspiratory time.

Indications for NIV

- Hypercapnic respiratory failure during an acute exacerbation of COPD with:
    - Arterial pH <7.35.
    - Arterial $PaCO_2$>6kPa (if acute onset).
    - Tachypnoea >25 breaths/min

Inclusion criteria for NIV

- Primary diagnosis of COPD exacerbation
- Able to protect the airway
- Conscious and cooperative
- Patient's wishes considered
- Potential for recovery of quality of life that will be acceptable to the patient
- NIV can be considered in the unconscious if within a critical care setting or intubation is inappropriate

Exclusion criteria for NIV

- Life-threatening hypoxaemia
- Intubation and ventilation are possible and would be in the patient's best interests
- Inability to protect the airway
- Confusion
- Agitation
- Undrained pneumothorax
- Fixed upper airway obstruction
- Facial burns/trauma
- Recent facial or upper airway surgery
- Vomiting
- Copious respiratory secretions
- Bowel obstruction
- Upper gastrointestinal surgery

- Severe co-morbidity
- Patient moribund

Pre-setting care

Before use, it is essential to prepare the equipment, including (Wheatley, 2021):

- Non-invasive ventilator.
- Hose (single- or dual-limb, depending on the device)
- Face mask and sizing gauge.
- Oxygen port if the NIV does not have piped oxygen
- Exhalation port for CO_2 clearance if this is not built into the face mask
- Bacterial and viral filter.
- If a patient is suspected or confirmed to have an infectious respiratory disease, such as Covid-19, increase the number of bacterial and viral filter placements.
- An oronasal facemask is recommended as a patient's initial interface (Davidson et al., 2016) the benefit of using this, or a full-face mask is that it reduces leakage from the mouth that would be experienced with a nasal mask.
- NIV settings should be prescribed by personnel who have had training and maintain competence appropriate for their role (Davies et al., 2018).
- Initial settings and any changes should be documented on a standardised proforma (NCEPOD, 2017).
- If a patient is receiving inhaled bronchodilators via NIV, a T-piece nebulisation adapter should be used as close to the NIV mask as possible and maintained in a horizontal position so that the nebuliser solution does not drain out.

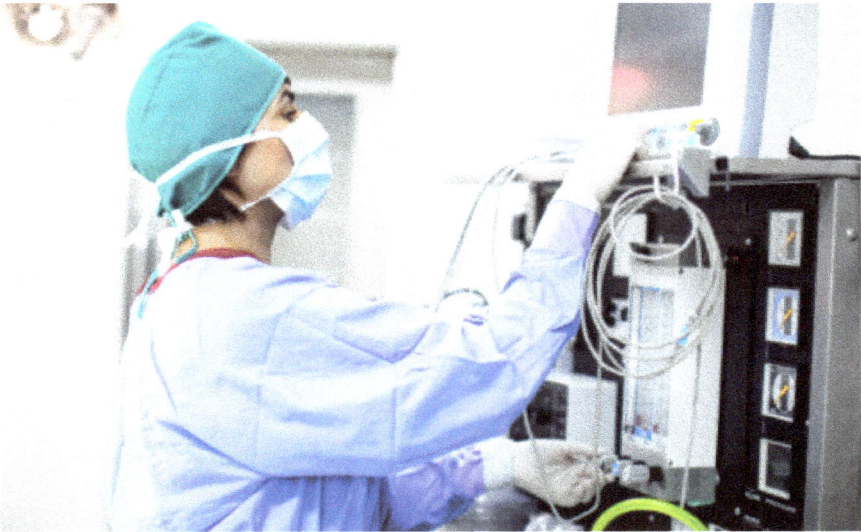

Fig.1.17.2. Setting up a ventilator

Setting up NIV treatment

- Consultant/Senior Decision-maker to commence NIV.
- Set EPAP at 4 – 5 cm H_2O and IPAP at 10 cm H_2
- Set back-up breathing frequency to 8 – 10 breaths/minute.
- Select appropriate size mask (full face in preference to nasal) to fit patient.
- Explain the procedure to the patient.
- Hold the mask in place to allow the patient to familiarise themselves.
- Attach pulse oximeter.
- Commence NIV, holding the mask in place initially.
- Secure mask in place with straps/headgear to prevent leaks – do not attach too tightly!
- Reassess the patient after a few minutes.
- Check for leaks and refit the mask if necessary.
- Add O_2 to maintain SpO_2 >85%.
- Instruct patient how to remove the mask and summon help.
- Increase IPAP gradually up to about 12 - 15 cmH_2O over 1 hr.
- Clinical assessment and, if appropriate, check ABG at 1 hour.

- If the procedure fails, institute an alternative management plan

Monitoring

- Initially, sit the patient up in a comfortable position, then repositioning to alleviate sacral pressure is possible.
- Ensure continuous electronic monitoring of oxygen saturation and electrocardiogram
- Ensure consistent observations for ACVPU (Alertness, Confusion, Voice, Pain, Unconsciousness), respiratory rate, temperature and blood pressure (Davidson et al., 2016).
- Ensure regular physiological monitoring using the National Early Warning Score (NEWS2) system (Wheatley, 2021).
- Set the NIV alarms to produce an audible alert of any issues.
- Ensure that the patient is reviewed by a specialist within four hours of starting acute NIV and by a consultant with expertise in NIV within 14 hours (Davies et al., 2018).
- Initial ABG is required in the first hour of starting NIV then repeated after four hours and if the patient shows signs of deterioration (Davies et al., 2018).
- Treatment is likely to be more successful if there are improvements in pH and $PaCO_2$ values and a reduction in respiratory rate after two hours of NIV (Roberts et al., 2011).
- If pH and $PaCO_2$ do not show any improvement, review the NIV treatment and, if appropriate, IPAP pressure titrated.
- Optimising a patient's tidal volume by altering IPAP to increase the pressure support range between IPAP and EPAP, to achieve 8ml/kg (based on ideal body weight), should help reduce $PaCO_2$ levels.
- An increase in IPAP pressure is often undertaken in $2cmH_2O$ increments. In acute settings, titration may be fast, with pressure increased over 10-30 minutes after the initial set-up.

Complications of NIV

- **Pressure ulcers or skin breakdown on the nasal bridge or cheeks:**
    - Result of tight mask seals used to attain adequate inspiratory volumes
    - Minimise pressure by intermittent application of non-invasive ventilation
    - Schedule breaks (30-90 min) to minimise effects of mask pressure
    - Balance strap tension to minimise mask leaks without excessive mask pressures
    - Cover vulnerable areas (erythematous points of contact) with protective dressings
- **Gastric distension or vomiting:**
    - Rarely a problem
    - Avoid by limiting peak inspiratory pressures to less than 25 cm of water
    - Nasogastric tubes can be placed but can worsen leaks from the mask
    - The nasogastric tube also bypasses the lower oesophageal sphincter and permits reflux
- **Aspiration of gastric contents:**
    - Especially if emesis during non-invasive ventilation
    - Avoid non-invasive ventilation in a patient with ongoing emesis or hematemesis
- **Non-compliance, fear or claustrophobia:**
    - Discuss treatment modalities and their benefits with the patients
    - Involve patients in decision making
    - Allow limited mask application time, then build-up
    - Arrange consultant review
    - Be persistent
    - Review ceiling of care

- **Dry mucous membranes and thick secretions:**
  - Seen in patients with extended use of non-invasive ventilation
  - Provide humidification for non-invasive ventilation devices
  - Provide daily oral care
- **Mask leak:**
  - Ensure appropriate mask interface
  - Accurate sizing and fit
- **Barotrauma:**
  - Significantly less risk with non-invasive ventilation
- **Discomfort:**
  - Consider using a nasal mask or full facial mask
  - Ensure appropriate mask interface
  - Reduce mask-strap tightness
- **Inadequate ventilation:**
  - Review NIV pressure and ABG
  - Adjust NIV settings
- **Hypotension related to positive intrathoracic pressure** (support with fluids):
  - Monitor BP and ECG
  - Provide IV fluid or adequate oral hydration

Weaning patients off NIV

- The duration of NIV therapy depends largely on the resolution or improvement of a patient's ABGs and clinical signs.
- NIV should be maximised in the first 24 hours and can be tapered thereafter, once the patient has stabilised.
- If a patient continues to be dependent on NIV, a common weaning protocol starts with breaks for meals and then works towards a routine of NIV only being used overnight and for two hours in the morning and two hours in the afternoon.

- If a patient is receiving oxygen via NIV, the British Thoracic Society/Intensive Care Society guidelines recommend reducing the oxygen gradually, but maintaining an arterial blood-oxygen level of 88-92% saturation in all causes of acute hypercapnic respiratory failure; the duration of NIV is individual to each patient, but normalisation of pH and a PaCO2 level of <6.5kPa are often used as a guide (Davidson et al., 2016).

Continuous Positive Airway Pressure (CPAP)

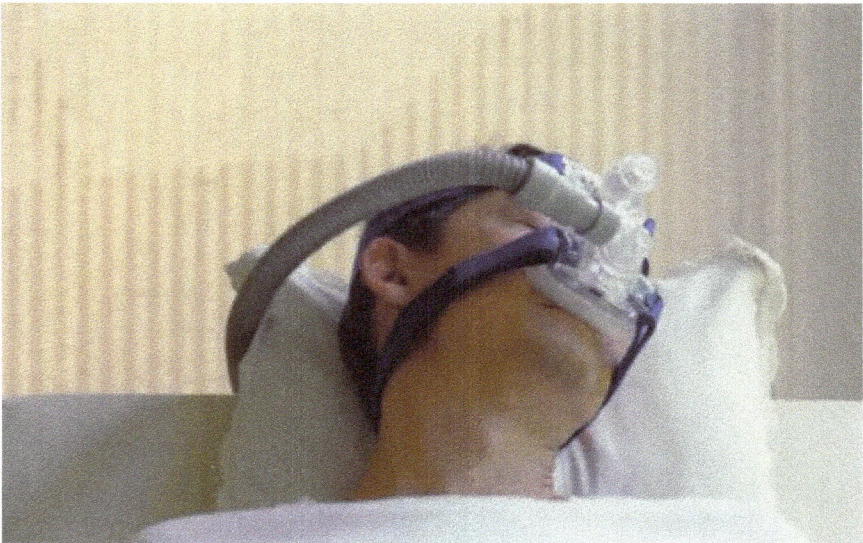

- **Indications:** Hypoxemia due to:
    - CCF, CPO, Pneumonia, asthma, COPD,
    - Near drowning
    - Obstructive Sleep Apnoea
- **Cautions**
    - Cardiogenic shock
    - Agitated patient
    - Right ventricular failure
    - Severe obstructive airways disease

- **Contraindications**
  - Immediate endotracheal intubation indicated
  - A respiratory arrest or inadequate spontaneous ventilation
  - Worsening life-threatening hypoxia
  - Unconscious patient unable to protect own airway
- **How to deliver NIV**
  - Correctly fitting mask
  - Supplemental O_2
  - Commence PEEP at 5-7.5 cm H_2O and increase to 10cm as tolerated
  - Continue for 30min/hr until the reduction in dyspnoea and saturations are maintained off NIV
- **Complications**
  - Dry mouth
  - Aspiration
  - Worsening right ventricular failure
  - Hyperpnoea,
  - Intolerance due to anxiety,
  - Pneumothorax
  - Skin/Eye discomfort.

Further reading

Medscape- Non-Invasive ventilation: https://emedicine.med-scape.com/article/304235-overview#a10

References

BMJ. (2002). Non-invasive ventilation in acute respiratory failure. Thorax, 57(3), 192. https://doi.org/10.1136/thorax.57.3.192

Davidson, A. C., Banham, S., Elliott, M., Kennedy, D., Gelder, C., Glossop, A., . . . Thomas, L. (2016). BTS/ICS guideline for the ventilatory management of acute hypercapnic respiratory failure in adults. Thorax, 71 Suppl 2, ii1-35. https://doi.org/10.1136/thoraxjnl-2015-208209

Davies, M., Allen, M., Bentley, A., Bourke, S. C., Creagh-Brown, B., D'Oliveiro, R., . . . Setchfield, I. (2018). British Thoracic Society Quality Standards for acute non-invasive ventilation in adults. BMJ Open Respir Res, 5(1), e000283. https://doi.org/10.1136/bmjresp-2018-000283

Imperial College Healthcare NHS Trust. (2018). Non-Invasive Ventilation – Improving patient experience and outcomes through understanding (INTU). NICE Guidelines. Retrieved 3 Dec. 2021 from https://www.nice.org.uk/sharedlearning/non-invasive-ventilation-improving-patient-experience-and-outcomes-through-understanding-intu

NCEPOD. (2017). Inspiring Change: A Review of the Quality of Care Provided to Patients Receiving Acute Non-invasive Ventilation . National Confidential Enquiry into Patient Outcome and Death. https://www.ncepod.org.uk/2017report2/downloads/InspiringChange_FullReport.pdf

Roberts, C. M., Stone, R. A., Buckingham, R. J., Pursey, N. A., & Lowe, D. (2011). Acidosis, non-invasive ventilation and mortality in hospitalised COPD exacerbations. Thorax, 66(1), 43-48. https://doi.org/10.1136/thx.2010.153114

Wheatley, I. (2021). Use of non-invasive ventilation for respiratory failure in acute care. Nursing Times, 117(3), 18-22.

| 18 |

Invasive Mechanical
Ventilation

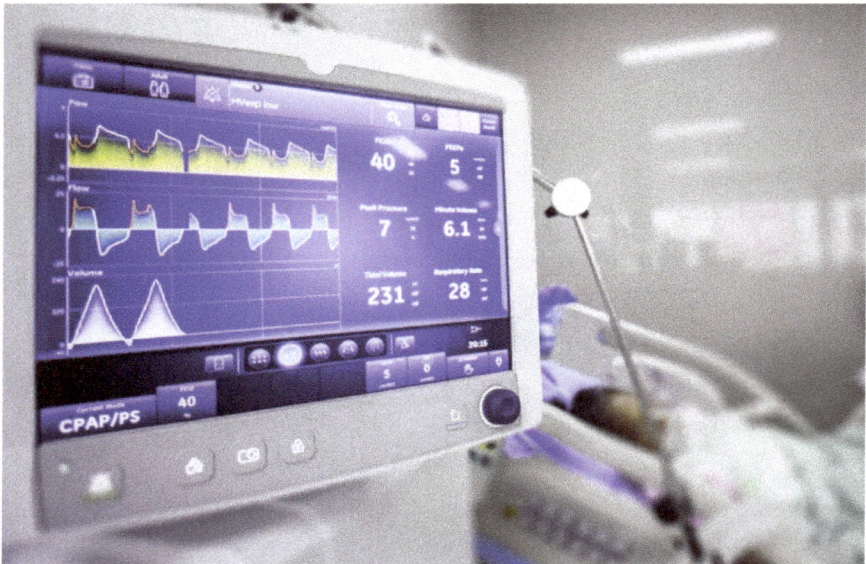

Overview

Mechanical ventilation is an indispensable component of critical care. Without mechanical support for respiration, many patients die due to acute hypoxemic and hypercapnic respiratory failure (Brochard, 2003). The emergency department (ED) length of stay of the patient's requiring admission to the intensive care units has increased gradually in recent years (Bayram & Şancı, 2019). Therefore, emergency physicians must maintain and monitor mechanically ventilated patients for longer than expected in the ED. Surprisingly, many ED physicians are not adequately equipped with mechanical ventilation in the resuscitation room. Therefore, the Royal College of Emergency Medicine emphasises the intensive care unit rotations to develop a comprehensive knowledge of mechanical ventilation.

Objectives

- By the end of this session, you should be able to:
  - Understand basic principles of an invasive mechanical ventilation
  - Essential modes used for mechanical ventilation of patients
  - Address acute changes in airway pressure and the diagnosis of auto-positive end-expiratory pressure.
  - Interpret the ventilator waveform

Indications for Invasive Mechanical Ventilation

- A decision to intubate and proceed with mechanical ventilation should normally be made within 4 hours of starting NIV, as improvements should usually be apparent during this time.
- Patients with COPD should be considered for ITU treatment, when necessary, especially if they are more unwell i.e., pH < 7.26.
- The Global Initiative for Chronic Obstructive Lung Disease 2013 guideline states the following may be indications for invasive mechanical ventilation:
  - NIV failure
  - Inability to tolerate NIV
  - Respiratory or cardiac arrest
  - Respiratory pauses with loss of consciousness or gasping for air
  - Reduced consciousness or uncontrolled agitation
  - Massive aspiration
  - Persistent inability to remove respiratory secretion
  - Heart rate <50 with loss of alertness
  - Haemodynamic instability unresponsive to fluid and vasopressors

○ Life-threatening hypoxaemia

Common Ventilator settings

Tidal Volume (VT)

This is the set amount of volume that will be delivered with each breath. Changing the VT will, in turn, change the minute ventilation (VT x RR); an increase in minute ventilation will result in a decrease in carbon dioxide (CO2), by the same token, a decreased VT will result in a decreased minute ventilation and increase in the patient's blood CO2 (Mora Carpio & Mora, 2021)

The fraction of inspired oxygen, FiO2

The fraction of inspired oxygen (FiO2) is the concentration of oxygen in the gas mixture. The gas mixture at room air has a fraction of inspired oxygen of 21%, meaning that the concentration of oxygen at room air is 21%. The percentage of oxygen at different altitudes remains the same, meaning the FiO2 of air in the atmosphere remains 21% irrespective of the altitude of an individual (Peacock, 1998).

Positive end-expiratory pressure (PEEP)

PEEP is a mode of therapy used in conjunction with mechanical ventilation. At the end of mechanical or spontaneous exhalation, PEEP maintains the patient's airway pressure above the atmospheric level by exerting pressure that opposes passive emptying of the lung.

This pressure is typically achieved by maintaining a positive pressure flow at the end of exhalation. This pressure is measured in centimetres of water (Jackson, 2020). The two types of PEEP are extrinsic PEEP (PEEP applied by a ventilator) and intrinsic PEEP (PEEP caused by an incomplete exhalation). The pressure that is applied or increased during inspiration is termed pressure support.

Respiratory Rate (RR) and Minute Ventilation

Minute & Alveolar Ventilation Minute ventilation (VE) is the total volume of gas entering (or leaving) the lung per minute. It is equal to the tidal volume (TV) multiplied by the respiratory rate (RR).

Minute ventilation = VE = TV x RR

Mechanical ventilation modes
- Mechanical ventilator modes are classified as (Bayram & Şancı, 2019):
  - Volume-targeted ventilation,
  - Pressure-targeted ventilation,
  - Dual-controlled modes.

Volume-Targeted Ventilation (VTV)

Also known as volume pre-set, volume control, volume assist or volume cycled ventilation. It is a "pressure control" mode of ventilation where tidal volume is a dependent variable to changes in pressure. Depending on the ventilator design or mode of VTV, the tidal volume may be measured at the flow sensor either during inspiration or during expiration or both. When volume-controlled ventilation is selected, each breath delivered by the ventilator is supplied with the pre-set inspiratory flow time.

Pressure-Targeted Ventilation

Also known as pressure-cycled, pressure-limited, pressure-control, pressure-assist, or pressure-targeted ventilation (Bayram & Şancı, 2019). It **lets the clinician control the airway pressure and helps the patient to influence the inspiratory flow rate and tidal volume**. Basically, the pressure control is determined by the user, and the device generates inspiration in the patient's airway and cuts off the gas flow when the pressure limit is reached.

Frequently Used MV Modes

1. Controlled Mechanical Ventilation (CMV)

It is classified as V-CMV, P-CMV depending on being volume targeted or pressure targeted. Volume controlled CMV is the simplest form of mechanical ventilation. The determined tidal volume is given to the patient with a set respiratory rate.

- **Disadvantages:**
  - This mode is time-triggered and time-cycled, ignoring spontaneous breathing. Consequently, it can only be applied in paralyzed, sedated, or apnoeic patients.
  - It generates problems such as coughing, incoordination with the mechanical ventilator ('fighting the vent') on the patients who are awake even slightly.
  - CMV is not fit for long-term ventilation because it may cause atrophy in the respiratory muscles (Bayram & Şancı, 2019).

2. Assist-Control Ventilation (A/C)

Assist-control (AC) mode is one of the most common methods of mechanical ventilation in the emergency department. AC ventilation is a **volume-cycled mode of ventilation**. It works by setting a fixed tidal volume (VT) that the ventilator will deliver at set intervals of time or when the patient initiates a breath.

- **Advantages:**
  - Its main feature is that each breath triggered or generated by the device is the same.

- The patient can determine his own respiratory rate, but the breaths are tidal volume or Paw controlled or supported.
- It guarantees the user-defined respiratory frequency when it is not triggered by the patient.
- For this reason, each breath is time-cycled (controlled) or volume/pressure-cycled (assisted).
- Since it can be triggered and supported by the patient, it requires less workload for the patient
- It is easy for the user to prevent respiratory acidosis and alkalosis.

- **Disadvantages**
  - It might cause breath stacking and auto-PEEP development on the patient with tachypnoea since there might not be enough time for an exhalation or respiratory alkalosis.
  - It requires strict monitoring to prevent plateau pressure and dynamic hyperinflation to prevent barotrauma (Chacko et al., 2015).

3. Synchronized Intermittent Mechanical Ventilation (SIMV)

Synchronized intermittent mandatory ventilation (SIMV) is a **type of volume control mode of ventilation**. With this mode, the ventilator will deliver a mandatory (set) number of breaths with a set volume while at the same time allowing spontaneous breaths (Lazoff & Bird, 2021).

- **Advantages:**
  - Its main feature is being synchronized.
  - In SIMV, when the patient-assisted breaths are in the assist window (in the number of frequencies that is set), it provides respiration guaranteeing the volume or pressure target.

○ If the patient does not have breathing effort in the time window determined by frequency, he guarantees the breath at the determined frequency.
○ Due to synchronization, the patients who are awake breath relatively more comfortably.

4. SIMV-PS

If no pressure support is additionally joined to SIMV, breaths greater than the frequency setting are not supported. In SIMV-PS respiration, a PS is determined in addition to the standard SIMV settings to enhance the volume of the patient's spontaneous breaths or to surmount the resistance of the endotracheal tube. In this case, the patient can adjust his own breathing rate and make pressure-assisted breaths. Apart from the weaning phase, the use of SIMV is often done with PS support (Bayram & Şancı, 2019).

5. Pressure-Support Ventilation (PSV)

Pressure support ventilation (PSV) is a **spontaneous mode of ventilation in which each breath is initiated by the patient but is supported by constant pressure inflation**. This method has been shown to increase the efficiency of inspiration and decrease the work of breathing.

- **Advantages:**
  ○ PSV is normally the favoured mode in the weaning phase.
  ○ When patients are not sedated, paralyzed, and retain their respiratory dynamics this mode is frequently used.
  ○ PSV prevents the development of atrophy of the respiratory muscles due to its little need for sedation.

○ Its main feature is that *the device only controls the pressure support level.*

Emergency Department ventilatory mode

The mode in the ED should be decided according to the physician's experience and the clinical presentation of the patients. VC-A/C ventilation might be the first choice in most EDs (Bayram & Şancı, 2019).

- **Numerous factors to consider:**
    - ○ The device to be used,
    - ○ The emergency physician's experience,
    - ○ The patient's clinical status
    - ○ The expected time for MV.

The A/C mode: is a useful initial mode in patients with metabolic and respiratory acidosis.

Volume controlled A/C ventilation: is the most preferred mode in EDs, ARDS patients and the other indications (Fuller et al., 2013).

A/C volume-controlled mode: is challenging for the patient if he wants to breathe more than the specified volume, or if the patient's inspiratory tendency is greater than the number of breaths determined (Spiegel & Mallemat, 2016).

SIMV: is the preferred mode of initial MV by some physicians, probably because it requires less sedation and allows the patient to have spontaneous respiratory efforts.

SIMV-pressure support ventilation: Additional pressure support to the patient's spontaneous breaths can help to cope with this problem.

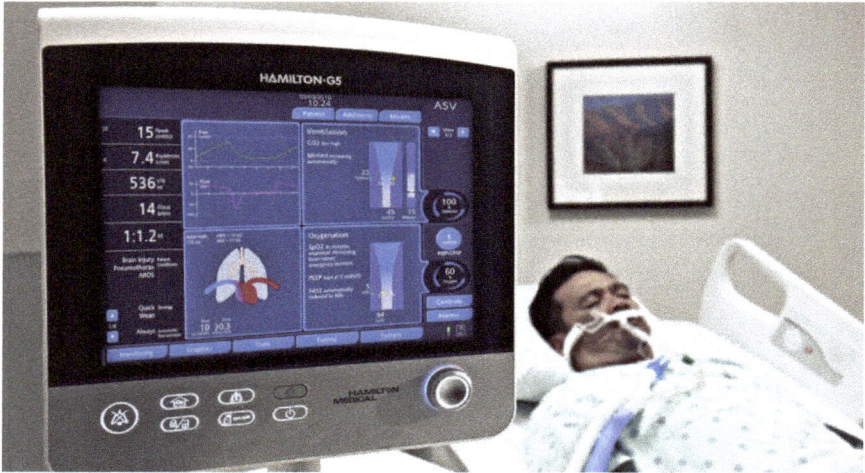

Fig.1.18.1. Setting up the ventilator

Setting a Ventilator

Normal Minute Ventilation

- **Indications:**
    - Intubated patients for upper airway obstruction (angioedema)
    - Altered mental status (ethanol intoxication),
    - Patients undergoing surgery.

Settings:

- The following settings are likely to achieve an adequate PaO2 (PaO2 8-10.6 Kpa, SpO2 >88%) and acceptable PaCO2 (4.0-6.5Kpa) in most adult patients (Walter et al., 2018):
    - Mode: AC-VC
    - RR: 14 breaths per minute
    - VT: 7 to 8 mL/kg ideal body weight
    - FiO2: 0.4 to 1.0, depending on the clinical scenario
    - PEEP: 5 cm H2O

○ Inspiratory flow rate and pattern: 80 LPM using a decelerating/ramp flow

Alternatively, in patients with normal lungs and an intact mental status, PS can be used. Reasonable initial settings include a PEEP of 5 cm H2O, Pi of 15 cm H2O, and a FiO2 of 0.4.

Subsequent adjustments to Pi should target an RR of roughly 14 breaths per minute and a VT of 8 to 10 mL/kg IBW (Bayram & Şancı, 2019).

ARDS

Apply lung-protective ventilation to prioritise low-tidal volumes and low plateau pressures and improve mortality (Hung et al., 2014).

- **Settings:**
    - ○ Mode: AC-VC
    - ○ RR: 20 breaths per minute
    - ○ VT: 7 to 8 mL/kg IBW
    - ○ FiO2: 1.0
    - ○ PEEP: 5 cm H2O
    - ○ Inspiratory flow rate and pattern: 80 LPM using a decelerating/ramp flow

A higher initial RR is needed to match the high minute ventilation of patients with ARDS.

The VT should be decreased over several hours to a goal of 6 mL/kg IBW. The RR is increased in parallel with the decrease in VT to maintain adequate minute ventilation and avoid progressive hypercapnia and acidaemia.

Tidal volume should be decreased further if necessary to achieve a Pplt <30 cm H2O.

PEEP and FiO2 are adjusted in a stepwise fashion to maintain a PaO2 of 55–80 mm Hg (Hung et al., 2014).

Severe Obstructive Lung Disease

- **Indications:**
  - Status asthmaticus
  - Chronic obstructive pulmonary disease

Ventilation for the above patients should allow for complete exhalation to prevent the development of auto-PEEP. This is most effectively accomplished by limiting RR and VT (Fuller et al., 2017).

- **Settings:**
  - Mode: AC-VC
  - RR: 10 to 14 breaths per minute
  - VT: 7 to 8 mL/kg IBW
  - FiO2: 1.0
  - PEEP: 5 cm H2O
  - Inspiratory flow rate and pattern: 60 LPM using a square waveform

Target minute ventilation of 6 to 8 L/minute to prevent auto-PEEP in patients with severe bronchospasm.

The use of deep sedation and neuromuscular blocking agents may be necessary (Fuller et al., 2017).

Elevations in PaCO2 are permitted to promote the reduction in minute ventilation provided the pH does not drop below 7.15.

The set flow rate can be raised above 60 LPM to further reduce the inspiratory time.

High flow rates will raise peak pressure because of an addition in airway resistive pressure.

Because these changes do not increase the distending pressure of the lung, isolated elevations in peak pressures are not necessarily harmful.

Risk factors for extubation

- Positive fluid balance
- Raised rapid shallow breathing index during spontaneous breathing trial
- Pneumonia or pulmonary disease as the cause requiring IMV
- Increased age
- Prolonged duration of IMV
- Anaemia
- Increased severity of illness
- Low albumin
- Previously failed extubation
- Bulbar dysfunction

Complications of Mechanical Ventilation

- **Complications of intubation**
  - Upper airway and nasal trauma
  - Tooth avulsion
  - Oral-pharyngeal laceration
  - Laceration or hematoma of the vocal cords
  - Tracheal laceration
  - Perforation
  - Hypoxemia
  - Intubation of the oesophagus
  - Inadvertent intubation of the right mainstem bronchus
  - Aspiration rates are 8–19% in intubations performed in adults without anaesthesia.
  - Sinusitis, tracheal necrosis or stenosis, glottic oedema,
  - Ventilator-associated Pneumonia may occur with prolonged use of endotracheal tubes.
- **Ventilator-induced lung injury (VILI)**
  - Barotrauma
  - Volutrauma

Further reading

Uptodate - Modes of Mechanical Ventilation: https://www.upto-date.com/contents/modes-of-mechanical-ventilation?search=mechan-ical-ventilation-&source=search_result&selectedTitle=2~150&usage_type=default&display_rank=2

Martin J. Tobin - Advances in Mechanical Ventilation. N Engl J Med 2001; 344:1986-1996. DOI: 10.1056/NEJM200106283442606

References

Bayram, B., & Şancı, E. (2019). Invasive mechanical ventilation in the emergency department. Turk J Emerg Med, 19(2), 43-52. https://doi.org/10.1016/j.tjem.2019.03.001

Brochard, L. (2003). Mechanical ventilation: invasive versus non-invasive. European Respiratory Journal (22), 31s-37s. https://doi.org/10.1183/09031936.03.00050403

Chacko, B., Peter, J. V., Tharyan, P., John, G., & Jeyaseelan, L. (2015). Pressure-controlled versus volume-controlled ventilation for acute respiratory failure due to acute lung injury (ALI) or acute respiratory distress syndrome (ARDS). Cochrane Database Syst Rev, 1(1), Cd008807. https://doi.org/10.1002/14651858.CD008807.pub2

Fuller, B. M., Ferguson, I. T., Mohr, N. M., Drewry, A. M., Palmer, C., Wessman, B. T., . . . Kollef, M. H. (2017). A Quasi-Experimental, Before-After Trial Examining the Impact of an Emergency Department Mechanical Ventilator Protocol on Clinical Outcomes and Lung-Protective Ventilation in Acute Respiratory Distress Syndrome. Crit Care Med, 45(4), 645-652. https://doi.org/10.1097/ccm.0000000000002268

Fuller, B. M., Mohr, N. M., Dettmer, M., Kennedy, S., Cullison, K., Bavolek, R., . . . McCammon, C. (2013). Mechanical ventilation and acute lung injury in emergency department patients with severe sepsis and septic shock: an observational study. Acad Emerg Med, 20(7), 659-669. https://doi.org/10.1111/acem.12167

Jackson, C. D. (2020). What is positive end-expiratory pressure (PEEP) therapy and how is it used with mechanical ventilation? Medscape. Retrieved 06 Dec. 2021 from https://www.medscape.com/answers/304068-104783/what-is-positive-end-expiratory-pressure-peep-therapy-and-how-is-it-used-with-mechanical-ventilation

Lazoff, S. A., & Bird, K. (2021). Synchronized Intermittent Mandatory Ventilation. StatPearls Publishing. Retrieved 04 Dec. 2021 from https://www.ncbi.nlm.nih.gov/books/NBK549846/

Mora Carpio, A. L., & Mora, J. I. (2021a). Ventilation Assist Control. StatPearls Publishing. Retrieved 04 Dec. 2021 from https://pubmed.ncbi.nlm.nih.gov/28846232/

Peacock, A. J. (1998). ABC of oxygen: oxygen at high altitude. Bmj, 317(7165), 1063-1066. https://doi.org/10.1136/bmj.317.7165.1063Hung, S. C., Kung, C. T., Hung, C. W., Liu, B. M., Liu, J. W., Chew, G., . . . Lee, T. C. (2014). Determining delayed admission to intensive care unit for mechanically ventilated patients in the emergency department. Crit Care, 18(4), 485. https://doi.org/10.1186/s13054-014-0485-1

Walter, J. M., Corbridge, T. C., & Singer, B. D. (2018). Invasive Mechanical Ventilation. South Med J, 111(12), 746-753. https://doi.org/10.14423/smj.0000000000000905 Spiegel, R., & Mallemat, H. (2016). Emergency Department Treatment of the Mechanically Ventilated Patient. Emerg Med Clin North Am, 34(1), 63-75. https://doi.org/10.1016/j.emc.2015.08.005

| 19 |

Pericardiocentesis

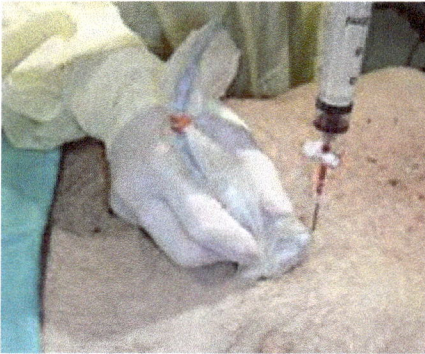

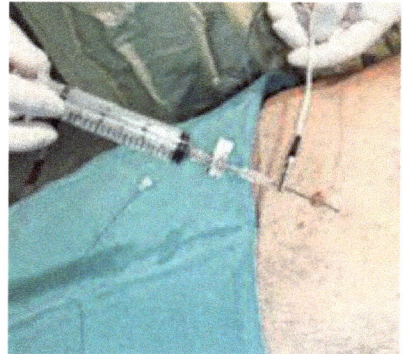

Overview

Pericardiocentesis is the aspiration of fluid from the pericardial space surrounding the heart. Pericardiocentesis is the most useful therapeutic procedure for the early management or diagnosis of large, symptomatic pericardial effusion and cardiac tamponade (Adler et al., 2015; Cruz et al., 2015). Pericardiocentesis can be performed blindly or under real-time transthoracic echocardiography (TTE) or fluoroscopy to reduce the risk of complications. The procedure may be performed at the bedside or in the cardiac catheterization lab (Willner & Grossman, 2021).

Objectives

- By the end of this chapter, you should be able to:
  - Outline the indications and contraindications for pericardiocentesis.
  - Learn the technique involved in performing pericardiocentesis.

- Highlight landmark for safely performing pericardiocentesis.
- Describe the complications of pericardiocentesis.

Indications

- **Emergent pericardiocentesis**
    - The presence of life-threatening hemodynamic changes in a patient with suspected cardiac tamponade (Juarez & Nemer, 2018)
- **Non Emergent pericardiocentesis**
    - The aspiration of pericardial fluid in hemodynamically stable patients for diagnostic, palliative, or prophylactic reasons, performed under ultrasonography, computerized tomography, or fluoroscopic visualization (Callahan & Seward, 1997; Klein et al., 2005).

Contraindications

- **Absolute**
    - In the hemodynamically unstable patient, no absolute contraindications exist to performing pericardiocentesis. Even withdrawal of a small amount of fluid in a very unstable patient can lead to an immediate improvement in hemodynamics (Willner & Grossman, 2021).
- **Relative**
    - Uncorrected coagulopathy
    - Anticoagulant therapy
    - Thrombocytopenia
    - Lack of knowledge about the anatomy of the chest.

Equipment

- Antiseptic (e.g., Chloraprep)
- 1 % lidocaine
- 25-gauge needle, 5/8-in. long

- 18-gauge catheter-type needle, 1½-nch long
- Syringes (10, 20, and 60 mL)
- Ultrasound (US) machine and cardiac/phased array probe
- Sterile US probe cover
- Cardiac monitor

Consent

- Informed Consent: should be obtained from the patient or parent if minor.
- Provide a focused set of risks and complications.
- Discuss how these risks can be avoided or prevented (e.g., proper positioning, ensuring that the patient remains as still as possible during the procedure, adequate analgesia).

Procedure

- Place at least one established intravenous access line, give supplemental oxygen and connect the patient to a cardiac monitor and continuous pulse oximetry.
- If possible, a nasogastric tube can be inserted to decompress the stomach and minimise the risk of gastric perforation. Identify the point of maximal effusion with the ultrasound.
- Identify the point of maximal effusion with US. Evaluate for hypoechoic or anechoic (dark) effusion around the heart, between the pericardial sac and the myocardium.
- A patient with hemodynamic compromise from a pericardial effusion or tamponade will have right ventricular collapse, septal bulging, and dilation of the inferior vena cava.
- Diastolic collapse of the right ventricular free wall can be absent in elevated right ventricular pressure and right ventricular hypertrophy or in right ventricular infarction.
- Measure the distance from the skin surface to the effusion border to assess the expected needle depth.
- Choose the needle trajectory based on the point of maximal effusion in the path with the fewest intervening structures.

- The most used approaches are left parasternal, apical, and subxiphoid. For complex loculated posterior pericardial effusions, optional techniques such as transatrial and transbronchial may be performed by specialists.
- These types of loculated effusions can occur in autoimmune diseases, infective pericarditis, after cardiac surgery, and after radiotherapy.
- Sterile preparation: prepare the skin of the entire lower xiphoid and epigastric area with antiseptic. Prepare the US transducer with a sterile sleeve.
- Local anaesthetic: if the patient is awake, anaesthetise the skin and planned route of the needle.
- Pericardial needle insertion depends on approach used.

1. Subxiphoid Approach

- The US transducer is placed just inferior to the xiphoid process and left costal margin.
- Insert the needle between the xiphoid process and the left costal margin at a 30–45° angle to the skin.
- Aim for the left shoulder.

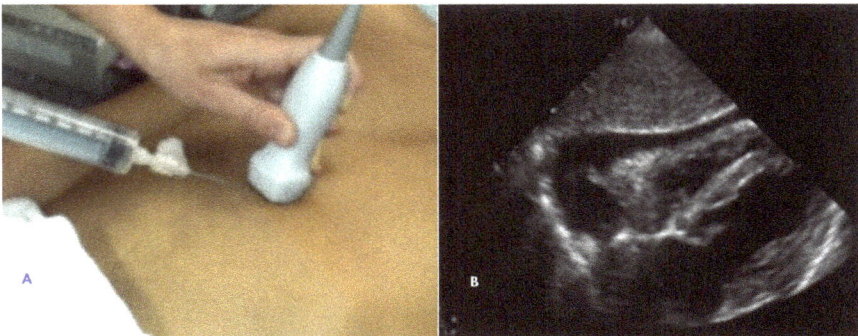

Fig.1.19.1. Pericardiocentesis- (A) Subxiphoid approach and (B) subxiphoid view of the heart demonstrating a moderate sized pericardial effusion.

2. Apical Approach

- The US transducer is placed at the patient's point of maximal impulse and aimed at the patient's right shoulder for a four-chamber view of the heart.
- Insert the needle in the fifth intercostal space 1 cm lateral to and below the apical beat, within the area of cardiac dullness.

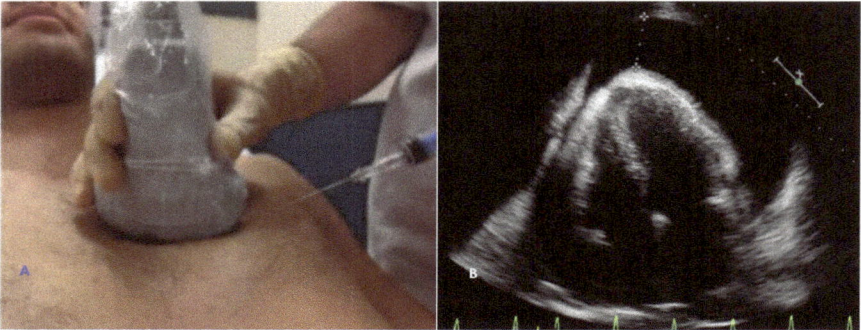

Fig.1.19.2. Pericardiocentesis - (A) apical approach and (B) Apical four-chamber ECHO demonstrating pericardial effusion

3. Parasternal Long-Axis Approach

- The US transducer is placed obliquely on the left sterna border between the fourth and fifth ribs with the transducer, indicator aimed at the right shoulder.
- Insert the needle perpendicular to the skin in the fifth intercostal space medial to the border of cardiac dullness.
- Visualize and feel a giving way as the needle penetrates the pericardium.
- Removal of fluid confirms successful entry. Remove fluid with the goal of restoring hemodynamic stability.
- Aspiration of fluid should result in improvement in blood pressure and cardiac output.
- Remove the catheter and apply a dressing.

- Optional: Place a pigtail catheter using the Seldinger technique for continued drainage.

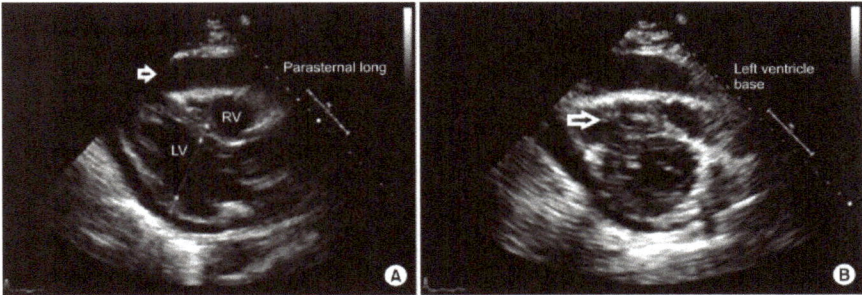

Fig.1.19.3. Pericardiocentesis- (A) along the parasternal long axis: the arrows show a large pericardial effusion. (B) along a short axis showing the right ventricular collapsed in diastole, suggestive of cardiac tamponade. LV, left ventricle; RV, right ventricle; TTE, transthoracic echocardiogram.
Credit- Mukul Bhattarai

Complications

- Blind techniques are associated with 20 % morbidity and 6 % mortality.
- The complication rate with US-guided approaches is less than 5 %.
- Any vital structure within reach of the pericardial needle has the potential for injury:
  - Pneumothorax and Haemothorax
  - Coronary vessel laceration
  - Hemopericardium
  - Heart chamber lacerations
  - Intercostal vessel injury
  - Dysrhythmias
  - Ventricular tachycardia.
  - Puncture of the liver, diaphragm, or gastrointestinal tract
  - Bacteraemia
  - Purulent pericarditis
  - Air embolisms
  - Pleuropericardial fistula

Table 1.19.1. Characteristics of the Different Pericardiocentesis Approaches

Place of Puncture	Disadvantages	Advantages
Apical	Risk of ventricular puncture due to the proximity to the left ventricle. Increased risk for pneumothorax for the proximity to the left pleural space.	The thicker left ventricle wall is more likely to self-seal after puncture. Due to ultrasound not penetrating air, using echocardiographic guidance ensures avoidance of the lung. The path to reach the pericardium is shorter.
Parasternal	Risk of pneumothorax and puncture of the internal thoracic vessels (if the needle is inserted more than 1 cm laterally).	Echocardiographic guidance, also with phase array probe, provides a good visualisation of pericardial structures.

Subxiphoid	A steeper angle may enter the peritoneal cavity, and a medial direction increases the risk of right atrial puncture. In some cases, the left liver lobe may be transverse intentionally if an alternative site is not available. The path to reach the fluid is longer.	Lower risk of pneumothorax.

Post-procedure care

After the procedure:

- Visualize the heart with ultrasonography to confirm the removal of the pericardial fluid and adequate cardiac function.
- Continue resuscitation as needed, depending on the patient's hemodynamic response to the procedure.
- Obtain a chest film after completing the procedure to assess for complications such as a pleural effusion or pneumothorax.
- Continue to monitor the patient for signs of hemodynamic instability and for physical findings that suggest fluid is continuing to accumulate in the pericardial sac.
- Definitive care may include the placement of a soft catheter in the pericardial space or surgical placement of a pericardial window to allow for continuous drainage.
- Consider consultation with an appropriate specialist to assist with the management of patient care after completing an emergency pericardiocentesis, as clinically indicated.

Further reading

Medscape- Pericardiocentesis: https://emedicine.medscape.com/article/80602-overview#a7

References

Adler, Y., Charron, P., Imazio, M., Badano, L., Barón-Esquivias, G., Bogaert, J., . . . Group, E. S. C. S. D. (2015). 2015 ESC Guidelines for the diagnosis and management of pericardial diseases: The Task Force for the Diagnosis and Management of Pericardial Diseases of the European Society of Cardiology (ESC)Endorsed by: The European Association for Cardio-Thoracic Surgery (EACTS). European Heart Journal, 36(42), 2921-2964. https://doi.org/10.1093/eurheartj/ehv318

Callahan, J. A., & Seward, J. B. (1997). Pericardiocentesis Guided by Two-Dimensional Echocardiography. Echocardiography, 14(5), 497-504. https://doi.org/10.1111/j.1540-8175.1997.tb00757.x

Cruz, I., Stuart, B., Caldeira, D., Morgado, G., Gomes, A. C., Almeida, A. R., . . . Pereira, H. (2015). Controlled pericardiocentesis in patients with cardiac tamponade complicating aortic dissection: experience of a centre without cardiothoracic surgery. Eur Heart J Acute Cardiovasc Care, 4(2), 124-128. https://doi.org/10.1177/2048872614549737

Juarez, M., & Nemer, J. (2018). Pericardiocentesis. In E. F. Reichman (Ed.), Reichman's Emergency Medicine Procedures, 3e. McGraw-Hill Education.

Willner, D. A., & Grossman, S. A. (2021). Pericardiocentesis. Statpearls. Retrieved 25 Nov. 2021 from https://www.ncbi.nlm.nih.gov/books/NBK470347/

Klein, S. V., Afridi, H., Agarwal, D., Coughlin, B. F., & Schielke, L. H. (2005). CT directed diagnostic and therapeutic pericardiocentesis: 8-year experience at a single institution. Emerg Radiol, 11(6), 353-363. https://doi.org/10.1007/s10140-004-0389-5

| 20 |

Procedural Sedation

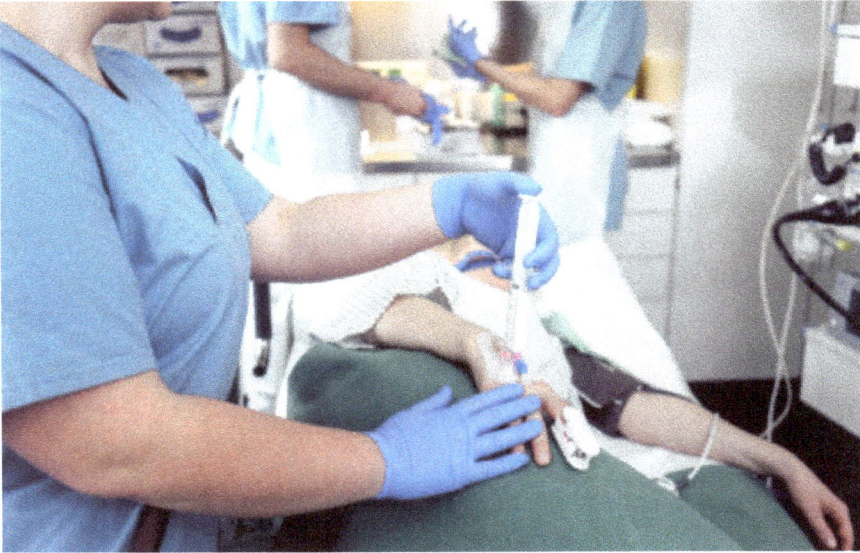

Overview

Patients presenting to the Emergency Department (ED) may require life or limb saving procedures as part of their management care. Often, such procedures may induce discomfort, pain, and anxiety. Performing the procedure in the ED may carry the advantage of preventing patient admission and helping hospitals by lessening admissions.

Procedural sedation is a well-established and safe practice in the Emergency Department that benefits patients by reducing pain and lowering the time to procedure. The drugs, dosages and techniques employed for the sedation are not intended to produce loss of consciousness. However, these drugs can cause severe and life-threatening complications (Benzoni & Cascella, 2022). These unfavourable consequences most often involve upper airway patency, ventilatory function or the cardiovascular system. Therefore, the procedure must follow recommended guidelines to avoid adverse effects through appropriate pre-sedation evaluation early identification of respiratory and cardiovascular function (Tobias & Leder, 2011).

Through this manual, the ED physician will comprehend the assessment of the airway by direct visual examination, tabulate risk factors by analysis of baseline risk, and will be able to correctly choose a medication that we will get the patient safely through the proposed procedure.

Objectives

- By the end of this module, you should be able to:
  - Outline the Indications and contraindications of procedural sedation in the ED
  - Administer proper medication for procedural sedation based on specific patient risks.
  - Describe the equipment, personnel, preparation, and technique regarding procedural sedation.
  - Review the potential complications and clinical significance of procedural sedation.

Indications

PS and PSA are indicated when the patient requires an intervention that will induce considerable pain and anxiety. The level of sedation required relies on the level of discomfort the patient is likely to experience, and the necessity of the patient remaining still during the procedure.

Contraindications

- Allergy or hypersensitivity to the relevant medications
- Lack of appropriately trained personnel to perform the sedation
- Patients have an ASA IV and above.

- Lack of appropriate monitoring and resuscitation equipment (for Potential GA.)
- High risk of aspiration, e.g., acute alcohol intoxication

Pre procedural care

Staff, Location, Equipment, Documentation

- Staffing: Minimum of three staff required for all procedural sedation. Sedation is only to be performed by trained clinicians.
- Location:
  - Level 2 moderate sedation (midazolam & opiate) minors theatre or resus.
  - Level 3 deep sedation (Propofol) or dissociative sedation (Ketamine) resus only.
- Equipment: Resus equipment available
- Documentation: ED sedation Pro-forma completed

Patient Assessment

- ASA Grade documented:
  - Only ASA I, II and selected grade III patients for sedation in the ED.
  - No ASA IV or V patients to be sedated without discussion with a senior anaesthetist
- Airway Assessment complete: No patient with a feature of the problematic airway to be sedated without discussion with a senior anaesthetist
- All patients must have a pre-procedure assessment performed and documented before procedural sedation. The pre-procedure assessment must include:
  - Weight, BMI
  - Complete medical history including present medical history, indication for the procedure, past medical history,

drug history, allergies, social history, recreational drugs and alcohol
- Anaesthetic history including previous general anaesthetics and sedation, complications during previous procedures, known airway problems, dentition
- History of reflux
- Date and time of last food and oral fluid intake
- Physical examination including vital signs and airway assessment

Equipment

The following equipment must be available in the location where procedural sedation is performed:

- Complete resuscitation equipment for basic and advanced life support (resus/ crash trolley)
- Difficult airway equipment/ trolley for deep sedation in resus
- Continuous high flow oxygen with appropriate devices of administration including non-rebreather masks, bag-valve-mask, Water's circuit with appropriately sized face masks
- High-pressure suction with appropriate suction catheters and yankhuers
- Trolley capable of being tilted head down
- Monitoring equipment (see below)
- An appropriate range of intravenous cannula and intravenous fluids
- Reversal agent if available (Flumazenil should be available when sedating with Midazolam)

ASA Grading

The most commonly used system for clinical assessment is the ASA Physical Status (Class) scoring:

ASA Class 1

- Normal healthy patient with no organic, physiologic, or psychiatric disturbance excludes the very young and old; healthy with acceptable exercise tolerance.

ASA Class 2

- Patients presenting with mild systemic disease: No functional limitations; has a well-controlled disease involving one body system; controlled hypertension or diabetes without systemic effects, cigarette smoking absent chronic obstructive pulmonary disease (COPD); mild obesity, pregnancy.

ASA Class 3

- Patients with severe systemic disease: Some level of functional limitation; has a controlled disease involving more than one body system or one major system; no immediate danger of death; controlled congestive heart failure (CHF), stable angina, prior heart attack, poorly controlled hypertension, morbid obesity, chronic renal failure; a bronchospastic disease with intermittent symptoms.

ASA Class 4

- Patients with severe systemic disease that represents a constant threat to life: Has at least one severe disease not well controlled or at end-stage; possible risk of death; unstable angina, symptomatic COPD, symptomatic CHF, hepatorenal failure.

ASA Class 5

• Moribund patients not expected to survive without the operation: Not expected to survive over 24 hours without surgery; imminent risk of death; multiorgan failure, sepsis syndrome with hemodynamic instability, hypothermia, poorly controlled coagulopathy.

ASA Class 6

• A patient declared brain-dead whose organs are being harvested for donor purposes.

The addition of "E" to physical status denotes an emergency procedure. The definition of an emergency exists when a delay in treatment of the patient would lead to a significant increase in the threat to life or body part.

Definitions and Depth of Sedation

Sedation is a continuum ranging from a normal level of consciousness to complete unresponsiveness.

The ASA defines four levels of sedation (Committee on Quality Management and Departmental Administration, 2019):

Level 1 minimal sedation (anxiolysis): patients normally respond to verbal commands. Cognitive function and coordination may be impaired. Ventilatory and cardiovascular functions are unaffected. In the ED, this is achieved with inhaled nitrous oxide.

Level 2 moderate/ conscious sedation: patients respond purposefully to verbal commands either alone or accompanied by light tactile stimulation. Protective airway reflexes and adequate ventilation are maintained without intervention. Cardiovascular function is usually maintained. In the ED, this is achieved with a combination of opioids and benzodiazepines.

Level 3 deep sedation: the patient cannot be easily roused but responds purposefully following repeated or painful stimulation. Assistance may be needed to ensure the airway is protected and adequate ventilation. Cardiovascular function is usually maintained. In the ED, this is achieved with the combination of opioids and Propofol.

Level 4 general anaesthesia: patients are not arousable, even by the painful stimulus. Require assistance to protect the airway and maintain ventilation. Cardiovascular function may be impaired.

Dissociative sedation is a separate sedation category produced by Ketamine. Ketamine causes a trance like cataleptic state characterised by profound analgesia and amnesia with retention of protective airway reflexes, spontaneous respirations and cardiopulmonary stability. As there is loss of verbal contact with patients during ketamine sedation and because of the risk of significant (although rare) complications, ketamine sedation is grouped with deep sedation (level 3).

Consent

Informed consent must be obtained and documented. Consent must include:

- Details of the procedure, including type and duration of sedation
- Indications for the procedure
- Potential risks of the procedure
- Potential for failure
- Alternatives
- Review of discharge criteria

Monitoring

All patients who require sedation will alter their consciousness and must be on full continuous monitoring:

- Cardiac monitor with alarm (Level 2,3),
- End-tidal CO2 Monitor (Level 2,3)
- NIBP every 5 min (Level 2,3)
- SpO2

Medication

Intravenous Analgesia/Sedative drugs should be given slowly – over 30 – 60 seconds and in small, incremental doses that are titrated to the desired endpoint of analgesia and sedation.

It is best to regard procedural sedation as a 2-step process - analgesia then sedation.

Most importantly, the team should choose an agent with whom they are familiar.

Choice of agent:

Level 1: We suggest nitrous oxide and or Opiate and anxiolytic doses of a Benzodiazepine. The analgesic is given first an inappropriate dose and then a bolus of Benzodiazepine. **Fentanyl** is the opioid, and **Midazolam** is the Benzodiazepine of choice; anxiolytic doses are 1 – 2 mg. Elderly patients might be deeply sedated on minimal doses of Midazolam; hence we suggest in the over 65 years old patients, Midazolam is considered as a level 3 sedation drug.

Level 2: The agents used for Level 2 sedation should preserve cardiorespiratory function and protective airway reflexes but alter consciousness. The drug of choice is **Ketamine.**

Level 3: The drugs used for this level of sedation may impair protective airway reflexes and depress respiratory function. These drugs include **Propofol, Etomidate** and higher doses of **Benzodiazepines**. A combination of Propofol and ketamine (0.5mg/kg of each) is an acceptable alternative.

Analgesic agents

Morphine

- Opiate analgesic
- Dose 0.05-0.1 mg/kg.
- Administered in a bolus of 1 – 2.5mg titrated to effect.
- Usual dose range 2.5-15mg. Onset: 5-10 min. Duration: 2-4 h
- Adverse effects: Respiratory depression, Hypotension, Nausea/vomiting

Fentanyl

- Opiate analgesic and first-line choice in the ED
- Dose 0.5-1 mcg/kg and administered in 25 mcg bolus titrated to effect.
- Usual dose range 25 – 150 mcg.
- Onset: 2-4 min. Duration: 45 min
- Adverse effects: Respiratory depression, Pruritus

Nitrous oxide

- Its analgesic and anxiolytic effect is reliable and dose-related, and the recovery is rapid once inhalation of the agent ceases.
- It is usually administered from cylinders containing the gas premixed with oxygen at a concentration of 50%, delivered via a demand valve which allows some patient control.
- It is useful as a sole analgesic for minor procedures or an adjunct to opiate analgesia for moderate to severe pain.

- When the inspired concentration of nitrous oxide reaches 70% (the usual anaesthetic dose), consciousness is lost, and the same standard of care as general anaesthesia is required.
- It is essential to be aware of this if a delivery method other than that described above is used, e.g., an anaesthetic machine. The oxygen concentration in the inspired gas must never be less than 30%.
- Nitrous oxide rapidly diffuses into closed air spaces causing volume expansion and pressure effects.
- It is contraindicated when there is any suspicion of pneumothorax, bowel obstruction, ruptured viscera, or decompression illness (potential air embolism).

Sedating agents

Midazolam

- Benzodiazepine
- Sedative, anticonvulsant, anxiolytic, amnesic
- Dose 1 mg bolus, titrated to the desired effect.
- Small doses will achieve anxiolysis and amnesia (1-2 mg), while sedation requires larger doses (3 – 8mg).
- Conscious sedation dose: 0.05mg/kg.
- Onset: 2-5 min. Duration: 30-120 min
- Adverse effects: Respiratory depression, unpredictable action, hypotension, poor sedative, long half time, so high risk of post-procedural sedation.
- Caution in the elderly patient
- Advantages: familiarity to most ED staff, excellent amnesic

Propofol

- Anaesthetic induction agent, which also hyperpolarises GABA receptors via the chloride channel.

- Sedative agent of choice in the ED
- Dose 0.5mg/kg bolus, then 0.25mg/kg top-ups repeated at 3 – 5 min intervals as required.
- Please half the bolus and the top-ups doses in an elderly patient
- Onset: 10-15 sec. Rapid onset of sedation within one arm-brain circulation.
- Duration: half time is by redistribution and is 3 – 8 minutes
- Adverse effects: profound hypotension especially in the depleted patient, respiratory depression, opisthotonus,
- Caution in the elderly patient
- Advantages: excellent sedation, excellent amnesia, rapid on/off-set

Ketamine

- The novel agent causes dissociative anaesthesia via NMDA receptors.
- It is a SNS stimulant and as such a bronchodilator and inotrope
- Dose 0.1mg/kg analgesic, 0.5-1.0mg/kg as sedation. The initial dose in young adults is 0.5-1 mg/kg with 0.5mg/kg top-ups as required every 5 – 10 minutes
- Onset: 30sec. Duration: 5-10 min
- Adverse effects: Can increase secretions and, as s such is, occasionally associated with laryngospasm. Hence, the emergence phenomenon considers pre-treating adults with 1 – 2 mg of Midazolam.
- Post use confusion – a particular problem in the elderly Advantages excellent analgesic, little CVS depression. The excellent safety profile in particular in pre-hospital and paediatric use

Etomidate

- Novel steroid-based induction agent.

- It is a second-line agent due to the high incidence of myoclonus and emesis.
- Dose 0.1 mg/kg for sedation. Onset: 30sec. Duration: 5-10 min
- Adverse effects: Myoclonus, Nausea and vomiting, steroid synthesis depression

Airway Evaluation

Table 1.20.1. Difficult Laryngoscopy and Intubation (LEMON)

Look externally	Use your clinical gestalt, evidence of lower facial disruption, bleeding, small mouth, agitated patient
Evaluate	Use the 3-3-2 rule: mouth open, mandible, glottis
Mallampati score	In order of increasing difficulty Class I-IV
Obstruction / Obesity	Four cardinal signs of upper airway obstruction: stridor, muffled voice, difficulty swallowing secretions, sensation of dyspnoea. Obese patients frequently have poor glottic views.
Neck mobility	May not be able to optimally move the head and neck due to trauma, arthritis, ankylosing spondylitis. Immobilize the neck and consider using video laryngoscopy.

Airway Evaluation is performed in anticipation of possible intubation. The patient's airway should be assessed; this includes identifying features associated with increased risk of difficult intubation and/or ventilation. Physical examination to identify features of the difficult airway using the LEMON mnemonic.

During the Procedure

The patient should have their analgesic requirements met as soon as possible:

- Fentanyl is the drug of choice, with morphine a close second.
- Boli should be given until the patient is comfortable or sedated (i.e. eyes closing, speech slurring) or there is respiratory depression (RR< 10 or ET CO_2 > 50 mmHg/6.5kPa)
- Wait 3 – 5 minutes post analgesic delivery, then add procedural sedation.
- Complete the procedure and allow the patient to return to alertness

The individual responsible for monitoring the patient should ascertain and record:

- All medication administered (route, site, time, drug, dose)
- All patients must be on oxygen at 15 l/minute via a nonrebreather
- The patient's vital signs were recorded every 3 minutes.
- The patient's head position should be checked frequently to ensure a patent airway.
- Appropriate medical consultation should be sought immediately if the patient becomes unstable during the procedure.
- The level of sedation was monitored and recorded as classified by the ASA.

Postprocedural care
- Continue oxygen saturation and ETCO2 monitoring.
- Record the patient's vital signs (as defined directly above) every 5 - 10 minutes for a minimum of 30 minutes following the last administered dose of IV sedation

Then if the patient is stable every 15-30 minutes until the patient returns to his/her pre-procedure state.

Discharge criteria should include:

- The patient has stable vital signs and oxygen saturation level
- The patient's swallow, cough and gag reflexes are present
- The patient is alert or appropriate to baseline
- The patient can sit unaided if appropriate to baseline and procedure
- The patient can walk without/with assistance if appropriate to baseline, and procedures
- Nausea and dizziness are minimal
- Hydration is adequate
- Adequate analgesia
- A physician has written discharge orders and instructions
- Responsible adult to accompany patient if discharged
- An appropriate follow up has been arranged.

Complications
- Possible Complication Although this may occur in level 2 and 3 sedation, they should never be encountered in level 1
- Laryngospasm/stridor
- Apnoea
- Hypoxia from respiratory depression (SpO2<90 mmHg).
- Transient hypotension
- Bradycardia

Further reading

RCEM- Procedural Sedation in adults: https://rcem.ac.uk/wp-content/uploads/2021/11/Procedural_Sedation_in_Adults_Clinical_Audit_2015_16.pdf

RCEM- Pharmacological Agents for Procedural Sedation and Analgesia in the Emergency Department: https://rcem.ac.uk/wp-content/uploads/2021/10/Pharmacological_Agents_for_Procedural_Sedation_and_Analgesia_October_2020_Revised_230421.pdf

References

Benzoni, T., & Cascella, M. (2022). Procedural Sedation. In *Stat-Pearls*. StatPearls Publishing. Copyright © 2022, StatPearls Publishing LLC.

Committee on Quality Management and Departmental Administration. (2019). *Continuum of Depth of Sedation: Definition of General Anesthesia and Levels of Sedation/Analgesia.* American Society of Anesthesiologists. Retrieved 03 Jan. 2022 from https://www.asahq.org/standards-and-guidelines/continuum-of-depth-of-sedation-definition-of-general-anesthesia-and-levels-of-sedationanalgesia

Tobias, J. D., & Leder, M. (2011). Procedural sedation: A review of sedative agents, monitoring, and management of complications. *Saudi journal of anaesthesia*, 5(4), 395-410. https://doi.org/10.4103/1658-354X.87270

| 21 |

Rapid Sequence Intubation

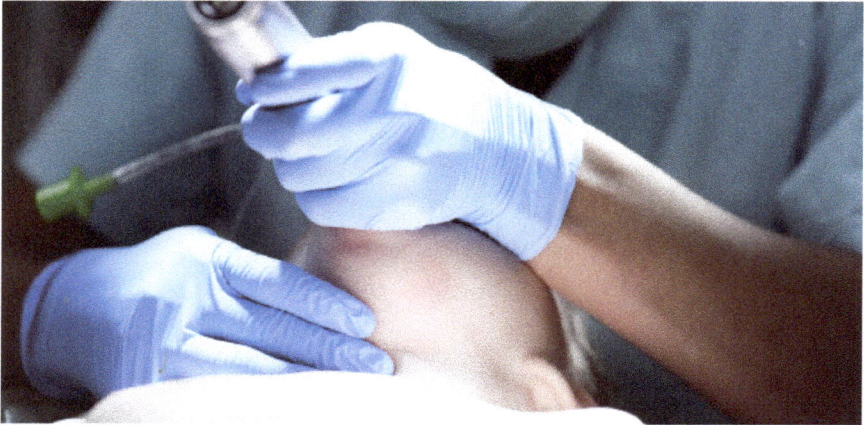

Overview

Airway control is one of the most crucial aptitudes for an emergency physician to master because failure to secure an adequate airway can quickly lead to death or disability (Reynolds & Heffner, 2005). The components of RSI are organised to protect the airway with a cuffed endotracheal tube through the vocal cords. Therefore, RSI is the cornerstone of emergency airway management (Lafferty, 2020; Sagarin et al., 2005). RSI requires administering paralytic drugs to a critically ill or injured patient supposed to have a full stomach. It aims to intubate the trachea as quickly and safely as possible (Sinclair & Luxton, 2005). It is instrumental in the patient with a complete gag reflex, a "full" stomach, and a life-threatening injury or illness requiring immediate airway control (Nickson, 2015)

A systematic process to RSI is crucial for the procedure's success. The emergency physician should consider the risk before the intervention and place the patient in an optimal position to understand the anatomy concerned. All required equipment must be available at the bedside, including alternative options to secure the airway in case of failure(Mosier et al., 2020).

Objectives

- By the end of this module, the reader should be able to:
  - Recognise the indications and contraindications of RSI
  - To describe equipment and drugs needed for RSI
  - To define steps for a successful RSI
  - To reiterate complications associated with RSI

Indications

- Unfasted patient or unknown fasting status e.g. trauma patients, emergency surgery, resuscitation situations and in patients with a reduced conscious level
- Known gastro-oesophageal reflux such as due to hiatus hernia
- Conditions leading to delayed gastric emptying e.g. autonomic gastroparesis (diabetes, Parkinson's disease), history of gastric banding surgery, patient in severe pain or with recent administration of opioids
- Pregnancy (from the second trimester onwards)

Contraindications

- **Absolute contraindications include the following:**
  - Total upper airway obstruction, which requires a surgical airway
  - Total loss of facial/oropharyngeal landmarks, which requires a surgical airway
- **Relative contraindications include the following:**
  - Anticipated "difficult" airway, in which endotracheal intubation may be unsuccessful, resulting in reliance on successful bag-valve-mask (BVM) ventilation to keep an unconscious patient alive.

- The "crash" airway, in which the patient is in an arrest situation, unconscious and apnoeic.
- Urgent need to OT and theatre are available anatomically or pathologically difficult airway (e.g., congenital deformity, laryngeal fracture)
- Proximity to OT
- Paediatric cases (especially <5 years of age)
- Hostile environment
- Poorly functioning team
- Lack of requisite skills among team
- The emergency surgical airway is not possible (e.g., neck trauma, tumour)

Pre-procedural Care

Preparation of the environment

- Clinical area e.g. resuscitation room
- Monitoring – ECG monitor, BP, SpO2, capnography
- Intravenous access – preferably two iv lines
- Position on trolley should optimise access for intubation
- Drugs – drawn up in labelled syringes + checked by medical staff

Preparation of the equipment

Suggested equipment (** optional) (Ross & Ellard, 2016):

- Oxygen supply (machine)
- Oxygen delivery device
  - Self-inflating bag with one-way valve
  - Nasal prongs**
- Standard airway equipment
  - Face mask
  - Laryngoscope handle x 2
  - Range of laryngoscope blades

- Cuffed oral endotracheal tubes of appropriate sizing, with a range of alternative sizes available
  - ET tube tie or tape
- Difficult airway equipment, as per the difficult airway plan. This may include:
  - Oro- and naso-pharyngeal airways
  - Bougie
  - Video laryngoscope (**)
- Supraglottic rescue device: Laryngeal mask airway or alternative supraglottic airway
- Suction
- Monitoring
  - Pulse oximeter
  - Waveform capnograph
  - Blood pressure cuff and sphygmomanometer, or arterial line
  - Electrocardiograph
- Drugs (see Drugs section for further detail)
  - Induction agent
  - Agent for maintenance of anaesthesia
  - Fast-acting neuromuscular blocking agent
  - Emergency drugs (vasopressor and adrenaline, atropine)
  - Fluids running to act as flush for rapidly delivering drugs to circulation

Induction agents

Five drugs are commonly used to induce anaesthesia: propofol, ketamine, etomidate, thiopentone and midazolam (Ross & Ellard, 2016).

Propofol (1-3 mg/kg) is commonly used in the operating theatre for haemodynamically stable patients. However, in elderly or hypovolaemic patients, the dose is drastically reduced: often 0.5-1mg/kg is sufficient, although time to effect is increased due to lower cardiac output.

Ketamine (1-2mg/kg) is increasingly used in unstable patients in pre-hospital settings. The usual effect is an elevation in heart rate and variable but modest blood pressure changes: secretions increase, which may necessitate suctioning or premedication with an anti-sialagogue such as atropine or glycopyrrolate.

Etomidate (0.3mg/kg) also has minimal haemodynamic effects. However, use has been limited by concerns of adrenal suppression, and there is limited availability in some countries.

Thiopentone (3-5mg/kg) has the most rapid and predictable effect, with less haemodynamic instability than propofol. However, there may be issues with poor availability and the harmful sequelae following extravasation, or intra-arterial injection should be considered.

Midazolam (0.1-0.2mg/kg) may be used, although the time to effect may be significantly prolonged. It is most suitable in patients who are already obtunded and primarily require amnesia rather than true anaesthesia.

Neuromuscular blocking agents:

- **Succinylcholine**
  - Dose: 1-2 mg/kg
  - It does have a rapid onset and offset of action, but unfortunately, there are many side effects, some of which are life-threatening.
  - Side effects of succinylcholine:
    - It can cause hyperkalaemia, muscle pains, bradycardia, and malignant hyperpyrexia.
    - It has a high incidence of anaphylaxis and histamine release.
    - Raised intraocular, intracranial and intragastric pressure can occur with resultant passive regurgitation in the presence of an incompetent lower oesophageal sphincter.
    - Succinylcholine apnoea may occur.

Non-depolarizing neuromuscular block:

- **Rocuronium**:
    - Dose: 0.6-1.2 mg/kg IBW
    - Advantage: has a more rapid onset than previous non-depolarizing blockers and is proposed as an alternative agent for RSI.
    - Disadvantage: the duration of action of rocuronium is much longer than that of succinylcholine.

Cricoid pressure

Cricoid pressure is the application of force to the cricoid cartilage of the patient. The justification is that the upper oesophagus is occluded by being compressed between the trachea and the cervical vertebrae, containing passive reflux of gastric contents and subsequent risk of aspiration pneumonitis. 10 Newtons of force is applied by the thumb and index finger of an assistant, increasing to 30N once consciousness is lost. Maintain the pressure until endotracheal tube placement is confirmed. Cricoid pressure should be reduced or released if laryngoscopy is challenging or if vomiting occurs (to reduce the chance of oesophageal rupture from active vomiting) (Ross & Ellard, 2016).

- **THE SELLICK MANOEUVRE**
    - It is cricoid pressure applied during endotracheal intubation.
    - It is used to reduce the risk of regurgitation of gastric contents and works by virtue of the cricoid pressure occluding the oesophagus, which passes directly behind it.
- **BURP MANOEUVRE**
    - It is used to improve the view of the glottis during laryngoscopy (not to prevent regurgitation like The Sellick Manoeuvre).

○ The 'BURP' manoeuvre requires an assistant to apply pressure of the thyroid cartilage posteriorly (1), then upwards (2), and finally laterally towards the patients right (3).

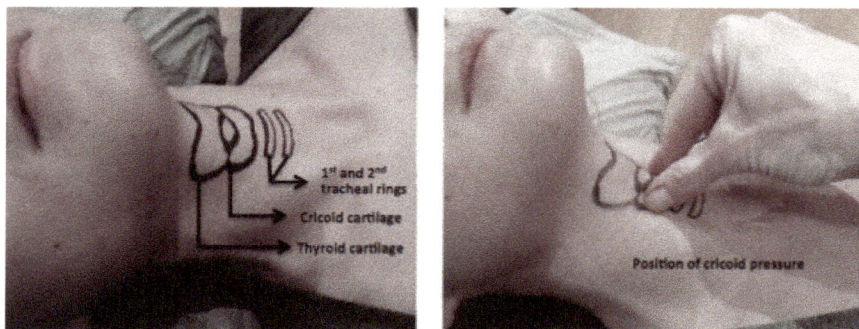

Fig.1.21.1. Cricoid pressure

Procedure

It is worth being aware of the '10 Ps' of ET intubation before you plan your procedure:

Preparation

You must have the right equipment and staff for the planned procedure. You should:

- Have a backup plan if you run into difficulties.
- Have the patient on complete monitoring (ECG/BP/pulse oximetry).
- Check all equipment (suction, laryngoscope, ET tube cuff).
- Ensure that there is IV access and the cannula is patent.
- Ensure that the emergency drugs are drawn up and labelled.
- Ensure that you have a trained assistant.

Plan for failure

- The importance of having a backup plan if you cannot intubate the patient cannot be overstressed.

- If you are not comfortable executing your backup plans B, C or even D, you should question whether you are the right person to be intubating the patient.

Positioning the Head

- The goal of positioning the head is to have the oral, pharyngeal and laryngeal inlets positioned in a straight line facilitating direct laryngoscopy.
- The ideal position is achieved by placing a pillow under the patient's head and extending the head on the neck in a **'sniffing the morning air' position.**
- This is the optimum position for intubation; however, a neutral position and in-line immobilisation must be maintained when you suspect a C-spine injury.

Pre-oxygenation

- Pre-oxygenation is performed with the patient breathing 100% oxygen through a tight-fitting non-rebreathing facemask **for 3 minutes.**
- This allows the replacement of nitrogen-containing air with oxygen and acts as an oxygen reservoir, delaying hypoxia onset in cases of prolonged apnoea or difficult intubation.
- After each failed attempt at intubation, the patient should be pre-oxygenated.

Pre-treatment

- Some situations require medications to attenuate the hypertensive response to laryngoscopy:
  - *Lidocaine*
  - *Opioids (e.g. Fentanyl or alfentanil)*

- These are generally not given in a crash induction, where the priority is securing the airway quickly and safely.

Protection of the airway

- Protection of the airway from aspiration of gastric contents is only achieved when a tube is positioned within the trachea, with no air leakage around the cuff.
- However, before the tube can be placed within the trachea, **cricoid pressure** must be applied to reduce the occurrence of passive regurgitation.
- Cricoid pressure (Sellick's manoeuvre) should be applied by a trained assistant using anteroposterior pressure on the cricoid cartilage at the onset of induction.
- The full 44 newtons of force should be applied when neuromuscular blocking agents are administered or when the patient is obtunded.
- The complete circumferential ring of the cricoid compresses the lumen of the oesophagus against the sixth cervical vertebra.
- **It does not prevent active vomiting**, and continued application in such circumstances can result in oesophageal rupture. Therefore, this is the only situation in which it should be released prematurely, and **the bed tilted head down with the patient on the left lateral position** to reduce aspiration.
- Otherwise, the cricoid should only be released after confirmed correct tube placement and adequate cuff inflation.

Paralysis with induction

- Only those trained in RSI and who routinely perform these techniques should administer muscle relaxants and anaesthetic agents, owing to contraindications and adverse complications associated with their use in the emergency setting.

- Give an appropriate intravenous induction agent: **thiopental or propofol**.
- These both cause hypnosis and amnesia.
- To ease laryngeal intubation, high-speed muscle relaxation is essential.
- The drug of choice in most circumstances is **suxamethonium**, although you should be aware of its contraindications.
- Suxamethonium is a depolarising muscle relaxant and causes muscle fasciculation before muscle relaxation.

Placement of the ET tube

- You will be asked to demonstrate this on the manikin.
- Stand behind the patient.
- Hold the laryngoscope with your **left hand** and insert it into the mouth over the **right side** of the tongue.
- Sweep the tongue **from right to left** and push it upwards so that the tip of the epiglottis comes into view. Ensure that teeth are not used as a fulcrum, and the lower lip does not get caught between the blade of the laryngoscope and the teeth.
- Advance the tip of the laryngoscope into the vallecula between the epiglottis and the tongue.
- To visualise the vocal cords, lift the oropharynx by moving the laryngoscope along the central axis of the handle.
- If you have a good view of the cords, you should insert the ET tube with your right hand so that it passes between the vocal cords into the trachea, ensuring that the cuff has passed beyond the vocal cords.
- In most adults, the tube will usually lie between **22 and 24 cm** at the level of the incisors.
- Stabilise the tube until it is taped or tied in place.
- Connect the tube via a catheter mount and ventilate the patient with 12–15 L of oxygen.

- The cuff should be inflated until no audible leak of ventilation gases is heard to pass around the cuff.

Proof of correct et tube placement

- It is imperative that you ensure that the ET tube is in the correct place and at the correct depth, by (in chronological order):
- Direct visualisation of the tube passing through the cords
- Compliance of the reservoir bag on manual ventilation and fogging of the tube
- Symmetrical expansion of the chest wall
- Auscultation of the chest bilaterally for breath sounds and auscultation over the epigastrium to exclude oesophageal intubation
- Attachment of an end-tidal CO_2 monitor (capnograph or calorimetric)
- Obtaining a chest X-ray to ensure placement of the tube above the carina and below the level of the cords

Post tube placement

- The tube should be secured, and the level at the central incisors noted in case of tube migration.
- The patient should be carefully monitored, and, once they have been stabilised, **a portable chest X-ray** should be performed to ensure that the main bronchus has not been inadvertently intubated.

Video-assisted laryngoscopy (VAL)

- VAL offers the advantage of abandoning the need for alignment of the optical axes in the mouth, pharynx, and larynx to visualise the glottis's entranced, therefore is more effective.

- VAL is now available as both a portable unit attached to a laryngoscope and a stand-alone unit that is wheeled to the bedside. Utilisation is often one of personal preference or institutional availability.

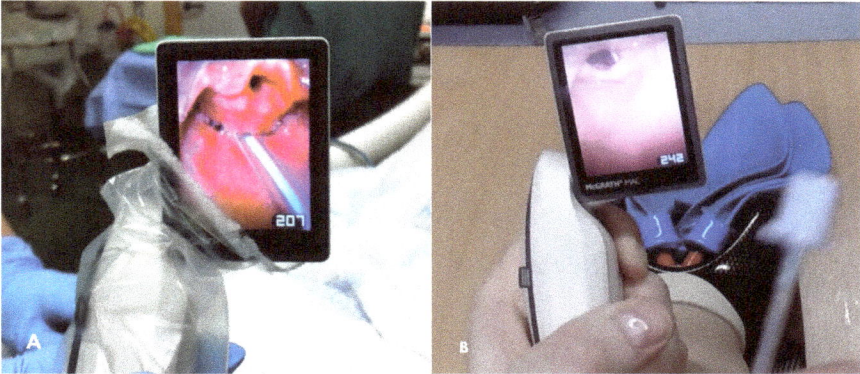

Fig.1.21.2. Video laryngoscope

Complications

- Failure to intubate
- Hypoxia
- Unrecognised oesophageal intubation
- Aspiration of stomach contents
- Hypotension
- Awareness
- Arrhythmias
- Cardiac arrest
- Aspiration of gastric content
- Inability to intubate, exacerbated by trauma from repeated attempted intubations
- Intubation of the oesophagus
- Dislodgement of the tube
- Bronchial intubation
- Tracheal stenosis
- Severe hypoxia if prolonged attempts are undertaken
- Chipping, loosening or dislodgement of teeth.

Difficult Airway Assessment

- Tools for rapid assessment of the difficult airway are the following:

LEMON assessment tool

- **L – Look externally**—four vital criteria: facial trauma, large incisors, beard or moustache, large tongue.
- **E – Evaluate**—evaluation by the 3-3-2 rule.
  - **Inter-incisor distance:** Adequately open the patient's mouth to allow the placement of three fingers between the upper and lower teeth
  - **Hyomental distance:** Use three finger breadths
  - **Thyromental distance:** Use two finger breadths

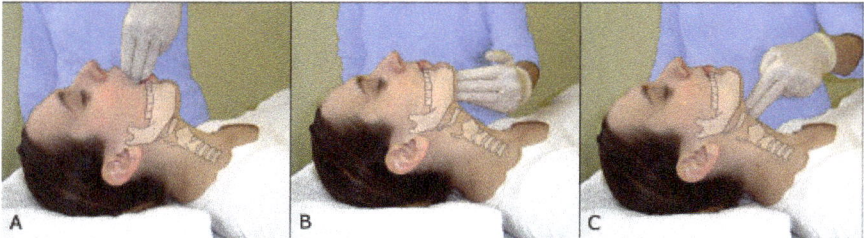

Fig.1.21.3. Evaluation of the 3-3-2

- **M – Mallampati:** Accomplished with the patient placed in a sitting position with the head in the neutral position and mouth completely open, and the tongue protruded maximally without phonation while the clinician looks from the front at the patient's eye level and inspects the pharyngeal structures with a pen torch without the patient phonating.

Mallampati grades:

- Class I: soft palate, uvula, fauces, and pillars visible.
- Class II: soft palate, uvula, fauces visible.

- Class III: soft palate, the base of uvula visible.
- Class IV: hard palate only visible.

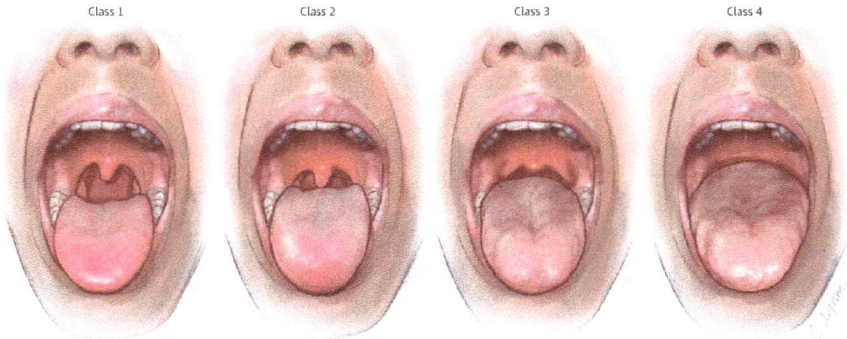

Fig.1.21.4. Mallampati grading tool

- **O– Obstruction:** Assess the patient for stridor, foreign bodies, and other forms of sub- and supraglottic obstructions, including tumours, abscesses, inflamed epiglottis, or expanding hematoma.
- **N – Neck mobility** is an essential condition for successful intubation. It is evaluated by the patient in the sitting position, placing their chin down onto their chest and then extending their neck, so they are looking towards the ceiling.

Cormack-Lehane grading scheme for laryngoscopy

- The hardship of direct laryngoscopy links with the best view of the glottis, as described by the Cormack-Lehane scale. With this scale, a grade I view connotes a full view of the entire glottic aperture, grade II denotes a partial glottic view, grade III describes a visualisation of the epiglottis only, and grade IV means the inability to visualise even the epiglottis (Hofmeyr, 2014).

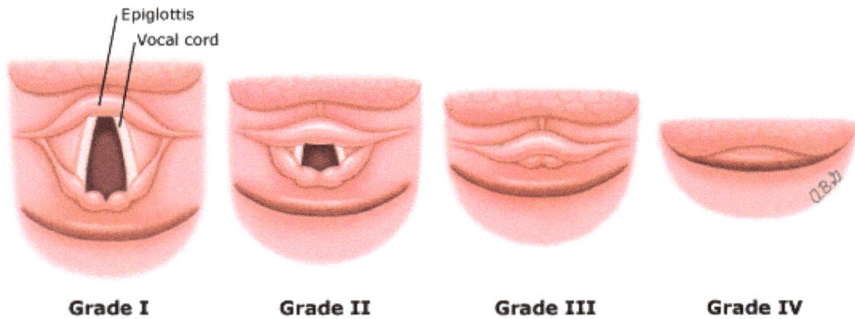

Fig.1.21.5. Cormack-Lehane grading system

Priorities in the failed airway situation

- Call for the most senior assistance available (Consultant in A&E, ICU, Anaesthetics, ENT +/- difficult airway trolley)
- Assess whether oxygenation is adequate:
    - If able to oxygenate and maintain saturation >90% with BVM then may be able to buy sufficient time to use alternative techniques e.g. fibreoptic scope
    - If unable to maintain saturation >90% then go back to GOOD basics while more help arrives/preparation for a surgical airway is occurring
        - High flow oxygen via anaesthetic circuit or BVM
        - Suction
        - OPA and NPA
        - Head positioning +/- pillow
        - person ventilation technique
        - Consider the use of an LMA

Further reading

Uptodate- Rapid sequence induction and intubation (RSII) for anesthesia: https://www.uptodate.com/contents/rapid-sequence-induction-and-intubation-rsii-for-anesthesia

StatPearls- Tracheal Rapid Sequence Intubation: https://www.ncbi.nlm.nih.gov/books/NBK560592/

References

Hofmeyr, R. (2014). *CORMACK-LEHANE GRADING EXAMPLES.* Open Airway. Retrieved 28 Dec. 2021 from https://openairway.org/cormack-lehane-grading-examples/

Lafferty, K. (2020). *Rapid Sequence Intubation.* Medscape. Retrieved 28 Dec. 2021 from https://emedicine.medscape.com/article/80222-overview

Mosier, J. M., Sakles, J. C., Law, J. A., Brown, C. A., 3rd, & Brindley, P. G. (2020). Tracheal Intubation in the Critically Ill. Where We Came from and Where We Should Go. *Am J Respir Crit Care Med, 201*(7), 775-788. https://doi.org/10.1164/rccm.201908-1636CI

Nickson, C. (2015). *Rapid Sequence Intubation (RSI).* Life in the fast lane. Retrieved 28 Dec. 2021 from https://litfl.com/rapid-sequence-intubation-rsi/

Reynolds, S. F., & Heffner, J. (2005). Airway management of the critically ill patient: rapid-sequence intubation. *Chest, 127*(4), 1397-1412. https://doi.org/10.1378/chest.127.4.1397

Ross, W., & Ellard, L. (2016). *Rapid Sequence Induction.* Anaesthesia Tutorials. Retrieved 28 Dec. 2021 from https://anaesthesiology.gr/media/File/pdf/-Rapid-Sequence-Induction.pdf

Sagarin, M. J., Barton, E. D., Chng, Y. M., & Walls, R. M. (2005). Airway management by US and Canadian emergency medicine residents: a multicenter analysis of more than 6,000 endotracheal intubation attempts. *Ann Emerg Med, 46*(4), 328-336. https://doi.org/10.1016/j.annemergmed.2005.01.009

Sinclair, R. C., & Luxton, M. C. (2005). Rapid sequence induction. *Continuing Education in Anaesthesia Critical Care & Pain, 5*(2), 45-48. https://doi.org/10.1093/bjaceaccp/mki016

| 22 |

Reduction of Dislocation/ Fracture

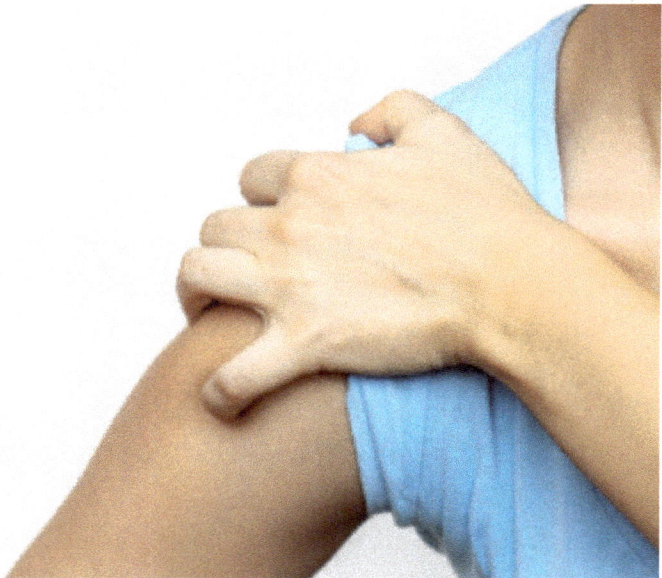

Overview

Shoulder dislocations represent half of all major joint dislocations, with the most common anterior dislocation (Abrams & Akbarnia, 2021). The shoulder joint is the most mobile joint of the human body. It can pivot in many directions; this makes it vulnerable for an easy dislocation (Athwa 2017). The instability of the shoulder joint is due to a shallow glenoid that only articulates with a small part of the humeral head. As a result, the shoulder can dislocate forward, backward, downward, and entirely or partially, though most occur anteriorly. This section will highlight diverse techniques commonly used to reduce shoulder dislocations in the emergency department.

Objectives

- By the end of this section, you should be able to:
    - Highlight the indications and contraindications of reducing shoulder dislocations
    - Describe the techniques commonly used to reduce diverse types of shoulder dislocations.
    - Explain advantages and disadvantages associated to each technique
    - List possible complications associated with this procedure

Indications

- Anterior dislocations (96 %)
- Posterior dislocations (4 %)
- Inferior dislocations (luxation erecta)

Contraindications

- Associated fracture warrants orthopaedic evaluation.
- Associated neurovascular deficit: May attempt reduction once but avoid multiple attempts.

Shoulder reduction techniques

- **Techniques to reduce anterior shoulder dislocations** (Borke, 2020):
    - Davos technique
    - External rotation
    - Milch technique
    - Scapular manipulation

- Spaso technique
- Stimson maneuverer
- Traction-countertraction
- **Techniques to reduce posterior shoulder dislocations** (Borke, 2020):
  - Traction-countertraction
- **Techniques to reduce inferior shoulder dislocations** (Borke, 2020):
  - Axial (inline) traction
  - Two-step reduction

Pre-procedural care

- Informed consent: The risks of the procedure and the specific risks of the agents to be used, if procedural sedation is planned must be clearly explained.
- Consider local anaesthesia or procedural sedation
- Bedsheet for traction-countertraction method
- Dangling weight for Stimson manoeuvre

Procedure

- **Physical examination**
  - Compare affected with the unaffected shoulder.
  - Perform a complete neurovascular examination: test axillary, radial, ulnar, and median nerves for sensory deficit and motor function.
- **Radiographs**
  - Useful before reduction to assess any possible fracture and type and position of dislocation.
  - Obtain three views: anteroposterior, scapular Y, and axillary lateral views.
    - Anterior dislocations: humeral head appears anterior to the glenoid fossa on lateral or Y views.
    - Posterior dislocations: vacant glenoid sign

- ○ **Pain management and sedation**
  - ■ Decide whether to use intra-articular lidocaine versus procedural sedation and analgesia.
- ○ **Reduction techniques:**
  - ■ It is important for the emergency department physician to be familiar with several different techniques:

1. Davos technique

- • **Technique**
  - ○ It is sometimes also referred to as the "**Boss-Holzach-Matter technique**".
  - ○ The patient sits upright on a stretcher and flexes the hip and knee on the ipsilateral side of the shoulder dislocation.
  - ○ Then clasps the fingers of both hands together around their flexed knee, after which the clinician binds the wrists together with an elastic bandage to allow the patient to relax their fingers.
  - ○ Next, the clinician puts weight on the patient's foot (e.g., sits on their foot) to hold it stationary.
  - ○ The patient is then instructed to relax their shoulder and arm muscles and then extend their head back and let the shoulders roll forward with the arms extended.
- • **Advantages**
  - ○ Without the need for sedation
  - ○ Safe, well-tolerated non-traumatic technique
  - ○ High success rate.

Davos technique is an easy, non-traumatic, very well-tolerated, and most of all, safe way to reduce a shoulder. It is complication-free and easy to apply, giving reproducible and comparable or superior results to other reduction tech-niques.

At the same time, it is well tolerated by a compliant patient, which makes it an ideal first-time reduction technique for anterior shoulder dislocations (Stafylakis et al., 2016).

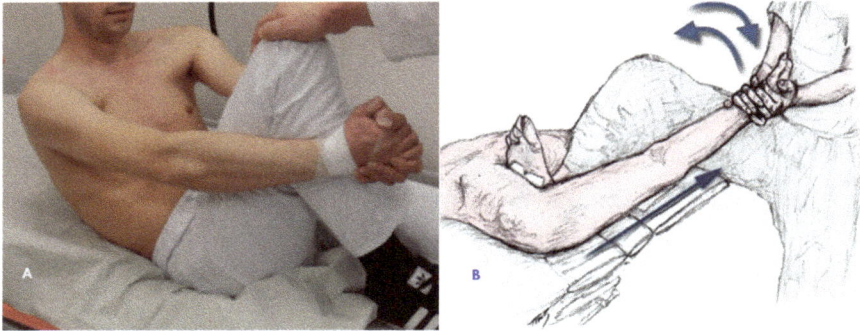

Fig.1.22.1. (A) Reduction of shoulder dislocation: Davos technique and (B) Reduction of shoulder dislocation: Hippocratic manoeuvre
Credit - (A) Reiner Wirbel and (B) Medscape

2. Hippocrates Method /Traction-Countertraction Technique

- **Technique**
    - With the patient is sitting up, have an assistant wrap a sheet around the upper chest and under the axilla of the affected shoulder.
    - Have the assistant wrap the sheet behind her or his back.
    - Now have the patient lay supine.
    - Wrap another sheet around the flexed elbow of the affected arm and behind the operator's back.
    - Both the operator and the assistant lean back, applying gentle traction.
- **Advantage:**
    - Many older physicians are familiar with this method and, therefore, have a high degree of success.

- **Disadvantages:**
  - ○ Requires two persons
  - ○ May cause skin tears on elderly patients.

3. Stimson Manoeuvre

- **Technique**
  - ○ The patient is placed in the prone position on an elevated stretcher.
  - ○ The affected shoulder should be off the edge of the stretcher, hanging downward in 90° of forward flexion.
  - ○ Attach 2.5–5 kg of weight hanging from the wrist.
  - ○ Reduction is usually achieved within 30 minutes.
- **Advantage:**
  - ○ Can be performed by one person only.
- **Disadvantages:**
  - ○ Requires time to gather materials.
  - ○ The danger involved in the patient falling off the stretcher
  - ○ Requiring staff to monitor the patient.

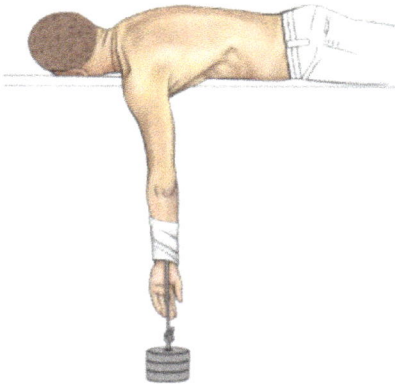

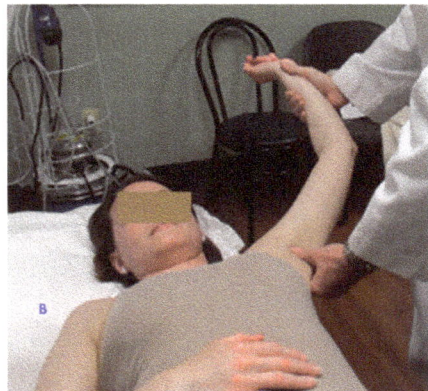

Fig.1.22.2. (A) Reduction of shoulder dislocation: Stimson manoeuvre and (B) Reduction of shoulder dislocation: Milch technique
Credit - (A) Musculoskeletal Key and (B) MDEdge

4. Milch Technique

- **Technique**
  - Abduct to fully externally rotate the injured arm into the overhead position
  - Maintain external rotation throughout the abduction.
  - Once in the overhead position, apply gentle vertical traction with external rotation.
  - An adjustment may need to be made if the reduction does not occur easily; push the humeral head upward into the glenoid fossa.
- **Advantages:**
  - Lack of complications
  - Patient tolerance
- **Disadvantage:**
  - Variable success rate reported: 70–90%

5. Spaso Technique

- **Technique**
  - Place the patient in the supine position.
  - Grasps the affected arm at the wrist and lifts the straight arm directly upward while applying longitudinal traction.
  - Apply external rotation.
- **Advantages:**
  - Single operator
  - High level of success
- **Disadvantage:**
  - It May require more time to allow the shoulder muscles to relax

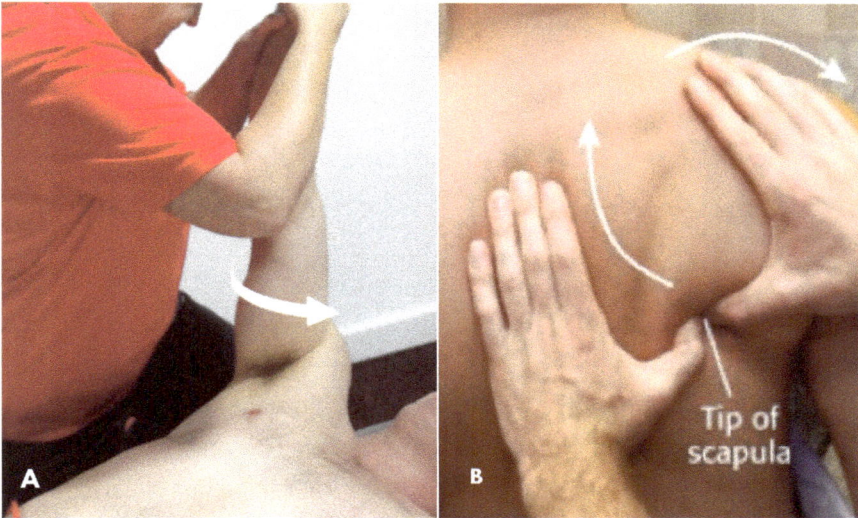

Fig.1.22.3. (A) Reduction of shoulder dislocation: Spaso technique and (B) Reduction of shoulder dislocation: Scapular manipulation technique
Credit - (A) Europe PMC and (B) NUEM Blog

6. Scapular Manipulation Technique

- **Technique**
  - Place the patient in the prone position with the affected arm hanging downward.
  - Apply traction down on the arm.
  - Locate the inferior tip of the scapula. Simultaneously push the inferior tip of the scapula medially toward the spine and use the other hand to push the superior scapula laterally.
- **Advantages:**
  - High success rate, greater than 90 %.
  - Very safe to perform.
- **Disadvantages:**
  - It requires the patient to assume the prone position
  - May require another person to perform traction.

7. External Rotation Method

- **Technique**
    - Place the patient in the supine position with the affected arm adducted directly next to the patient's side with the elbow flexed to 90°.
    - The operator uses one hand to direct downward traction on the affected arm while maintaining it next to the patient's side.
    - The operator uses the other hand to hold the patient's wrist and guide the arm into slow external rotation.
    - Reduction usually takes place between 70° and 110° of external rotation.

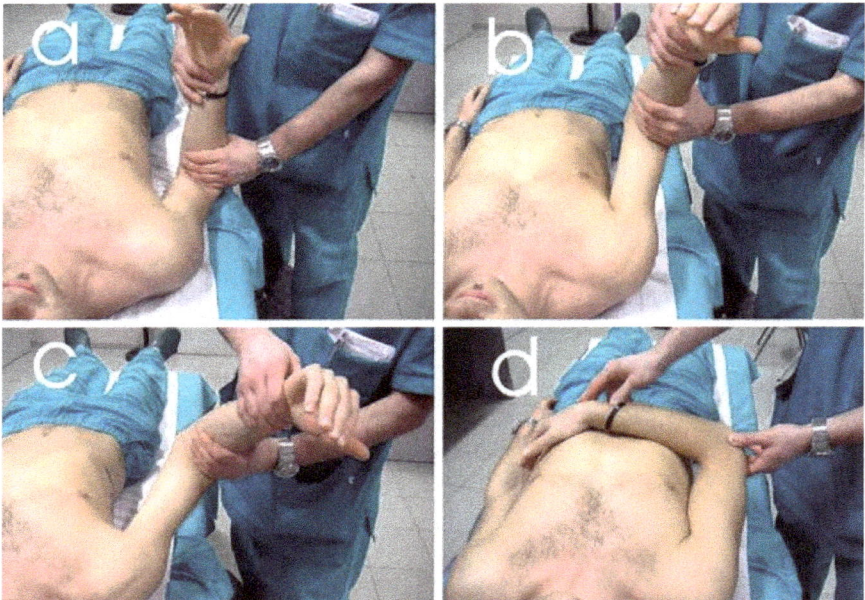

Fig.1.22.4. Reduction of shoulder dislocation: external rotation technique
Credit - Journal of Orthopaedics and Traumatology

- **Advantages:**
    - Requires no strength by the operator
    - Well-tolerated by patients.

- **Disadvantage:**
  - The patient may have persistent dislocation during the procedure,
  - Requiring operator to adjust.

8. Reduction of posterior shoulder dislocation

- **Technique**
  - Give adequate premedication.
  - Place the patient supine and apply lateral traction on the proximal humerus.
  - Have an assistant apply anterior pressure to the posteriorly located humeral head.
- **Advantage:**
  - Logical methods for reduction
- **Disadvantages:**
  - Require sufficient premedication because often posterior dislocations present late
  - May require open reduction

Post-reduction

- It is imperative to document the pre-and post-reduction neurovascular status in the medical record.
- If unsure whether the reduction was successful, attempt to place the palm of the injured extremity on the contralateral shoulder.
- Obtain post-reduction x-rays.
- There is some literature on using ultrasound to confirm adequate reduction, which allows repetitive assessments throughout the procedure, as well as reduce radiation
- Do a post-reduction neurovascular examination.
- Sling and swath or shoulder immobiliser for 2–3 weeks.
- Orthopaedic follow-up in 1 week.

- **Signs of a successful reduction include the following** (Borke, 2020):
  - Palpable or audible clunk
  - Return of rounded shoulder contour
  - Relief of pain
  - Increase in range of motion (e.g., the patient can touch the opposite shoulder with the palm of the affected arm)

Complications

- Fractures
- Adhesive capsulitis, or frozen shoulder; especially a concern in the elderly with prolonged immobilization in a sling
- Brachial plexus injury, especially of the axillary nerve
- Vascular laceration, most commonly of the axillary artery
- Rotator cuff tears

Further reading

MSD Manual- How To Reduce Anterior Shoulder Dislocations Using the Stimson Technique: https://www.msdmanuals.com/en-gb/professional/injuries-poisoning/how-to-reduce-dislocations-and-subluxations/how-to-reduce-anterior-shoulder-dislocations-using-the-stimson-technique

References

Abrams, R., & Akbarnia, H. (2021). Shoulder Dislocations Overview. In *StatPearls*. StatPearls Publishing. Copyright © 2021, StatPearls Publishing LLC.

Athwa, G. S. (2017). *Dislocated Shoulder*. OrthoInfo. Retrieved 12 Dec. 2021 from https://orthoinfo.aaos.org/en/diseases--conditions/dislocated-shoulder/

Borke, J. (2020). *Reduction of Shoulder Dislocation Technique*. Medscape. Retrieved 12 Dec. 2021 from https://emedicine.medscape.com/article/109130-technique

2. Reduction of Elbow Dislocation

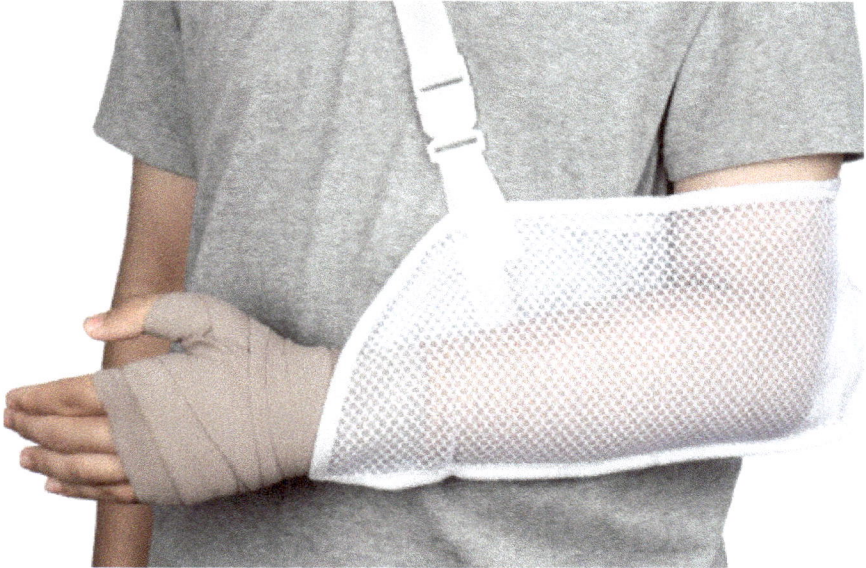

Overview

Dislocations of the elbow joint are common and can be classified as simple or complex depending on associated injury to neighbouring structures. Simple dislocations occur in the absence of fracture since there is only ligamentous injury and are more likely to be successfully managed without surgery. Complex dislocations have one or more fractures in addition to soft tissue injury. Posterior dislocations of the elbow joint are more common than anterior dislocations and are more frequently seen in the emergency department because of the increasing public participation in sports. Posterior elbow dislocations are the most common type of joint dislocation in children under-10 (Uhl et al., 2000). In adults, posterior elbow dislocations are the second most dislocated joint, proceeded by shoulder dislocations (de Haan et al., 2010). This section will highlight in detail diverse techniques commonly used to reduce elbow dislocations in the emergency department.

Objectives

- By the end of this section, you should be able to:
  - Highlight the indications and contraindications of reducing elbow dislocations
  - Describe the techniques commonly used to reduce diverse types of elbow dislocations.
  - Explain the advantages and disadvantages associated with each technique
  - List possible complications associated with this procedure

Indications

- Any dislocation of the elbow joint.
- The direction of the dislocation (i.e., anterior, posterior, lateral and divergent radius, and ulnar dislocations) is determined by the position of the ulna relative to the joint space.

Contraindications

- Compound fracture-dislocation (Relative)

Pre-procedural care

- Parenteral sedation and analgesia medications
- Local anaesthetic for local and intra-articular anaesthesia
- Splinting material
- Stockinette
- Padding
- Elastic bandage
- Tape
- Sling

Procedure

- Obtain a true lateral and anteroposterior radiograph of the affected elbow.
- Ensure adequate sedation and analgesia.
- Consider intra-articular analgesia.

- Check the neurovascular status of the affected extremity.
- Follow a selected method for reduction as detailed later.
- Following successful reduction gently flex the elbow to ensure a full range of motion.
- Place a long-arm posterior splint with the elbow in at least 90° flexion and secure the arm in a regular sling.
- Check neurovascular status.
- Obtain a post-reduction radiograph of the elbow.

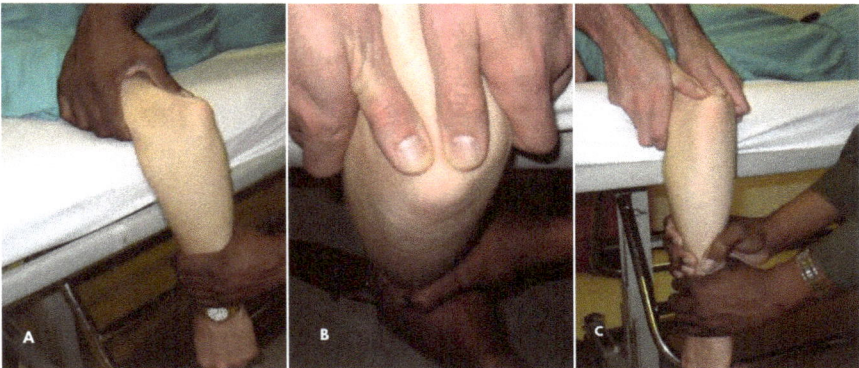

Fig.1.22.5. (A) Reduction of posterior elbow dislocation. Prone (one-person) technique, (B) Reduction of posterior elbow dislocation. Prone (two-person) technique. Positioning of fingers against posterior olecranon and (C) Reduction of posterior elbow dislocation. Prone (two-person) technique.
Credit - Medscape

METHOD A

- Position the patient on a stretcher in the supine position.
- Apply steady traction at the supinated distal forearm keeping the elbow slightly flexed, while an assistant applies countertraction to the mid-humerus with both hands.

METHOD B

- Position the patient on a stretcher in the supine position.
- Extend the affected extremity over the edge of the stretcher.

- Apply traction to the supinated forearm slightly flexed at the elbow, while an assistant holds the distal humerus with both hands and uses thumbs to apply pressure to the olecranon as if pushing it away from the humerus.

METHOD C

- Position the patient on a stretcher in the prone position.
- Hang the affected extremity over the side of the stretcher toward the floor.
- Apply downward traction to the pronated distal forearm and with the other hand just above the patient's antecubital fossa lift the humerus toward you.

Procedure for anterior dislocations

- Follow pre-and post-procedure steps as documented for the posterior dislocation.
- Position the patient on a stretcher in the supine position.
- With one hand, apply traction to the supinated distal forearm with the elbow extended, while an assistant applies countertraction with both hands around the distal humerus.
- Using the other hand, apply downward and backward pressure over the proximal forearm just below the antecubital fossa.

Complications
- Concomitant fractures
- Vascular injury, most commonly to the brachial artery
- Median nerve injury/entrapment
- Recurrent dislocation—rare

Radial head subluxations - Pulled elbow

- **Technique**
    - This procedure can normally be performed without any sedation or parenteral analgesia.
    - Position the patient, most commonly a child aged 1–3 years, facing forward on the caretaker's lap.
    - Hold the flexed elbow of the affected extremity placing your thumb firmly over the radial head.

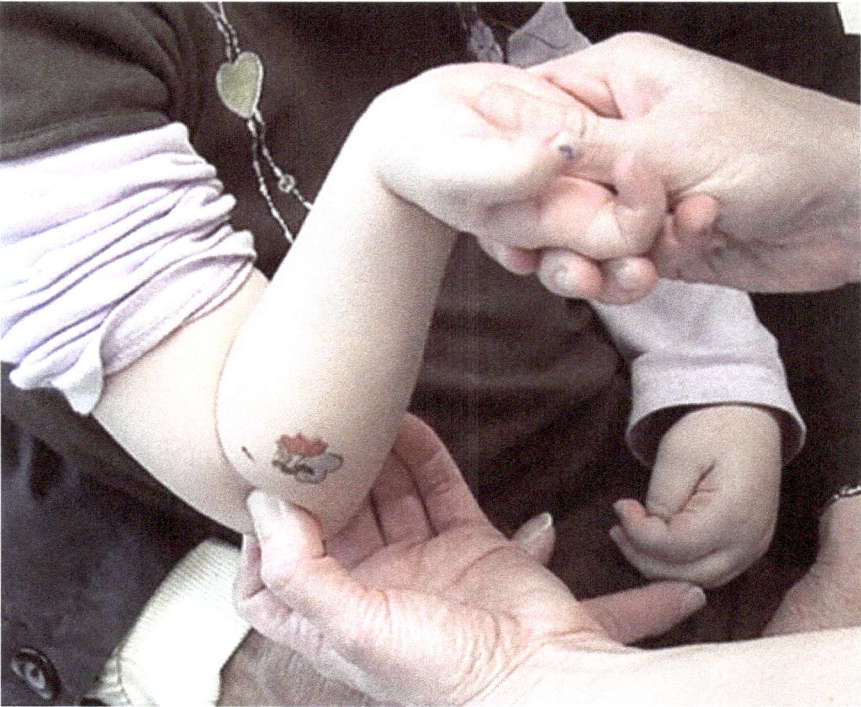

Fig.1.22.6. Reduction of pulled elbow
Credit - NEJM

- With the other hand, take the child's hand and wrist, and in one continuous movement, hyper-pronate and flex the Forearm.
- Another method is to supinate and flex the forearm instead of hyper-pronating it.

- Leave the room, encourage the caretaker to engage the child with distracting activities and re-examine the child in 10–20 min, at which stage, if the reduction was successful, the child should be using the extremity normally again.
- No post-reduction radiograph or immobilisation is required.

Further Reading

MSD Manual-How To Reduce a Posterior Elbow Dislocation: https://www.msdmanuals.com/en-gb/professional/injuries-poisoning/how-to-reduce-dislocations-and-subluxations/how-to-reduce-a-posterior-elbow-dislocation

References

de Haan, J., Schep, N. W., Tuinebreijer, W. E., Patka, P., & den Hartog, D. (2010). Simple elbow dislocations: a systematic review of the literature. Arch Orthop Trauma Surg, 130(2), 241-249. https://doi.org/10.1007/s00402-009-0866-0

Uhl, T. L., Gould, M., & Gieck, J. H. (2000). Rehabilitation after posterolateral dislocation of the elbow in a collegiate football player: a case report. J Athl Train, 35(1), 108-110.

3. Reduction Distal Interphalangeal Joint Dislocation

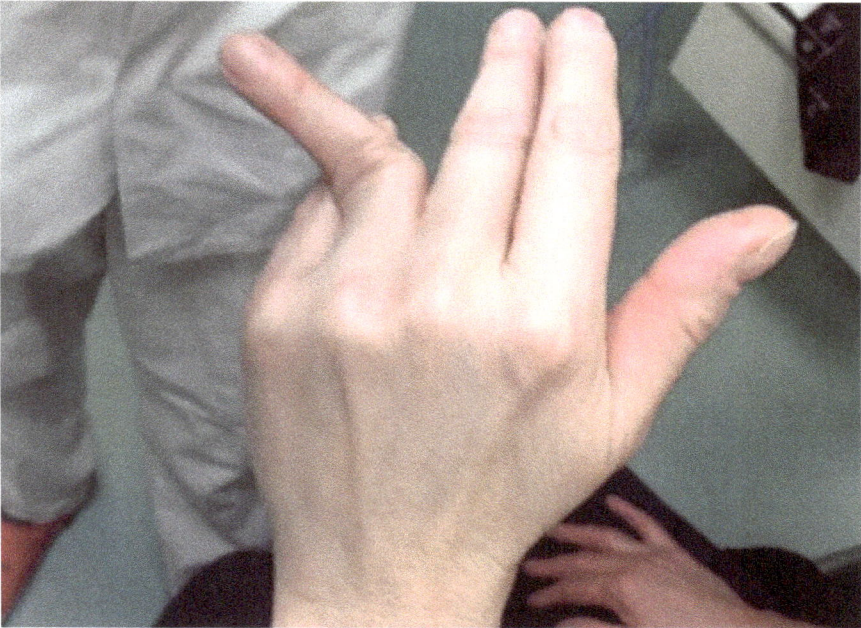

Overview
- Distal interphalangeal (DIP) joint dislocation is rare.
- It occurs when an axial force is applied to the distal phalanx

Indications
- DIP joint reduction is performed to alleviate functional and anatomical derangements resulting from DIP joint dislocation, commonly dorsal, from axial compression.

Contraindications
- **Absolute**
  - Absence of radiographic confirmation (anteroposterior, true lateral, and oblique) of simple DIP joint dislocation, especially in paediatric cases

- **Relative**
  - Open joint dislocation, associated fracture, or entrapped volar plate
  - Digital neurovascular compromise

Procedure

- Place the patient in the seated position with the arms at rest on a bedside table or supported by an assistant.
- Pronate the patient's hand, remove rings if present, and rest on a flat surface.
- Insert a 25-gauge needle at the dorsolateral aspect of the base of the finger to form a wheal to reduce patient discomfort.

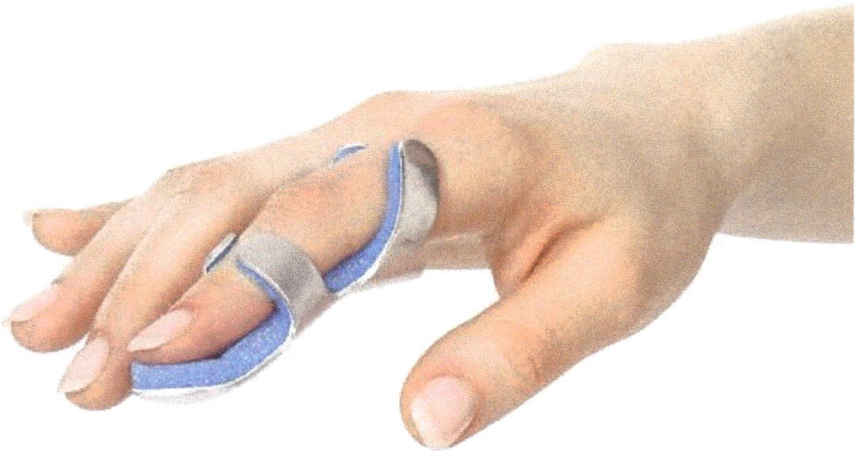

Fig.1.22.7. Padded aluminium splint applied to block the DIP joint

- Advance the needle and direct anteriorly toward the phalangeal base.
- Inject 0.5–1 mL of local anaesthetic as the needle is withdrawn 1–2 mm from the point of bone contact.
- Inject an additional 1 mL of local anaesthetic continuously as the needle is withdrawn.

- The injection should never render the tissue tense nor be circumferential.
- Hyperextend the DIP joint while applying longitudinal traction, followed by immediate joint flexion at the base of the distal phalanx.
- Place finger(s) in an aluminium digital dorsal splint in slight flexion for 2 weeks.
- A Post-reduction radiograph is recommended for confirmation.

Complications
- Irreducible dislocations
- Stiffness
- Recurrent dislocation
- Extensor lag in joints with residual subluxation
- Associated with dorsal joint prominences, swan-neck/ boutonnière deformity, and degenerative arthritis

Post-procedure
- Place finger(s) in an aluminium digital dorsal splint in slight flexion for 2 weeks.
- A Post-reduction radiograph is recommended for confirmation.
- Irreducible DIP joint dislocations may be due to entrapment of an avulsion fracture, the profundus tendon, or the volar plate.

4. Reduction of Hip Joint Dislocation

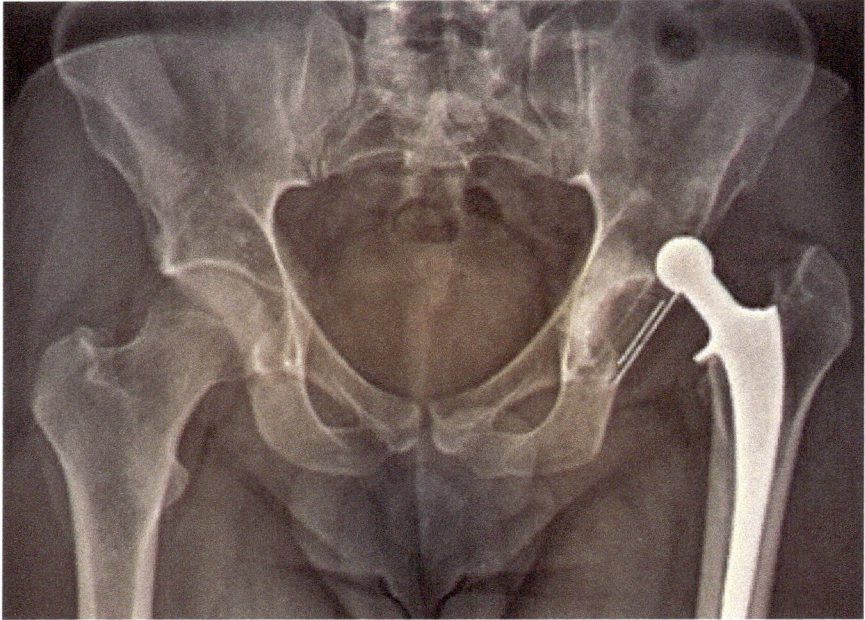

Overview

Hip dislocations are a common presentation in the Emergency Department (ED) and require urgent reduction to reduce the risk of avascular necrosis (Gottlieb, 2018). A traumatic hip dislocation happens with the dislodgement of the head of the femur out of the acetabulum. It generally requires significant power to dislocate the hip, thus causing damage to the surrounding hip tissues. The common causes are road traffic accidents and fall from heights. Over 90% of all dislocations can successfully be reduced in the ED, and there is evidence that cases are awaiting operative reduction result in significant delays (Gottlieb, 2018). This section will highlight in detail diverse techniques commonly used to reduce hip dislocations in the emergency department.

Objectives

- By the end of this section, you should be able to:
  - Highlight the indications and contraindications of reducing hip dislocations
  - Describe the techniques commonly used to reduce diverse types of hip dislocations.
  - Explain the advantages and disadvantages associated with each technique
  - List possible complications associated with this procedure

Indications

- Displacement of the femoral head in relation to the acetabulum without concomitant femoral neck, head, or acetabulum fractures:
  - Posterior hip dislocations make up 80–90 % of cases.
  - Anterior hip dislocations make up 10–15 % of cases.
    - These are classified into obturator, pubic, iliac, central, or inferior types.
    - Central dislocations are associated with comminuted acetabulum fractures, and inferior dislocations are a rare occurrence normally occurring in children younger than 7 years of age.
  - Prosthetic hip dislocations

Contraindications

- **Absolute**
  - Femoral neck fracture: attempted reduction may increase the displacement of the fracture and increase the probability of avascular necrosis.
- **Relative**
  - Fractures in other parts of the affected lower extremity: these may limit the pressure that can be applied necessary for traction during reduction.

Materials and Medications
- Parenteral sedation and analgesia medications
- Sheet or belt to fix the pelvis to the stretcher
- Knee immobilizer
- Abduction pillow

Procedure
- Check the neurovascular status of the affected extremity.
- Obtain anteroposterior (AP) views of the pelvis and lateral views of the hip.
- Ensure adequate parenteral sedation and analgesia.
- Decide upon a technique, as detailed later, and position the patient accordingly.
- Once the hip has been successfully reduced, test the joint for stability by moving it gently through its range of motion.
- Place a knee immobilizer and an abduction pillow between the knees.
- Check the neurovascular status.
- Obtain repeat AP films of the pelvis.

1. Stimson's Manoeuvre

- Place the patient prone on the stretcher with the affected extremity hanging over the edge and the hip flexed to 90° (Stimson, 1883).
- Flex the knee and the foot to 90°.
- Apply downward pressure to the area just distal to the popliteal fossa with a hand or knee while using the opposite hand to internally and externally rotate the hip at the ankle.
- Have an assistant simultaneously manipulate the displaced femoral head into position with both hands, applying downward pressure over the affected buttock.

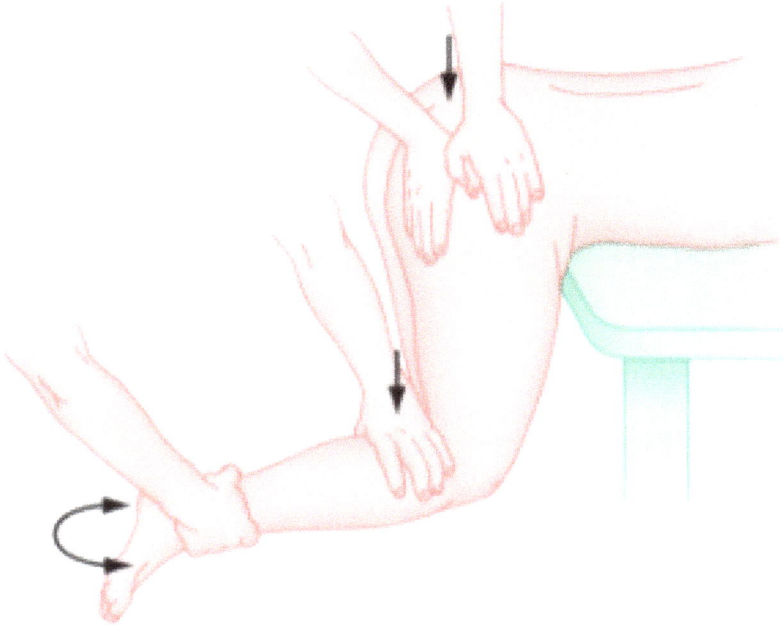

Fig.1.22.8. Reduction of hip joint dislocation: Stimson's manoeuvre with hand and Knee
Credit - CanadiEM

2. Allis Manoeuvre

- Position the patient supine on the stretcher.
- The operator should stand on the stretcher to achieve maximum leverage or have the patient on a backboard on the ground.
- Have an assistant apply downward pressure to both iliac crests.
- Apply constant, gentle upward traction in line with the deformity while manoeuvring the hip to 90° flexion and through internal and external rotation.
- Have a second assistant provide lateral traction to the midthigh.
- Once the femoral head has cleared the outer lip of the acetabulum, continue traction while keeping the hip in external rotation and gently abducting and extending the hip.

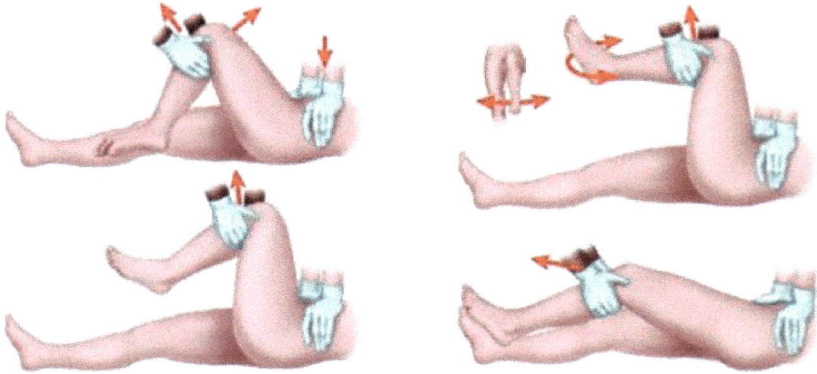

Fig.1.22.9. Reduction of hip joint dislocation: Allis technique
Credit - Mohammed Lahfaoui

3. Whistler Technique

- Position the patient supine on the stretcher with the knee and hip flexed to 45°.
- Have an assistant stabilise the pelvis with downward pressure on both iliac crests.
- Stand on the side of the affected extremity and place one arm under the knee, resting the hand on the flexed knee of the unaffected extremity.
- Secure the ankle of the affected extremity with the other hand and elevate the shoulder of the opposite arm, providing upward traction at the distal thigh and a strong fulcrum to reduce the dislocation. Internal and external rotation can be achieved with the opposite hand at the ipsilateral ankle

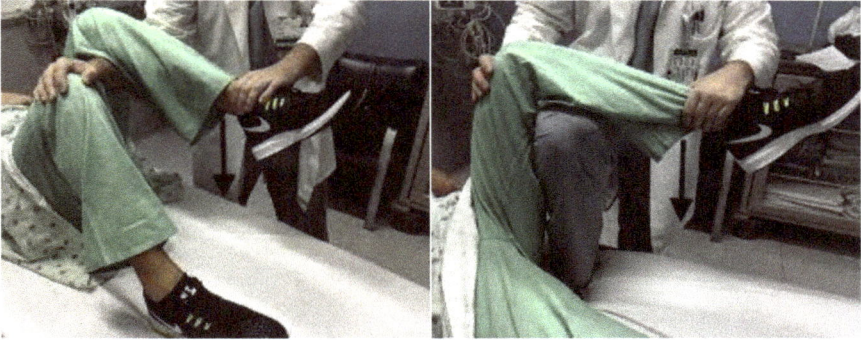

Fig.1.22.10. (A) Reduction of hip joint dislocation: Whistler technique and (B) Captain Morgan technique
Credit - Michael Gottlieb

4. Captain Morgan Technique

- Position the patient supine on the stretcher with the knee and hip flexed to 90°.
- Stabilise and fix the pelvis with a sheet tied securely over the pelvis and under the stretcher.
- Standing on the side of the affected extremity, the operator's foot should be resting perpendicular on the stretcher with the knee placed under the patient's knee.
- With the opposite hand, apply downward pressure to the ankle and provide a sustained upward force to the patient's thigh by elevation of the knee through plantar flexion of the toes and the upward pressure of the other hand placed behind the patient's knee.
- Internal and external rotation can be applied simultaneously, if necessary, by gently twisting the ankle.

5. Bigelow manoeuvre

- Place the patient in the supine position. Holds the ankle of the affected leg with one hand and puts your opposite forearm under the patient's knee (Bigelow, 1870).

- The hip is flexed to 90 degrees, ensuring the affected leg is kept in an adducted and internally rotated position.
- While a helper stabilises the pelvis with downward pressure, apply traction in line with the femur while abducting, externally rotating, and extending the affected hip.
- Preferably, the clinician should perform this manoeuvre while standing at the side of the bed; however, at times, entering the bed is a necessity.

6. Skoff manoeuvre

- Place the patient in the lateral decubitus position with the injured leg facing up (Skoff, 1986).
- The assistant places the affected leg into 90-100 degree hip flexion, 40-45 degree internal rotation, and 40-45 degree adduction and flexes the knee to 90 degrees.
- The assistant then tilts back, providing lateral traction in line with the femur.
- Simultaneously, palpate the deformity in the gluteal region and force the femoral head until reduction into the acetabulum is achieved.

Complications

- Sciatic nerve injury
- Avascular necrosis of the femoral head due to delay inadequate reduction
- Inability to perform reduction due to occult fractures and fracture fragments, incarceration of the joint capsule, or associated tendons
- Unstable or irreducible dislocations
- Traumatic arthritis and joint instability

Further reading

Larry Mellick - Hip Dislocation Emergency: https://www.youtube.com/watch?v=eMVsjwAukU4

References

Bigelow, H. J. (1870). Luxations of the hip-joint. The Boston Medical and Surgical Journal, 82(4), 65-67.

Gottlieb, M. (2018). Hip Dislocations in the Emergency Department: A Review of Reduction Techniques. The Journal of Emergency Medicine, 54(3), 339-347. https://doi.org/https://doi.org/10.1016/j.jemermed.2017.12.002

Skoff, H. (1986). Posterior hip dislocation, a new technique for reduction. Orthopaedic review, 15(6), 405-409.

Stimson, L. A. (1883). A treatise on fractures. Henry C. Lea's Son & Company

5. Reduction of Knee Dislocation

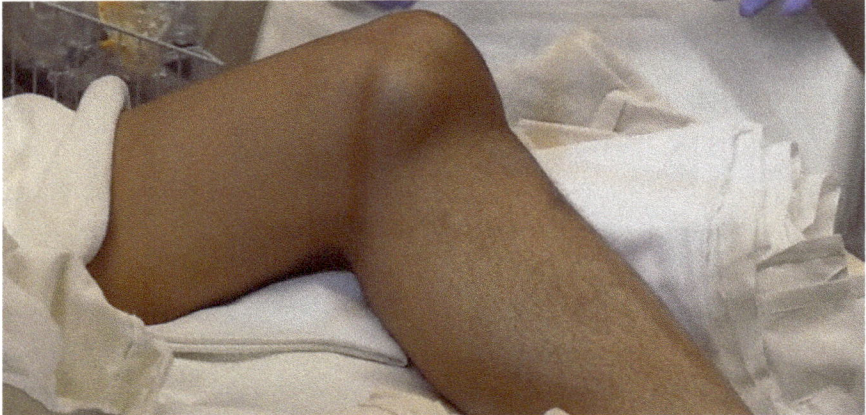

Overview

A dislocated knee is an overwhelming injury and is frequently considered a limb-threatening emergency and requires prompt identification and assessment with proper imaging and consultation with specialities for definitive management (Mohseni & Simon, 2021). The diagnosis is clinical with careful assessment of limb neurovascular status. Vascular damage and compartment syndrome should never be missed in assessing a knee dislocation. The knee dislocation with its incidence of 0.02% of orthopaedic injuries is presumably underreported as approximately 50% self-reduce and are misdiagnosed. *Dislocations of the knee* are defined in terms of the tibia's position concerning the femur. All knee dislocations require orthopaedic evaluation at the earliest possible opportunity. Knee dislocations are frequently associated with popliteal artery and peroneal nerve injury; therefore, a neurovascular examination is mandatory before and after any attempts at reducing or manipulating the knee. *Dislocations of the head of the fibula* are often anterolateral, but these do not result in neurovascular compromise. Anterior dislocations typically result from a fall on the flexed, adducted leg, often combined with ankle inversion. While superior fibula head dislocation is associated with interosseous membrane damage and proximal shift of the lateral malleolus, posterior fibular head dislocations usually result from direct trauma to the flexed knee and may be accompanied by peroneal nerve injury. *Patellar dislocation* occurs most frequently among adolescents, often in external rotation combined with a strong valgus force and quadriceps contraction. These dislocations are described in the patellar relationship to the normal knee joint. The most common patellar dislocations are lateral. Dislocations tend to be recurrent, particularly in patients with patellofemoral anatomical abnormalities.

This section will highlight diverse techniques commonly used to reduce knee dislocations in the emergency department.

Objectives

- By the end of this section, you should be able to:
    - ○ Recognise potential complications of a knee dislocation
    - ○ Highlight the indications and contraindications of reducing knee dislocations
    - ○ Describe the techniques commonly used to reduce diverse types of knee dislocations.
    - ○ Explain the advantages and disadvantages associated with each technique

Indications

- Dislocation of the knee/fibular head/patella

Contraindications

- **Absolute**
    - ○ None
- **Relative**
    - ○ Immediate availability of orthopaedic consultation

Materials and Medications
- Parenteral sedation and analgesia medications
- Knee immobiliser or splinting materials

Procedure

1. Knee (femur/tibia) dislocation reduction

- Assess neurovascular function.
- Pre-treat the patient with sedation or analgesia as appropriate. Position the patient supine with the affected leg fully extended.
- Instruct an assistant to stand near the patient's hip and, facing the patient's affected knee, grasp the distal femur firmly with both hands to fix it in place.
- Stand near the patient's foot and face the patient's affected knee, grasp the distal tibia and apply straight traction in a distal direction.
- Longitudinal traction-countertraction alone, as described previously, will usually reduce the dislocation. If reduction does not occur, proceed with the following steps.

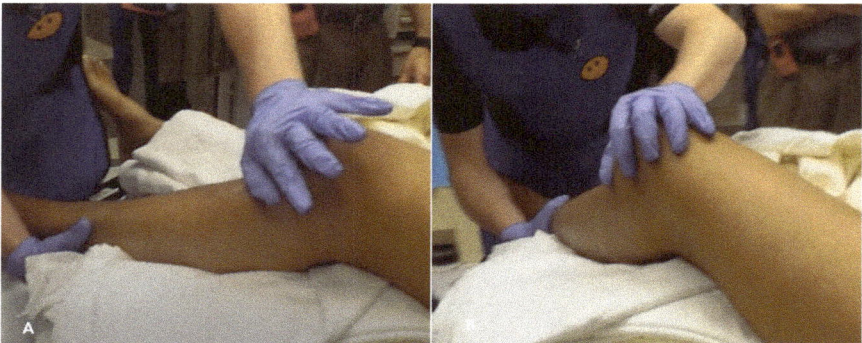

Fig.1.1.22.11. Reduction of Knee joint dislocation

- While applying straight traction in a distal direction to the tibia with the dominant hand, with the non-dominant hand:

- ○ **Anterior dislocation:** push the proximal tibia in a posterior direction.
- ○ **Posterior dislocation:** lift the proximal tibia in an anterior direction.
- ○ **Lateral dislocation:** push the proximal tibia in a medial direction.
- ○ **Medial dislocation:** push the proximal tibia in a lateral direction.
- ○ **Rotary dislocation:** rotate the proximal tibia into proper linear alignment with the femoral condyles.
- Reduction may be facilitated using two assistants rather than just one.
- The second assistant grasps the distal tibia and applies straight traction in a distal direction, freeing the operator to manipulate the proximal tibia as described previously using both hands.
- After reduction, reassess neurovascular function and, if available, obtain angiography.
- Immobilise the knee in 15° of flexion in a knee immobiliser or long-leg posterior splint.

2. Fibular head dislocation reduction

- Assess neurovascular function. pre-treat the patient with sedation or analgesia as appropriate.
- Position the patient supine.
- Flex the knee to 90° to relax the biceps femoris tendon.
- Instruct an assistant to stand near the patient's hip and, facing the patient's affected knee, grasp the distal femur firmly with both hands to fix it in place.
- Stand near the patient's foot and, facing the patient's affected knee, grasp the distal tibia and apply straight traction in a distal direction with the dominant hand and with the non-dominant hand.

○ **Anterior dislocation:** push the fibular head in a posterior direction.

○ **Posterior dislocation:** push the fibular head in an anterior direction.

- Reduction may be facilitated using two assistants rather than just one.
- If a second assistant is available, instruct the second assistant to stand near the patient's foot and, facing the patient's affected knee, grasp the distal tibia and apply straight traction in a distal direction.
- This enables the operator to grasp and move the proximal fibula as described previously using both hands.
- Reduction is often signified by a palpable and audible click as the fibula snaps back into position.
- After reduction, reassess neurovascular function and, if available, obtain angiography.
- After reduction, patients should receive an orthopaedic referral, avoid weight-bearing for the first 2 weeks, and then gradually increase weight-bearing over the next 6 weeks.
- Typically, immobilisation is not required following reduction of an isolated fibular head dislocation

3. Lateral patellar dislocation reduction

- Pre-treat the patient with sedation or analgesia as appropriate.
- Stand at the side of the affected knee and facing the knee, grasp the distal tibia and slowly extend the knee with one hand, and with the other hand simultaneously apply gentle pressure to the patella in a medial direction.
- The lateral edge of the patella may be lifted slightly to facilitate its travel over the femoral condyle during reduction.

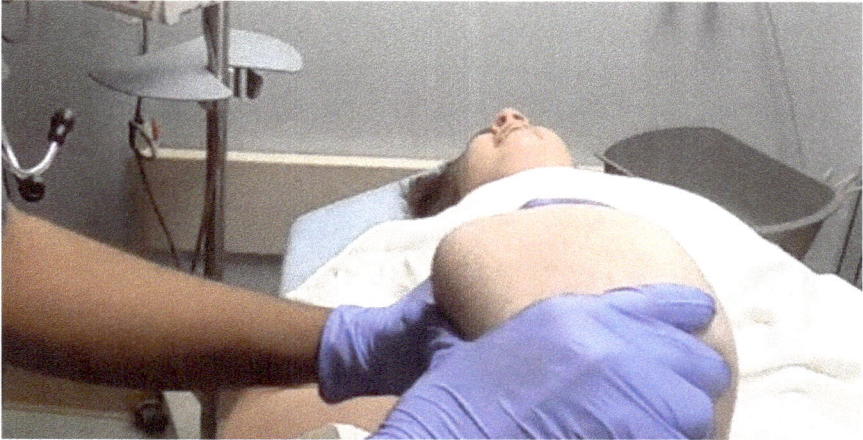

Fig.1.22.12. Reduction of the lateral patellar dislocation

Post-reduction care

After reduction, the knee should be immobilised in full extension in a knee immobiliser or long-leg posterior splint, and the patient should receive an orthopaedic referral, avoid weight-bearing for the first 2 weeks, and then gradually increase weight-bearing over the next 6 weeks.

Complications

- **Knee (femur/tibia) dislocations**
  - Distal ischaemia (even requiring amputation)
  - Degenerative arthritis
  - Joint instability due to ligamentous injury
- **Fibular head dislocations**
  - Peroneal nerve injury
  - Fibular head instability/subluxation
  - Degenerative arthritis
- **Patellar dislocations**
  - Failure of reduction
  - Degenerative arthritis
  - Recurrent dislocation/subluxation

Further reading

PEMBlog - Reduction of the dislocated patella: https://www.youtube.com/watch?v=57dGvS4JL4k

Dr. Nabil Ebraheim - Knee Dislocation - Everything You Need To Know: https://www.youtube.com/watch?v=BRy4DmCiDEw

Larry Mellick – Traumatic knee dislocation reduction: https://www.youtube.com/watch?v=aN7zDxtyHy8

References

Mohseni, M., & Simon, L. V. (2021). Knee Dislocation. In *StatPearls*. StatPearls Publishing. StatPearls Publishing LLC. Available at: https://www.ncbi.nlm.nih.gov/books/NBK470595

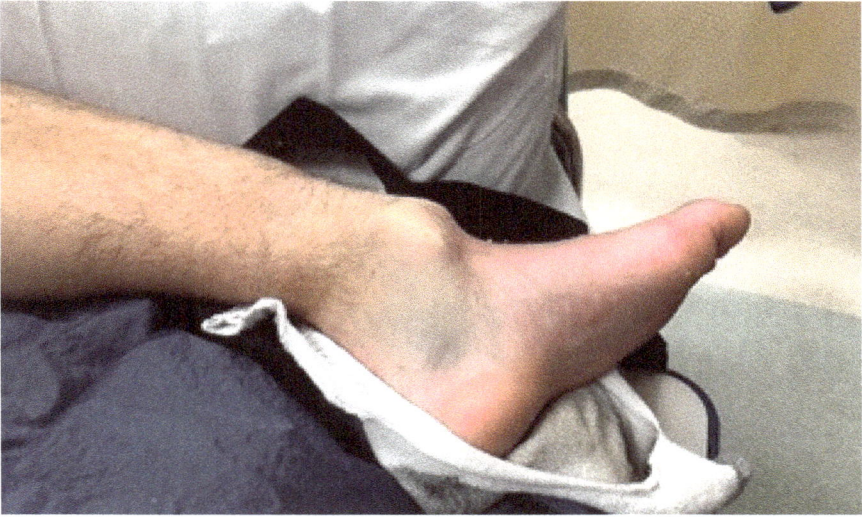

6. *Reduction of Ankle Dislocation*

Overview

The ankle joint stability is provided by the close articulation of the talus with the tibia and fibula. The mortise structure further improves the stability of the configuration (Keany, 2016). Rarely, the ankle dislocates without associated fractures. Ankle dislocations in the absence of fracture happen when a powerful force is applied to the joint, resulting in loss of opposition of the articular surfaces (Thangarajah et al., 2008). Ankle dislocation is an orthopaedic emergency, and reduction should not be delayed by imaging if there is evidence of neurovascular impairment. Complications exacerbated by a delay in management include concomitant fractures, gross deformity of the ankle, severe stretching and tenting of the skin with resultant skin blisters, skin necrosis, and possible conversion to a compound fracture. Always check the radiograph carefully for commonly associated fractures, particularly images of the malleoli. This section will highlight diverse techniques commonly used to reduce ankle dislocations in the emergency department.

Objectives

- By the end of this section, you should be able to:
  - Highlight the indications and contraindications of reducing ankle dislocations
  - Describe the techniques commonly used to reduce diverse types of ankle dislocations.
  - Explain the advantages and disadvantages associated with each technique
  - List possible complications associated with this procedure

Indications

- Dislocation of the ankle joint.
- This is defined by the articulation of the talus with the mortise that is formed by the distal tibia and fibula.
- Dislocations can be posterior, anterior, superior, or lateral and are classified by the position of the talus in relation to the tibial mortise.

Contraindications

- **Relative**
  - Open dislocations where there is no evidence of acute neurovascular compromise are better managed definitively in the operating room to avoid further contamination.

Materials and Medications

- Parenteral sedation and analgesia medications
- Local anaesthetic for local and intra-articular anaesthesia
- Splinting material
- Stockinette
- Padding
- Elastic bandage
- Tape
- Sheet

Procedure

- Check the neurovascular status of the affected foot and ankle.
- If there is no evidence of critical neurovascular compromise, obtain a lateral and an anteroposterior radiograph of the affected ankle.
- Ensure adequate parenteral sedation and analgesia to maximise success and limit pain and suffering.
- Position the patient on a stretcher with the knee flexed at 90° over a folded pillow or rolled-up sheet or with the lower leg and knee hanging over the edge of the stretcher.

1. Posterior dislocations

- Hold the heel in one hand and pull with longitudinal traction.
- With the other hand, hold the top of the foot and gently plantarflex it downward, while an assistant provides countertraction at the back of the midcalf.
- Continue longitudinal traction at the heel and countertraction at the calf.
- Dorsiflex the foot while another assistant applies downward pressure to the distal anterior leg.
- Examine the foot for restoration of normal anatomy and for any new lacerations or defects to the skin.
- Recheck neurovascular integrity.
- Place the leg in a sugar-tong splint with the foot at 90°.
- Recheck neurovascular integrity.

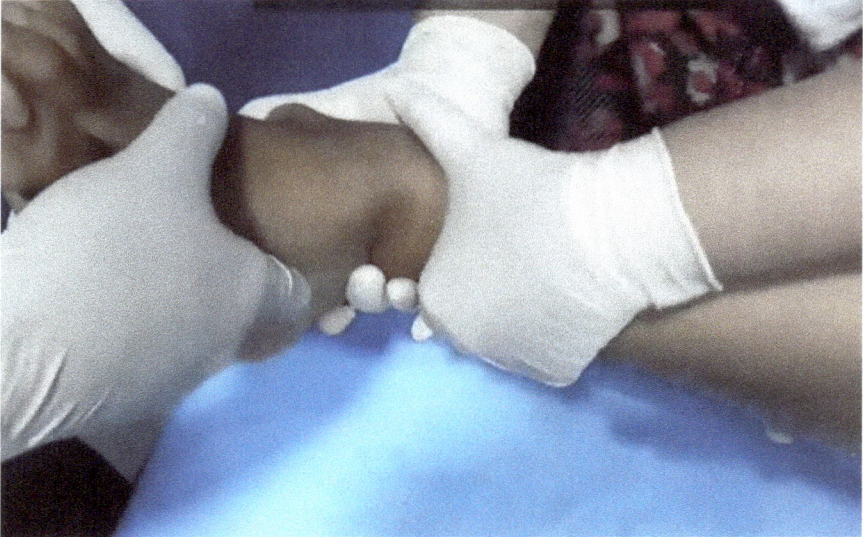

Fig.1.22.13. Reduction of ankle dislocation

2. Anterior dislocations

- Hold the heel in one hand and pull with longitudinal traction.
- With the other hand, hold the top of the foot and dorsiflex, while an assistant provides countertraction at the back of the midcalf.
- Continue longitudinal traction at the heel and countertraction at the calf.
- Keeping the foot at 90° to the leg, hold the foot firmly and push the foot downward toward the floor while another assistant applies upward pressure to the distal posterior leg.
- Examine the foot for restoration of normal anatomy and for any new lacerations or defects to the skin.
- Recheck neurovascular integrity.
- Place the leg in a sugar-tong splint with the foot at 90°.
- Recheck neurovascular integrity.

Post-procedure care

- Confirm the successful reduction by a restoration of a normal calcaneal contour and by decreased pain.

- Reassess neurovascular status. A post-procedure neurovascular deficit implies emergency orthopaedic evaluation.
- Apply a long leg posterior splint with 90° of foot dorsiflexion along with a stirrup splint to provide additional stability.
- Request control x-rays to ensure proper reduction and identify any initially hidden fractures.
- Elevate the limb elevated
- Recheck for any neurovascular deficits and development of compartment syndrome.
- Arrange orthopaedic follow-up.

Complications
- Compound fractures
- Neurovascular injury
- Skin and soft tissue damage
- Compartment syndrome

Further reading
Larry   Mellick   –   Ankle   fracture-dislocation   reduction: https://www.youtube.com/watch?v=peSuuAOXVaQ

References

Keany, J. E. (2016). *Ankle Dislocation in Emergency Medicine*. Medscape. Retrieved 17 Dec. 2021 from https://emedicine.medscape.com/article/823087-overview#a5

Thangarajah, T., Giotakis, N., & Matovu, E. (2008). Bilateral ankle dislocation without malleolar fracture. *J Foot Ankle Surg, 47*(5), 441-446. https://doi.org/10.1053/j.jfas.2008.05.004

| 23 |

Regional Nerve Block

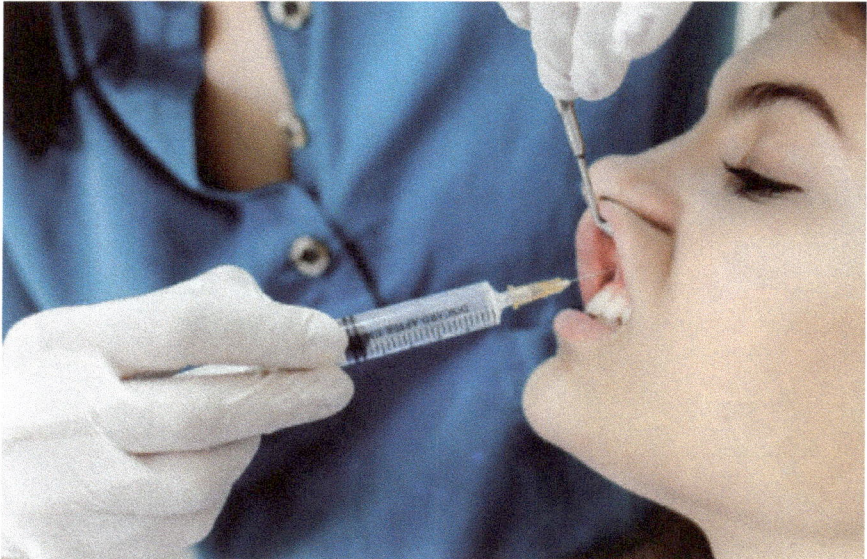

Overview

Systemic effects of local anaesthetic (LA) commonly occur because of a therapeutic error. Circumstances leading to toxicity include accidental venous or arterial injection and too high a dose of ingested or topically administered local anaesthetic-containing preparations. Lidocaine toxicity has been reported after subcutaneous administration, oral administration, and intravascular injection (Smith et al., 1992). Adding a vasoconstrictor (e.g., adrenaline) can decrease the systemic absorption of an anaesthetic, thus raising the maximum safe dosage.

For lidocaine, the maximum safe dose is 3 mg per kg of body weight; 7 mg/kg are needed if an adrenaline solution is used. There are few reports of local anaesthetic toxicity in infants and children. However, seizures, arrhythmias, cardiac arrest, and transient neuropathic symptoms have been reported (Gunter, 2002). The progression of lidocaine toxicity is directly proportional to the ascending serum levels, with initial benign symptoms developing at 5μg/ml, worsening into life-threatening cardiac arrest at levels above 25μg/ml. Therefore, symptoms such as tinnitus, light-headedness, circumoral numbness, diplopia and a metallic taste in the mouth suggest the onset of toxicity and possible impending development of severe symptoms. Cardiovascular toxicity is often revealed as tachycardia and hypertension; bradycardia and hypotension occur with increased toxicity. In addition, ventricular arrhythmias and cardiac arrest are well-documented side effects (Brown & Skiendzielewski, 1980).

Complications of Local Anaesthesia

- **Technique-related**
    - Direct nerve trauma
    - Bleeding
    - Haematoma
    - Infection
    - Intravascular injection
    - Damage to surrounding structures (tendons, pneumothorax)
- **Drug-related**
    - Anaphylactoid
    - Methaemoglobinuria (prilocaine)
    - Toxicity by intravascular injection
    - Toxicity by overdose and systemic absorption

Table 1.23.1. lignocaine toxicity according to the specific doses

Dose of lignocaine (mcg/ml)	Presenting symptoms
5	Light-headedness Circumoral paraesthesia Slurred speech Tinnitus
10	Convulsions Loss of consciousness
15	Coma Myocardial depression
20	Respiratory arrest Cardiac arrhythmia
25	Cardiac arrest

Emergency Management of severe LA toxicity

According to the Association of Anaesthetists of Great Britain and Ireland (AAGBI (AAGBI, 2010)), the emergency approach to local anaesthetics toxicity can be summarised as below:

- **Recognition of signs of severe toxicity:**
    - Sudden alteration in mental state, severe agitation, or loss of consciousness, with or without tonic-clonic convulsions
    - Cardiovascular collapse: sinus bradycardia, conduction blocks, asystole and ventricular tachyarrhythmias may occur
    - Local anaesthetic (LA) toxicity may occur sometime after an initial injection

- Consider the use of Intralipid in local-anaesthetic-induced cardiac arrest or circulatory failure that is unresponsive to standard therapy.

- **Immediate management**
  - Stop injecting the LA
  - Call for help
  - Maintain the airway and, if necessary, secure it with a tracheal tube
  - Give 100% oxygen and ensure adequate lung ventilation (hyperventilation may help by increasing plasma pH in the presence of metabolic acidosis)
  - Confirm or establish intravenous access
  - Control seizures: give a benzodiazepine, thiopental or propofol in small incremental doses
  - Consider drawing blood for analysis, but do not delay definitive treatment to do this

- **Treatment**
  - **In circulatory arrest**
    - Start cardiopulmonary resuscitation (CPR) using standard protocols
    - Manage arrhythmias using the same protocols, recognising that arrhythmias may be very refractory to treatment
    - Consider the use of cardiopulmonary bypass if available
    - Give intravenous lipid emulsion (see below)
    - Continue CPR throughout treatment with lipid emulsion
    - Recovery from LA-induced cardiac arrest may take >1 h
    - Propofol is not a suitable substitute for lipid emulsion

■ Lidocaine should not be used as an anti-arrhythmic therapy

○ **Without circulatory arrest**

■ Use conventional therapies to treat hypotension, bradycardia, tachyarrhythmia

■ Consider intravenous lipid emulsion (see below)

■ Propofol is not a suitable substitute for lipid emulsion

■ Lidocaine should not be used as an anti-arrhythmic therapy

Intralipid Emulsion

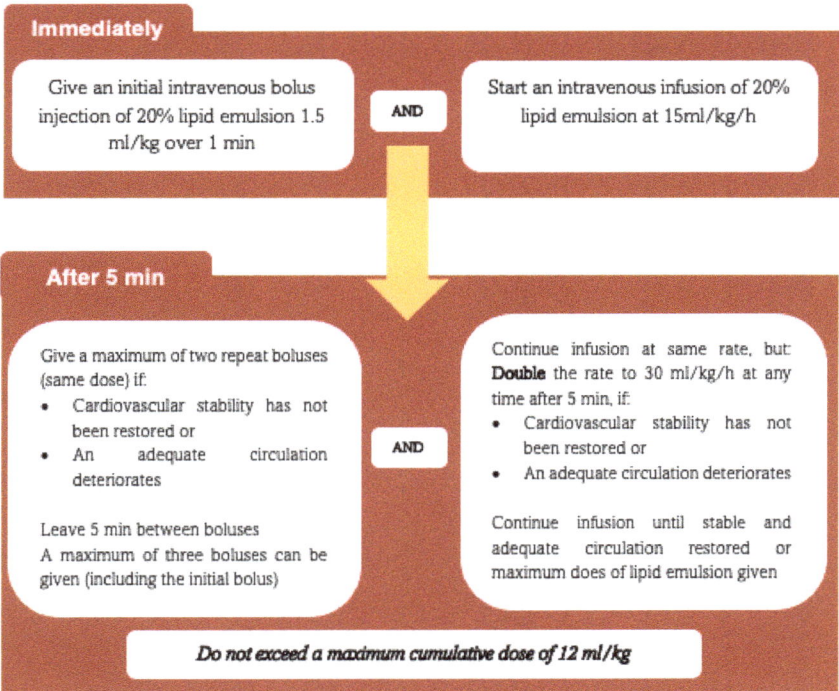

Immediately

Give an initial intravenous bolus injection of 20% lipid emulsion 1.5 ml/kg over 1 min

AND

Start an intravenous infusion of 20% lipid emulsion at 15ml/kg/h

After 5 min

Give a maximum of two repeat boluses (same dose) if:
• Cardiovascular stability has not been restored or
• An adequate circulation deteriorates

Leave 5 min between boluses
A maximum of three boluses can be given (including the initial bolus)

AND

Continue infusion at same rate, but: **Double** the rate to 30 ml/kg/h at any time after 5 min, if:
• Cardiovascular stability has not been restored or
• An adequate circulation deteriorates

Continue infusion until stable and adequate circulation restored or maximum does of lipid emulsion given

Do not exceed a maximum cumulative dose of 12 ml/kg

Fig.1.23.1. AAGBI Safety Guidelines Management of Severe Local Anaesthetic Toxicity
Credit - AAGBI, 2010

- **Follow-up**
  - Arrange safe transfer to a clinical area with appropriate equipment and suitable staff until sustained recovery is achieved
  - Exclude pancreatitis by regular clinical review, including daily amylase or lipase assays for two days
  - Report cases as follows: in the United Kingdom to the National Patient Safety Agency (via www.npsa.nhs.uk).
  - In the Republic of Ireland to the Irish Medicines Board (via www.imb.ie).
  - If Lipid has been given, please also report its use to the international registry at www.lipidregistry.org.

2. Supratrochlear Nerve Block

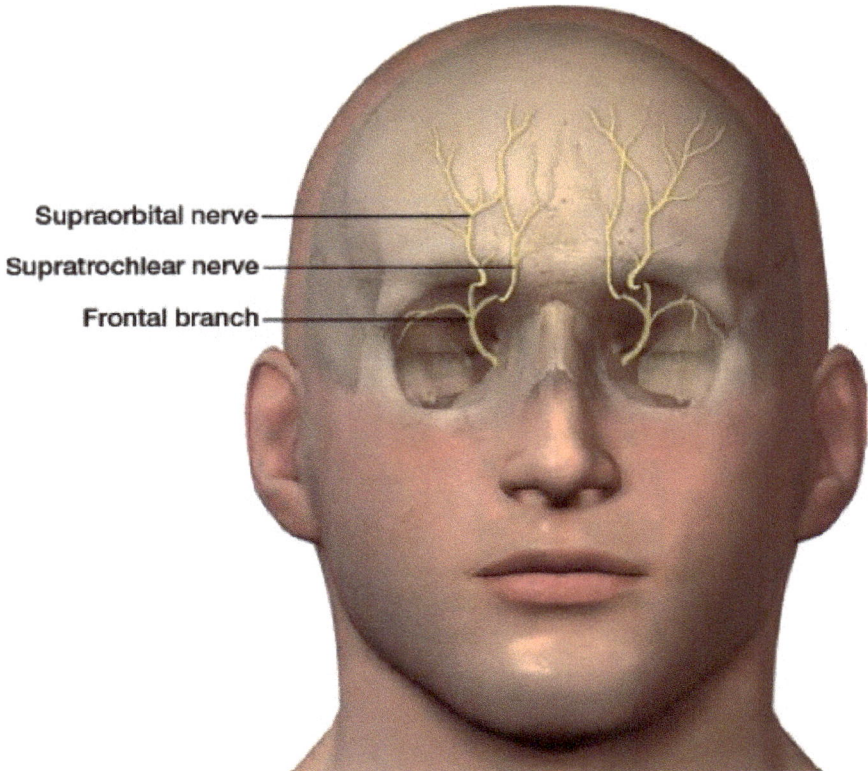

Supraorbital nerve

Supratrochlear nerve

Frontal branch

Overview

The supratrochlear nerve also is a branch of the ophthalmic division of the trigeminal nerve and exits through the superior medial aspect of the orbit. A regional block allows for minimal anaesthetic use, which permits the operator to obtain the intended anaesthesia over a larger surface area than local infiltration (Napier et al., 2021). This section will provide you with the essentials of supratrochlear nerve block in the emergency department.

Objectives

- By the end of this module, you should be able to:

○ Describe the indications and contraindications for a supratrochlear nerve block.
○ Identify the common complications associated with a supratrochlear nerve block.
○ Explain step by step how to perform this procedure

Indications

- Relief from neuropathy (Macario, 2021).
- Analgesia for wound closure or debridement
- Analgesia for local excision or biopsy

Contraindications

- Patient refusal or inability to obtain consent
- Allergy to available local anaesthetics
- The inability of the patient to cooperate with or tolerate the procedure
- Infection at the injection site
- Distortion of surface or bony anatomy

Procedure

- Inject local anaesthetic solution over the midline of the forehead at eyebrow level.
- Inject a 25- or 27-gauge needle through skin wheal aimed laterally while injecting 3–5 mL local anaesthetic subcutaneously.
- Stop infiltrating when the needle reaches the midline of the orbit.

3. Supraorbital Nerve Block

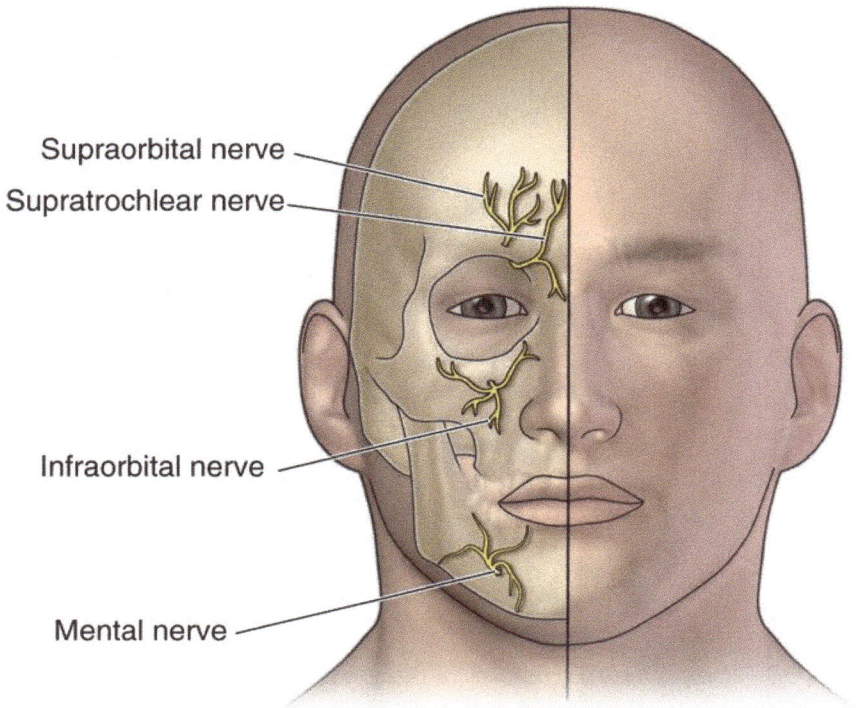

Supraorbital nerve

Supratrochlear nerve

Infraorbital nerve

Mental nerve

Overview

The supraorbital nerve emerges from the supraorbital foramen/ notch and is a branch of the ophthalmic division of the trigeminal nerve. The supraorbital nerve block procedure is indicated for immediate localised anaesthesia for injuries such as complex lacerations to the forehead, upper eyelid laceration repair, debridement of abrasions or burns to the forehead, removal of foreign bodies from the forehead, or pain relief from acute herpes zoster. A regional block allows for minimal anaesthetic use, which permits the operator to obtain the intended anaesthesia over a larger surface area than local infiltration (Napier et al., 2021). This section will provide you with the essentials of supraorbital nerve block in the emergency department.

Objectives

- By the end of this module, you should be able to:
  - Describe the indications and contraindications for a supra-orbital nerve block.
  - Identify the common complications associated with a supraorbital nerve block.
  - Explain step by step how to perform this procedure

Indications

- Wound closure (Byrne, 2019)
- Pain relief
- Anaesthesia for debridement

Contraindications

- Any allergy or sensitivity to the anaesthetic agent
- Evidence of infection at the injection site
- Distortion of anatomical landmarks
- Uncooperative patient

Anaesthesia

- A supraorbital nerve block requires 1-3 mL of the chosen anaesthetic agent.
- Lidocaine (Xylocaine) is the most used agent.
  - The onset of action for lidocaine is approximately 4-6 minutes.
  - The duration of effect is approximately 75
- Bupivacaine (Marcaine) is another frequently used anaesthetic agent.
  - The onset of action of bupivacaine is slower than that of lidocaine.
  - The duration of anaesthesia of bupivacaine is about 4-8 times longer than that of lidocaine.
- The dose of anaesthetic used in typical volumes for this procedure is not toxic.

4. Infraorbital Nerve Block

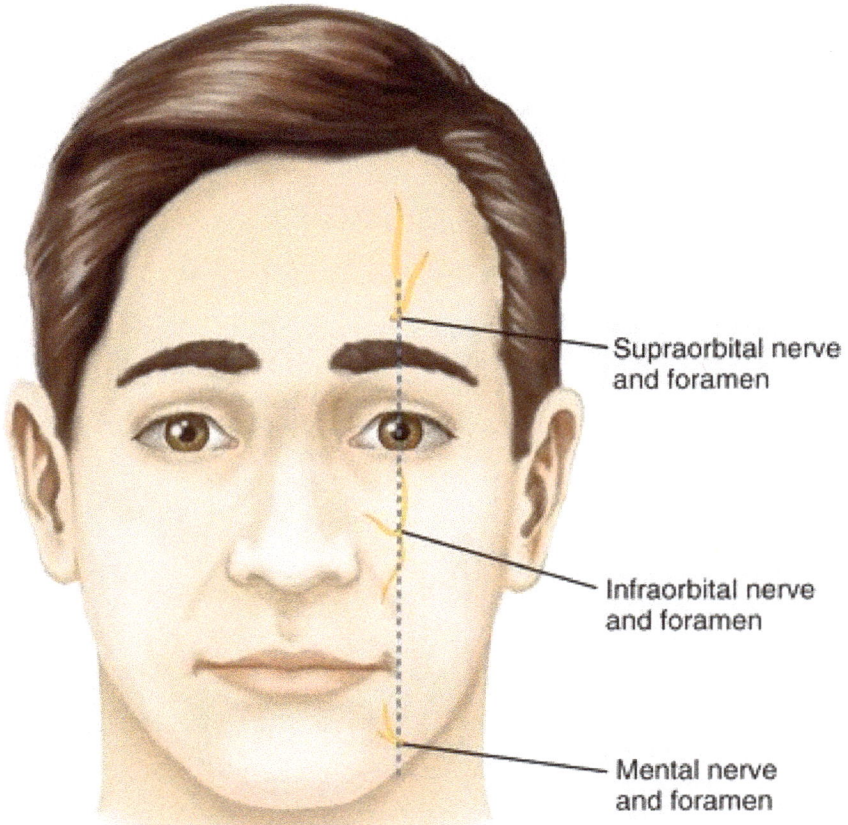

Supraorbital nerve and foramen

Infraorbital nerve and foramen

Mental nerve and foramen

Overview

The infraorbital nerve emerges from the infraorbital foramen and is a branch of the maxillary division of the trigeminal nerve. Anaesthesia to the infraorbital nerve will also provide anaesthesia to its terminus, the superior alveolar nerves. A regional block allows for minimal anaesthetic use, which permits the operator to obtain the intended anaesthesia over a larger surface area than local infiltration (Napier et al., 2021). This section will provide you with the essentials of infraorbital nerve block in the emergency department.

Objectives

- By the end of this module, you should be able to:
  - Describe the indications and contraindications for an infraorbital nerve block.
  - Identify the common complications associated with an infraorbital nerve block.
  - Explain step by step how to perform this procedure

Indications

- Wound closure
- Pain relief
- Anaesthesia for debridement
- Contraindication to general anaesthesia

Contraindications

- Any allergy or sensitivity to the anaesthetic agent (Byrne, 2019)
- Evidence of infection at the injection site
- Distortion of anatomical landmarks
- Uncooperative patient

Procedure

- **Extraoral Approach**
  - Palpate the inferior orbital foramen in its midline position.
  - The infraorbital nerve is often tender on palpation as it exits the foramen.
  - Inject a 25- or 27-gauge needle just above the infraorbital foramen injecting 1–2 mL of local anaesthetic.
  - Take care not to inject into the foramen because there is an increased risk of intraneural injection.
  - Hold a finger on the inferior orbital rim to avoid ballooning of the lower eyelid with injection.
  - The intraoral approach is possible and preferred because it is less painful.

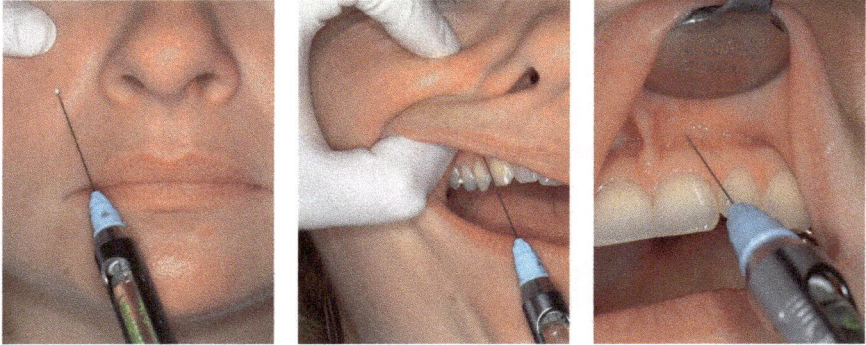

Fig.1.23.2. Infraorbital nerve block extra and intraoral approaches
Credit - Pocket Dentistry

- **Intraoral Approach**
    - Apply topical benzocaine or lidocaine gel to the point of insertion, which is the height of the mucobuccal fold over the first premolar, which is the site of insertion.
    - Wipe off after 1–3 min.
    - Palpate with the finger of the non injecting hand over the inferior border of the inferior orbital rim.
    - Retract the lip with the non injecting hand.
    - Using a long 25- to 27-gauge needle, with the bevel toward the bone, advance the needle at the insertion site toward the infraorbital foramen.
    - Once the target is reached, aspirate and inject 1 mL of local anaesthetic.
    - Exert pressure on the foramen for 1 min after injection to force the anaesthetic through the infraorbital foramen.
    - If the needle is difficult to advance and the patient experiences pain on insertion, redirect the needle laterally and advance.
    - If analgesia is attained for the lip but not the eyelid, the analgesia was placed inferior to the foramen, and if analgesia is attained for the eyelid but not the lip, placement was superior to the foramen.

5. Mental Nerve Block

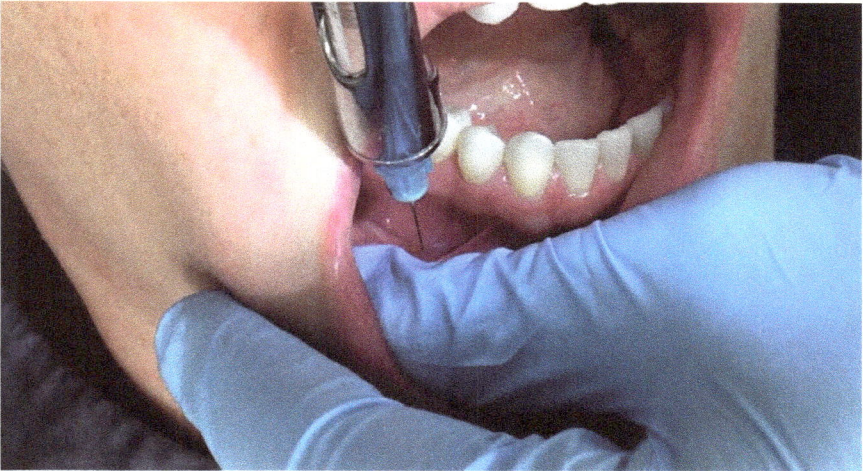

Overview

The mental nerve arises from the mental foramen and is a branch of the mandibular division of the trigeminal nerve. It lies in the vertical plane with the midpoint of the pupil and sits in the middle of the body of the mandible. A nerve block of the mental nerve anaesthetises the ipsilateral lower lip and skin of the chin and the lateral (buccal) gingiva and mucosa anterior to the mental foramen up to the midline. In addition, a regional block allows for minimal anaesthetic use, which permits the operator to obtain the intended anaesthesia over a larger surface area than local infiltration (Napier et al., 2021). This section will provide you with the essentials of mental nerve block in the emergency department.

Objectives

- By the end of this module, you should be able to:
  - Describe the indications and contraindications for a mental nerve block.

○ Identify the common complications associated with a mental nerve block.

○ Explain step by step how to perform this procedure

Indications

- Lacerations of the lower lip, especially if the vermillion border is involved (Fishman, 2019)
- Lacerations to the soft tissue of the chin that extends from the lip anteriorly to the alveolar process and caudally to the mid-body of the mandible
- Surgical removal of facial tumours/lesions
- Relief from post-herpetic neuralgia

Contraindications

- Noncooperative patient
- Overlying infection
- Allergic reaction to local anaesthetic
- Patient refusal
- Distorted anatomy

Procedure: extraoral approach

- Inject local anaesthetic solution over the identified location of the mental foramen, creating a skin wheal.
- Advance a 25- or 27-gauge needle through the skin wheal until the mandible is contacted, injecting 1–2 mL of local anaesthetic.
- The intraoral approach is possible and preferred because it is less painful.

Procedure: Intraoral Approach

- Apply topical benzocaine or lidocaine gel to the point of insertion, which is the mucobuccal fold between the apices of the first and the second premolars.
- Wipe off after 1–3 min.

- Insert a 25- to 27-gauge needle, with the bevel toward the mandible, aimed toward the mental foramen.
- After advancing one-third the depth of the mandible and contacting the mandible, inject 1–2 mL of local anaesthetic.
- By pressing firmly on the mental foramen for 2–3 min after the mental foramen has been blocked, an incisive nerve block is also created.
- This is useful if anaesthesia to the lower anterior teeth is also desired.

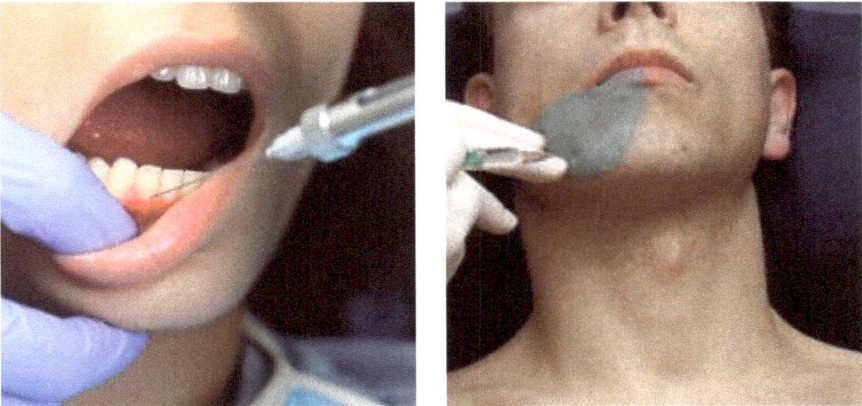

Fig.1.23.3. Mental nerve block intraoral and extraoral approaches

6. External ear nerve block

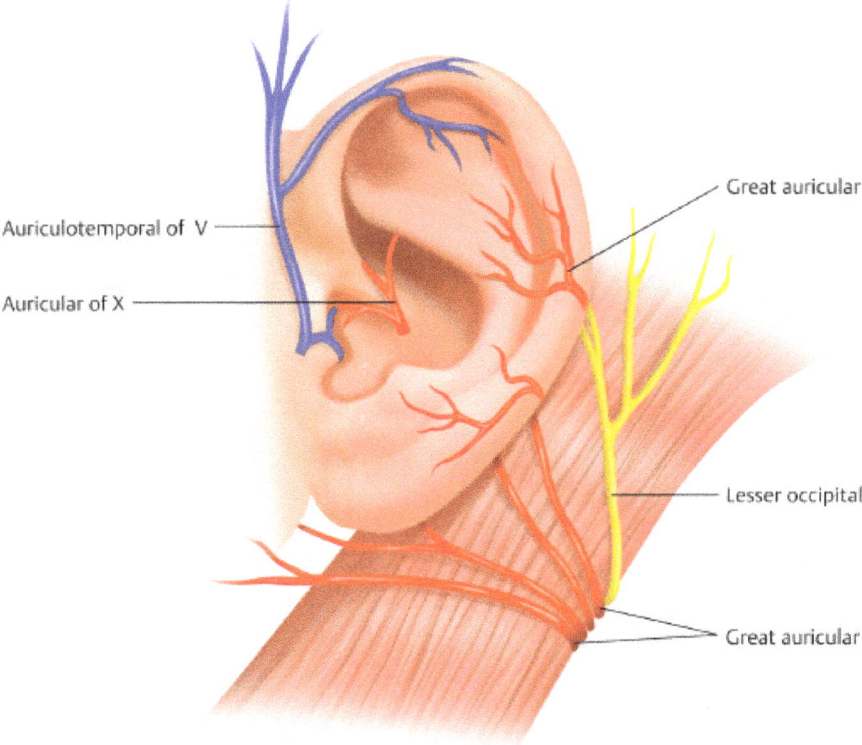

Auriculotemporal of V

Auricular of X

Great auricular

Lesser occipital

Great auricular

Overview

Patients often present to the emergency department (ED) with different ear complaints ranging from trauma (lacerations and avulsions), auricular collections requiring incision and drainage (hematomas and abscesses) and entrenched foreign bodies (earrings and earring backings) (Kravchik et al., 2021). Anaesthesia of the ear is helpful for the repair of lacerations, hematoma incision and drainage, and other painful procedures of the ear (Hutchens, 2018). Auricular block anaesthetises four nerves that innervate the auricle: lesser occipital nerve, greater auricular nerve, the auricular branch of the vagus nerve and auriculotemporal nerve. A regional block allows for minimal anaesthetic use, which permits the operator to obtain the intended anaesthesia over a larger surface area than local infiltration (Napier et al., 2021). This section will provide the reader with the essentials of auricular nerve block in the emergency department.

Objectives
- By the end of this module, you should be able to:
    - Describe the indications and contraindications for an auricular nerve block.
    - Identify the common complications associated with an auricular nerve block.
    - Explain step by step how to perform this procedure

Indications
- In the emergency department, a nerve block of the external ear is most suitable for, but not limited to the following situations (Jeon & Kim, 2017):
    - Analgesia to allow for a more thorough exam and repair of the external ear in trauma
    - Patients with contraindications to general anaesthesia and procedural sedation
    - Incision and drainage, followed by packing of an auricular hematoma
    - Incision and drainage of abscesses and cysts
    - Laceration repair
    - Foreign body removal
    - Red ear syndrome
    - Great auricular neuralgia

Contraindications
- Known anaesthetic agent allergy
- Uncooperative patient

- Cellulitis or erythema overlying the injection site (relative contraindication due to the theoretical risk of spreading the infection)
- Coagulopathy

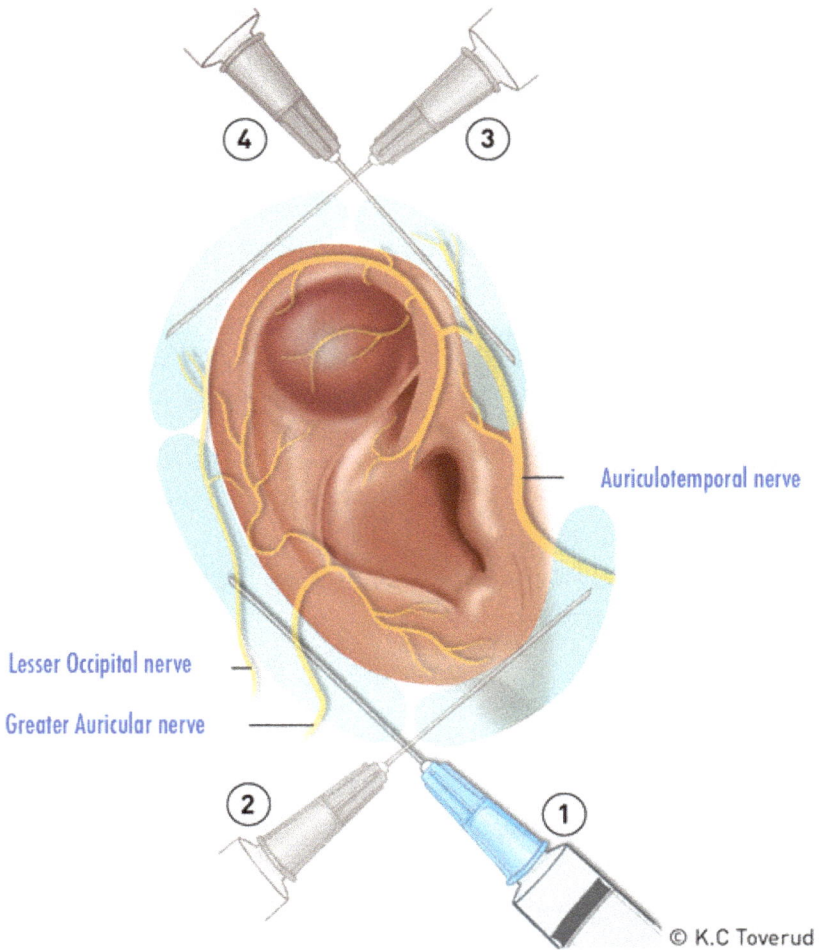

Fig.1.23.4. Auricular nerve block approach

Equipment

- Sterile gloves
- Surgical mask with eye protection/goggles

- Local anaesthetic agent: 0.5% bupivacaine or 1% lidocaine with or without epinephrine
- 25 or 27 gauge 1.5-inch needle and 10 mL syringe
- Chlorhexidine 2%
- Sterile 4 x 4 gauze

Procedure

- Using a 25- to 27-gauge needle, insert the needle just inferior to the earlobe directing it toward the tragus.
- Aspirate and advance the needle superiorly subcutaneously injecting 3–4 mL of local anaesthetic.
- Withdraw the needle without fully removing it and redirect it postero-superiorly along the inferior posterior auricular sulcus, aspirating and injecting as before.
- Remove the needle and insert it just superior to the point of helix insertion into the scalp.
- Advance the needle and aspirate and inject in the direction of the tragus.
- Inject into the subcutaneous tissue while avoiding the ear cartilage.
- Withdraw and redirect the needle posteriorly and inferiorly toward the skin behind the ear, injecting as before.
- Beware of inadvertent cannulation of the superficial temporal artery, which crosses the zygomatic arch and crosses medial to the ear.
- If the artery is violated, it requires 20–30 min application of firm pressure.

7. Wrist & Hand Nerve Blocks

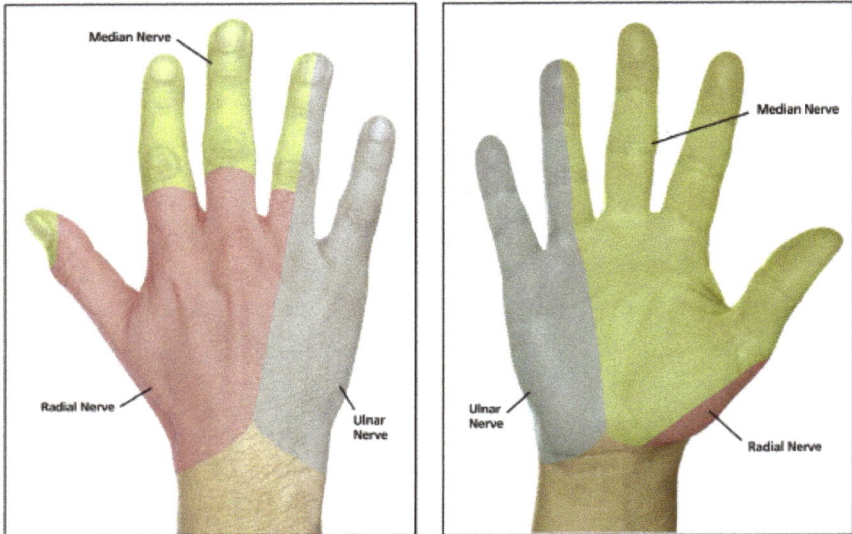

Overview

A wrist block is a procedure of blocking terminal branches of some or all the six nerves that supply the wrist, hand, and fingers. Wrist or elbow blocks may deliver adequate anaesthesia for minor hand interventions; hence, sparing the patient the complications of general anaesthesia and delivering excellent postoperative analgesia with less need for opioid analgesics (Brown, 2002). Digital Nerve Blocks (Ring, Web Space & Tendon Sheath) are indicated to anaesthetise the digits in preparation for laceration repair, nail bed repair, joint reduction, or pain relief.

Objectives

- By the end of this module, you should be able to:
  - Describe the indications and contraindications for hand nerve block.

- ○ Identify the common complications associated with a wrist nerve block.
- ○ Explain step by step how to perform this procedure

Indications

- To anaesthetise the hand in preparation for laceration repair, fracture or dislocation reduction, or pain relief.

Procedure

Median Nerve Block

- Advance the needle at 45° to the skin towards the wrist (McCahon & Bedforth, 2007).
- The median nerve runs 1–1.5 cm deep; 3–5 ml of LA is injected.
- Paraesthesia of the thumb or index finger warrants withdrawal of the needle by 1–2 mm.
- To block the palmar cutaneous branch of the median nerve, the needle is advanced subcutaneously towards the flexor retinaculum and a further 3–5 ml of LA is injected as the needle is withdrawn.
- Note that in patients with carpal tunnel syndrome, a block of the median nerve at the wrist could cause pressure-induced neuropraxia in the tight carpal tunnel.

Radial Nerve Block

- At the wrist, the radial nerve is separated into numerous terminal branches.
- LA is injected subcutaneously between the radial styloid and the midpoint of the dorsum of the wrist.
- This should be confluent with the LA infiltration of the dorsal cutaneous branch of the ulnar nerve (McCahon & Bedforth, 2007).

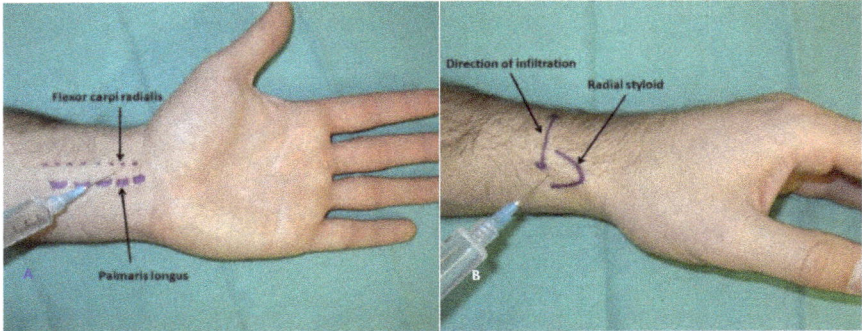

Fig.1.23.5. (A) Median nerve block and (B) Radial nerve block

Ulnar Nerve Block

- To block the ulnar nerve, the same needle can be advanced beneath the tendon of FCU towards the radial border of the forearm, to a depth of 1–1.5 cm.
- The needle is redirected subcutaneously around the ulnar aspect of the wrist to block the dorsal cutaneous branch of the ulnar nerve.
- This medial approach to the ulnar nerve reduces the risk of intra-arterial needle placement.
- The alternative is to make an anterior approach, medial to the ulnar artery and lateral to the tendon of FCU.
- This approach may require a second injection around the ulnar border of the wrist. Using either method, 3–5 ml of LA is injected at each site (McCahon & Bedforth, 2007)

Ring Block

- Insert a 25-gauge needle on the dorsal surface of the proximal phalanx of the digit to be anaesthetised. Inject 1 mL along the dorsal surface and withdraw the needle.
- Reinsert the needle again perpendicular to the last injection and run on the lateral surface of the phalanx.
- Inject 1–1.5 mL of a local anaesthetic to just past the phalanx base

- Repeat the injection in the same fashion on the medial aspect of the phalanx.
- Do not inject more than 5 mL into a digit.
- Toe blocks are like finger ring blocks, except that the great toe requires plantar surface injection as well, owing to its unique nerve supply.

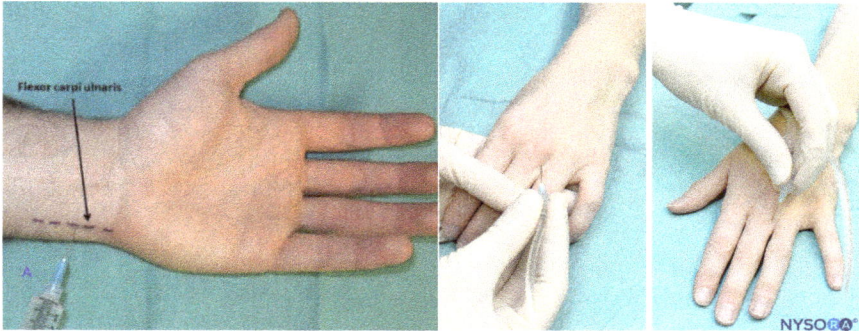

Fig.1.23.6. (A) Ulnar nerve block and (B) Digital Ring block
Credit - Nysora

Web Space Digital Block

- Have the patient abduct the fingers.
- Palpate the metacarpophalangeal joint and then insert a 25- to 27-gauge needle into the lateral webspace subcutaneously, directing it dorsally.
- Aspirate then inject 1 mL of local anaesthetic. Withdraw the needle but before the exiting skin, redirect toward the palmar aspect until the tip is next to the metacarpophalangeal joint, and inject 1 mL of local anaesthetic.
- Repeat the procedure on the medial webspace of the digit.
- Each digit blocked requires injection on both the lateral and the medial web spaces.

Intrathecal Digital Block: Flexor Tendon Sheath Procedure

- Inject anaesthetic directly into the flexor tendon sheath.
- Palpate on the palmar surface over and proximal to the metacarpophalangeal joint.
- Gentle flexion of digits may better reveal the sheath.
- Have the patient abduct the fingers.
- Insert a 25-gauge needle at a 45° angle to the skin and along the long axis of the digit directly into the flexor tendon sheath at the level of the distal skin crease.
- Inject 2 mL of local anaesthetic.
- The anaesthetic should flow freely if it is in the sheath.
- If it does not, it is likely in the tendon and should be withdrawn slightly.
- Contraindications to intrathecal block are local infection and pre-existing flexor tendon injury.
- Risk of tenosynovitis; sterilize the skin before introducing the needle.
- If laceration has involved the tendon, an anaesthetic may leak from the wound.

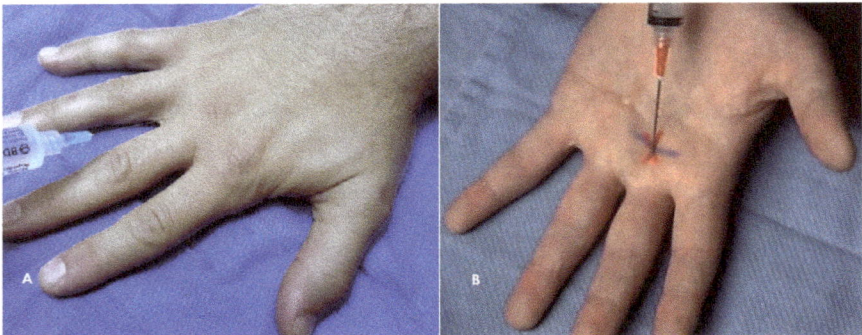

Fig.1.23.7. (A) Webspace digital nerve block and (B) Intrathecal nerve block

8. Intercostal Nerve Block

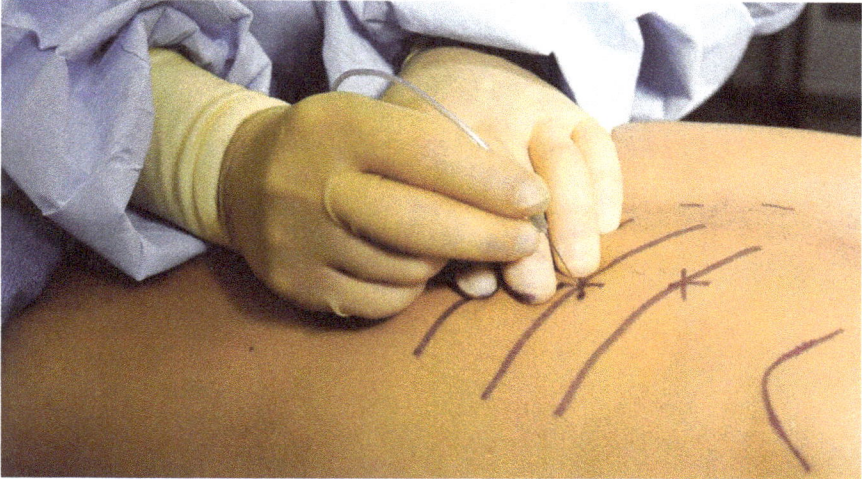

Overview

The intercostal nerves supply significant parts of the skin and musculature of the chest and abdominal wall (Ho et al., 2021). Intercostal nerve blocks are indicated to manage pain in the chest wall and upper abdomen. In addition, a regional block allows for minimal anaesthetic use, which permits the operator to obtain the intended anaesthesia over a larger surface area than local infiltration (Napier et al., 2021). This section will provide you with the essentials of intercostal nerve block in the emergency department.

Objectives

- By the end of this module, you should be able to:
    - Describe the indications and contraindications for an intercostal nerve block.
    - Identify the common complications associated with an intercostal nerve block.
    - Explain step by step how to perform this procedure

Indications

- Thoracic or upper abdominal surgery
- Rib fractures (Hwang & Lee, 2014)
- Breast surgery
- Incisional pain from thoracic surgery
- Analgesia for thoracostomy
- Herpes zoster or post-herpetic neuralgia
- Differentiating between visceral and somatic pain

Contraindications

- **Absolute:**
  - Local infection
  - Patient refusal
- **Relative**
  - Coagulation disorder
  - Patient on anticoagulants
  - Lack of skills
  - Lack of resuscitating equipment

Equipment

- Catheter placement: 18- to 20-gauge Tuohy needle (adults)
- Local anaesthetic
- Sterile gloves
- Syringe and needle for local infiltration
- Needle: Single shot: 20- to 22-gauge 4- to 5-cm needle (adults)
- Ultrasound machine
- Marking pen
- ECG monitor and Blood pressure monitor
- Pulse oximetry

Procedure

- An intravenous line should be ready, and resuscitation drugs should be readily available.
- Clean the skin with an antiseptic,

- Inject 1 to 2 mL of local anaesthetic, the fingers of the palpating hand should be utilised to lift the skin up so that the needle will contact the middle of the rib to be blocked.
- As the skin is fixed with the palpating hand, the needle is positioned through the skin wheal at an approximately 20-degree angle cephalad until it makes contact with the rib, which should be made within 1cm.
- The palpating hand then allows the skin to return to its normal position as the needle is "walked-off," the inferior border of the rib.
- Progress the needle further approximately 1 to 3 mm anteriorly, where a subtle "pop" may be appreciated as the needle advances through the fascia of the internal intercostal muscle.
- After negative aspiration, 3 to 5 mL of local anaesthetic can be injected (Bhatia et al., 2013).

Complications
- Pneumothorax
- Tension pneumothorax and the subsequent need for tube thoracostomy (rare).
- Penetration of the peritoneum and abdominal viscera

9. Femoral Nerve Block & Fascia Iliaca Compartment Block

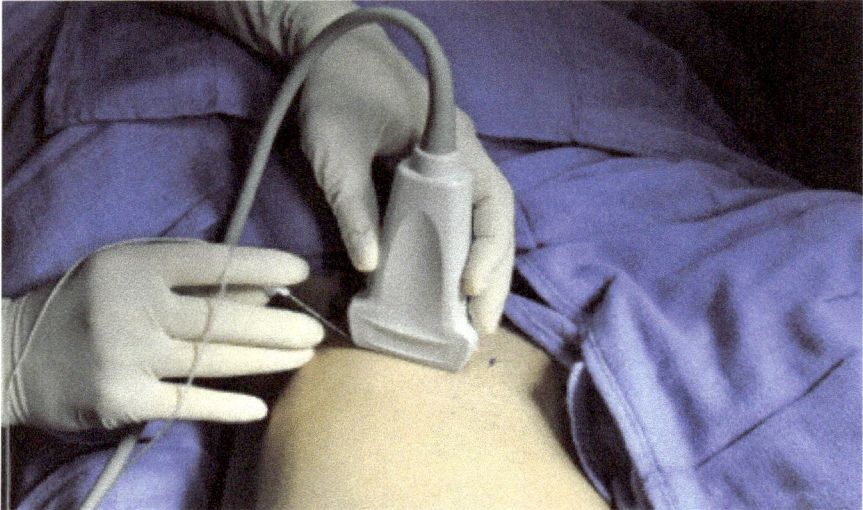

Overview

The femoral nerve originates from the lumbar plexus, consisting of branches from L2 to L4. It provides motor innervation to the extensors of the knee (Quadriceps Femoris and Sartorius), sensory innervation to the anterior thigh, anteromedial aspect of the knee, medial lower leg and the medial aspect of the ankle and foot (via its terminal sensory branch, the saphenous nerve) and supplies the periosteum of the femur. Historically, the femoral nerve block technique was called the "3 in 1 block" because it was thought a single injection could block the femoral, lateral femoral cutaneous and obturator nerves. The femoral nerve block is recommended to be performed under ultrasound guidance with secured IV access and complete cardiac monitoring. There is a low but definite risk of local anaesthetic toxicity, and the maximum recommended dose of Bupivacaine is 2 mg/kg (= 0.4 ml/kg of 0.5% bupivacaine). A mixture of lignocaine and Bupivacaine is often used with a maximum dose of 2mg/kg in total.

Currently, Fascia Iliaca Compartment Block (FICB) is preferred over the Femoral Nerve Block (FNB) by Emergency Departments (ED) as it carries a lower risk of intraneural and intravascular injection and blocks the lateral cutaneous nerve of the thigh. The FICB may be thought of as an anterior approach to the lumbar plexus where local anaesthetic (LA) is infiltrated proximally beneath the fascia iliaca, aiming the blockage of the femoral nerve (FN), obturator nerve (ON), and lateral cutaneous nerve of the thigh (LCNT) simultaneously. Unlike the FN block, the needle is not directed to lie adjacent to the FN, thus lessening the risk of neuropraxia. The FICB provides a safe and relatively simple alternative to femoral and lumbar plexus blocks (O'Reilly et al., 2019). In addition, a regional block allows for minimal anaesthetic use, which permits the operator to obtain the intended anaesthesia over a larger surface area versus that of local infiltration (Napier et al., 2021). This section will provide you with the essentials of the emergency department of femoral and fascia iliaca nerve blocks.

A. Femoral Nerve Block

Indications
- The femoral nerve block (FNB) is indicated for surgery on the anterior aspect of the thigh.
- It may also be combined with a sciatic nerve block to provide complete lower extremity coverage below the knee, and additionally with an obturator block to provide complete lower extremity anaesthesia.
- Both single injection and continuous infusions provide pain relief following total knee replacement (Ilfeld et al., 2008).
- A femoral nerve block is also useful for analgesia in femoral neck fractures, femur fractures, and patellar injuries.
- A femoral nerve block may be utilised alone or as part of a multimodal pain management plan (Chan et al., 2014).

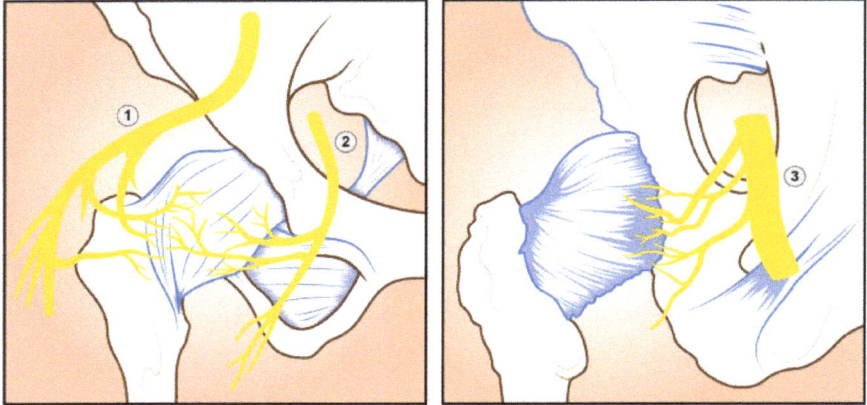

Fig.1.23.8. Innervation of the hip. Anterior portion of the joint capsule: (1) branch of the femoral nerve (L1–L4) along with the iliopsoas muscle. Anteromedial portion: (2) a branch of the obturator nerve (L1–L4). Posterior portion: (3) branches of the sciatic nerve *(O'Reilly et al., 2019)*

Contraindications

- **Absolute:**
  - ○ Patient refusal
  - ○ Inability to cooperate,
  - ○ Severe allergy to local anaesthetic agents.
- **Relative:**
  - ○ Current infection at the site of local injection
  - ○ Patients on anticoagulation and antithrombotic medications
  - ○ Patients with bleeding disorders.

The Emergency Physician should discuss the possibility of further nerve damage in patients with pre-existing nerve damage or those who may be susceptible to nerve injury (such as severe diabetes, trauma to nerves, etc.) (Kasibhatla & Russon, 2009).

Landmarks & Surrounding Structures

- *Important landmarks include the femoral crease, ASIS, pubic tubercle, femoral artery (palpable) and veins (not palpable), both located medially.*
  - A line is drawn from the ASIS to the pubic tubercle, in order to outline the inguinal ligament.
  - The femoral artery is marked.
  - A 4 cm 22 ga. needle is inserted just lateral to the femoral artery.
  - The femoral nerve is often found within a triangular hyperechoic region, lateral to the femoral artery and superficial to the iliopsoas muscle.

B. Fascia Iliaca Compartment Block

This section is based on the 2020 Royal College of Emergency Medicine (RCEM) guideline published on Fascia Iliaca block (RCEM, 2020):

Indications

- The aim is to reduce the requirement for systemic analgesics such as opioids and non-steroidal anti-inflammatories, along with their side effects.
- This is particularly important in elderly patients, who form by far the largest group admitted with the neck of femur fractures.
- Pre-operative analgesia for patients with neck of the femur or femoral shaft fractures
- Analgesia for the application of plaster in children with femoral fractures (the following discussion with a senior clinician).

Contraindications

- The patient refuses procedure/unable to comply with the procedure
- Allergy or intolerance to local anaesthetic

- Coagulopathy (anticoagulants, INR>1.5, platelets< 100)
- Infection at the injection site
- Patient unable to report possible analgesia complications/side-effects due to e.g. confusion/dementia/learning difficulties
- Inability to identify landmarks
- Previous femoral vascular surgery

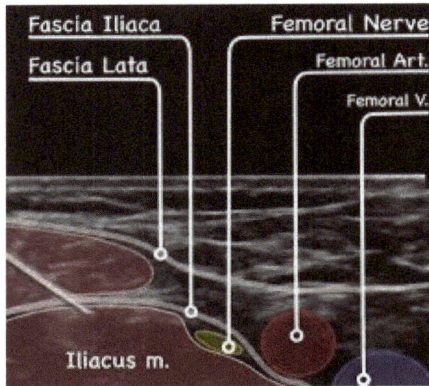

Fig.1.23.9. Ultrasound anatomy of the femoral nerve
Credit - Embeds.co.uk

General preparation

- Obtain consent
- Position patient supine
- This is a sterile procedure
- Prepare equipment, and drugs (0.5ml/kg (ideal bodyweight) of 0.25% Bupivacaine drawn up in anaesthetic 20ml syringes) -1ml of 0.25% Bupivacaine contains 2.5mg
- Ensure you do not exceed the maximum safe dose of **2mg per kg**
- Complete proforma
- If no pain relief after 30 minutes offer alternate analgesia
- Do not repeat block

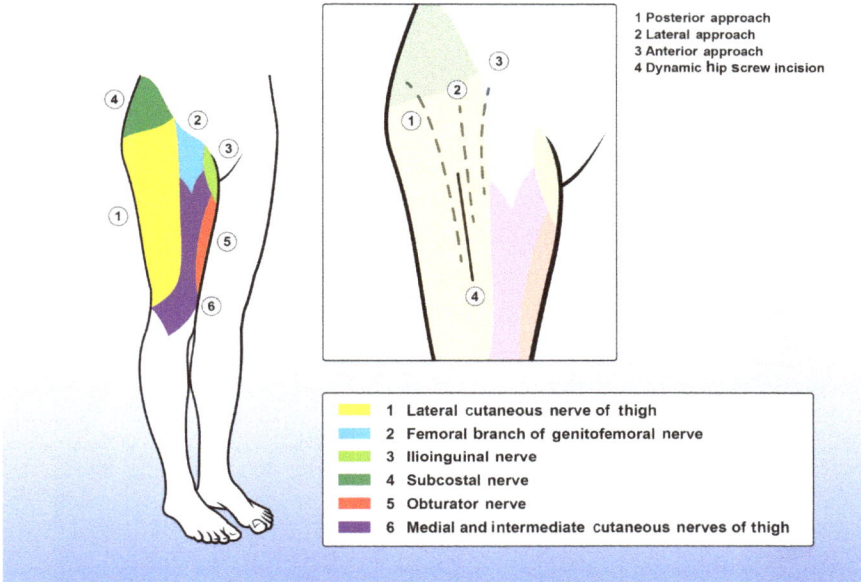

Fig.1.23.10. Cutaneous innervation of the hip and relation to surgical incision sites for (1) THR posterior approach, (2) THR lateral approach, (3) THR anterior approach, (4) dynamic hip screw incision. Note that the posterior incision extends beyond the territory of the lateral cutaneous nerve of the thigh to the subcostal territory and may also involve the lateral cutaneous branch of the iliohypogastric nerve (origin L1) not shown here. THR, total hip replacement
(O'Reilly et al., 2019)

Landmark Procedure

- The landmarks for the procedure are the anterior superior iliac spine (ASIS) and the ipsilateral pubic tubercle.
- Ensure patient has iv access, and that resuscitation equipment is nearby (RCEM, 2020)
- Ensure that patient is monitored (3L ECG, NIBP, SpO2, RR, GCS)
- Find line joining anterior superior iliac spine and pubic tubercle (line of the inguinal ligament).
- Find and mark junction where lateral 1/3 and medial 2/3 meet and move inferiorly 1cm from this point. This is to be the point of injection.
- Palpate to ensure you are not close to the femoral artery.

- If you are, recheck landmarks and if still over the artery abandon procedure.
- Chlorhexidine/Betadine skin prep, sterile gloves, drape the area.
- Raise a small bleb of Lignocaine at the intended skin puncture site.
- Pierce the skin with a large gauge needle.
- Change to a blunt-ended needle (BD Integra™ - Blunt Fill Needle 18G) connected via a short extension tube to your syringe of local anaesthetic (LA).
- Advance the needle (aspirating intermittently) perpendicular to the skin and feel for two "pops" indicating you have crossed the fascia lata followed by the fascia iliaca.
- Aspirate again and slowly inject the LA whilst asking the patient how they feel throughout, being vigilant for signs of LA toxicity or accidental injection into a nerve (severe pain/paraesthesia). Stop injecting if adverse effects occur.
- After injection, withdraw the needle and apply 30secs of pressure distal to the injection site to direct the local anaesthetic proximally.
- Dress the injection.

Complications
- Intravascular injection
- Local anaesthetic toxicity
- Temporary or permanent nerve damage
- Infection
- Block failure
- Injury secondary to numbness/weakness of
- Allergy to any of the preparations used

10. Bier's Block

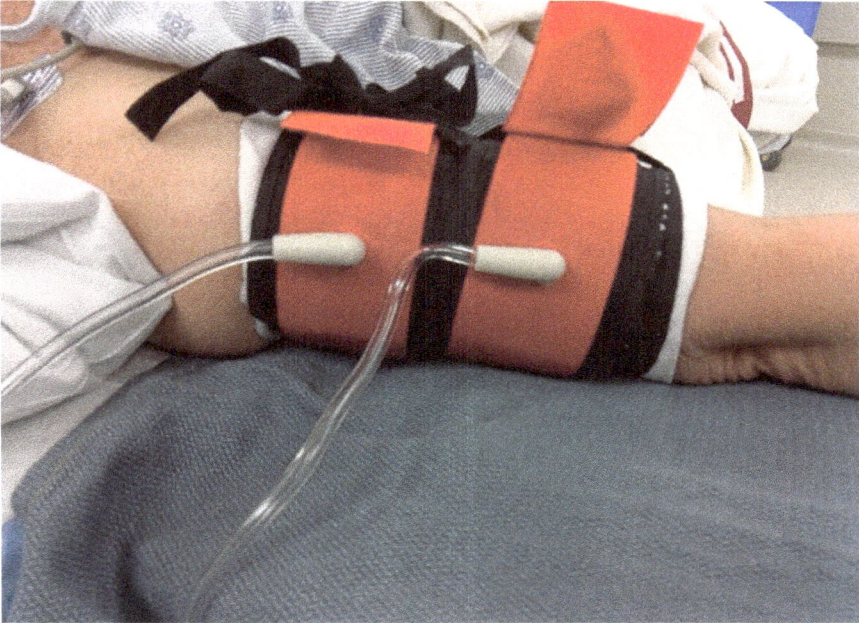

Overview

Fractures of the distal forearm are very common to our Emergency Departments. From the age of 35 and above, they hold a prevalence of 9/10,000 in men and 37/10,000 in women (McGlone, 2017). Compared to the haematoma block, Bier's block has more efficacy, offers better radiological results, and leads to less re-manipulation. Bier's block is the anaesthetic management of choice for Colles' fractures requiring manipulation within the A&E department (Kendall et al., 1997). A regional block allows for minimal anaesthetic use, which permits the operator to obtain the intended anaesthesia over a larger surface area than local infiltration (Napier et al., 2021). This section will provide you with the essentials of Bier's block in the emergency department.

Objectives

- By the end of this module, you should be able to:
  - Describe the indications and contraindications for Bier's block.
  - Identify the common complications associated with Bier's block.
  - Explain step by step how to perform this procedure

Indication

- Reduction of wrist fractures, most commonly Colles' fracture (McGlone, 2017).

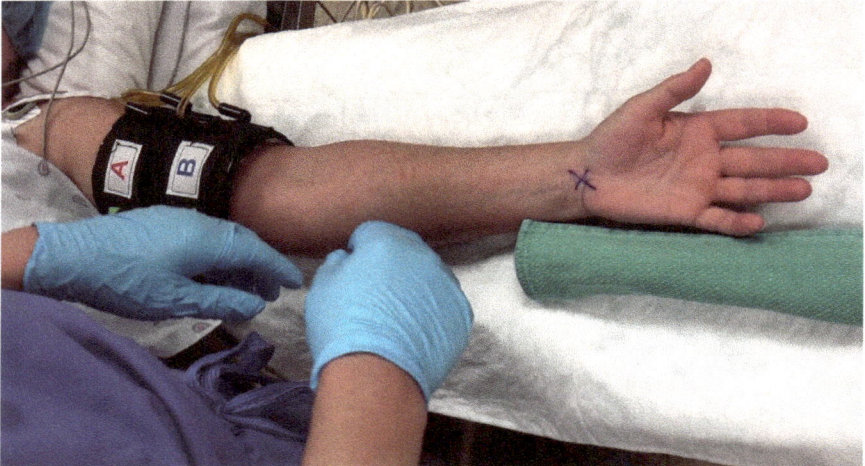

Fig.1.23.11. Bier's block
Credit - Henry Hu

Contraindications

- Allergy to local anaesthetic
- Children – consider whether appropriate on an individual basis
- Hypertension >200mm Hg
- Infection in the limb
- Lymphoedema
- Methaemoglobinaemia
- Morbid obesity (as the cuff is unreliable on obese arms)

- Peripheral vascular disease
- Procedures needed in both arms
- Raynaud's phenomenon
- Scleroderma
- Severe hypertension
- Sickle cell disease or trait
- Paget's Disease
- An uncooperative or confused patient

Drugs

According to the 2017 RCEM best practice guideline on intravenous regional anaesthesia (IRVA or Bier's block) (McGlone, 2017):

- 5% or 1% prilocaine without preservative
- No preparation with adrenaline
- Prilocaine 3mg/Kg
- If 0.5% prilocaine is unavailable, use half volume of 1% plain prilocaine and the same volume of normal saline (e.g. instead of 40ml 0.5% plain prilocaine, use 20 ml 1% plain prilocaine and dilute with 20ml normal saline)
- Bupivacaine should NOT be used
- During a period of prilocaine shortage in the UK, the following regime was found to be an acceptable alternative; 0.5% plain lidocaine at a dose of 3 mg/kg up to a maximum of 200 mg (40 ml) (McGlone, 2017).

Pre-procedural care

Immediately prior to the procedure, an invasive procedures checklist should be completed (McGlone, 2017):

- Check for the Consent
- Ensure that the patient is weighed in kilograms
- Fasting not required

- Assure that the patient is transferred to resus or appropriately sited, well lit, and fitted with resuscitative equipment available in the department
- Connect the ECG, BP and pulse oximeter to monitor the patient throughout the procedure
- Check that the air cylinder holds at least 1/4th full if the electronic machine is not used.
- Electronic machines must be kept on charge when being stored between procedures.
- Check cuff for leaks
- Prepare the drug to be used (prilocaine), the dosage and preparation
- Be aware of the location of stocked emergency drugs
- Insert an IV access on normal side 22G
- IV access, distal to the cuff, with small-bore cannulae (22G) on the side to be anaesthetised.
- The proximal vein can be used but injection should be slow and wait 13 mins for effect
- Radiographer must be informed about the requirement of post-reduction X-ray
- There is some evidence to support the use of ultrasound guidance to aid the reduction

Procedure

- Ensure patient is on a cardiac monitor,
- Ensure that two doctors are present throughout the procedure (one of which should have adequate airway management training).
- Elevate the injured arm for three minutes to exsanguinate the limb
- Apply and inflate the double-cuff tourniquet and inflate to 100mmHg above the systolic BP or to 300mmHg (whichever is greater)

- Check for the absence of radial pulse, Inject the 0.5%/1% plain prilocaine
- Warn the patient about the cold/hot sensation and mottled appearance of the arm
- Check for anaesthesia, may have touched but not pain, after five minutes
- If anaesthesia is inadequate, flush cannula with 10-15 ml normal saline
- Remove the cannula, Lower arm onto a pillow and check tourniquet not leaking
- Perform the reduction of the fracture and obtain check x-ray,
- Watch for signs of toxicity.
- The cuff must be inflated for a minimum of 20 minutes and a maximum of 45 minutes.
- If satisfied with the post-reduction position of fracture, deflate the cuff, observing the patient and monitor.
- Observe the patient and limb closely for signs of delayed toxicity until fully recovered.
- Check limb circulation prior to discharge.
- Arrange patient follow up and analgesia as appropriate.

Further reading

EMCage.net- How to perform Bier's block: https://emcage.net/perform-biers-block

Leicester Pain education - Supra Orbital, Infra Orbital and Mental Nerve Blocks: https://www.youtube.com/watch?v=UcWEcf3MFUA

Michael Bemtley - Intercostal nerve Block: https://www.youtube.com/watch?v=BOLdHJC6_50

NEJM - Peripheral Nerve Blocks for Hand Procedures: https://www.youtube.com/watch?v=NThhhrdhC84

Regional Anesthesiology and Acute Pain Medicine - Femoral and lateral femoral cutaneous nerve blocks: https://www.youtube.com/watch?v=TOcvCKr9J18

References

AAGBI. (2010). Management of severe local anaesthetic toxicity. In. Internet: Association of Anaesthetists.

Bhatia, A., Gofeld, M., Ganapathy, S., Hanlon, J., & Johnson, M. (2013). Comparison of anatomic landmarks and ultrasound guidance for intercostal nerve injections in cadavers. Reg Anesth Pain Med, 38(6), 503-507. https://doi.org/10.1097/aap.0000000000000006

Brown, A. R. (2002). Anaesthesia for procedures of the hand and elbow. Best Practice & Research Clinical Anaesthesiology, 16(2), 227-246.

Brown, D. L., & Skiendzielewski, J. J. (1980). Lidocaine toxicity. Ann Emerg Med, 9(12), 627-629. https://doi.org/10.1016/s0196-0644(80)80475-6

Byrne, K. M. (2019). Supraorbital Nerve Block. Medscape. Retrieved 17 Dec. 2021 from https://emedicine.medscape.com/article/82641-overview#a1

Chan, E. Y., Fransen, M., Parker, D. A., Assam, P. N., & Chua, N. (2014). Femoral nerve blocks for acute postoperative pain after knee replacement surgery. Cochrane Database Syst Rev, 2014(5), Cd009941. https://doi.org/10.1002/14651858.CD009941.pub2

Fishman, I. (2019). Mental Nerve Block. Medscape. Retrieved 17 Dec. 2021 from https://emedicine.medscape.com/article/82603-overview#a3

Gunter, J. B. (2002). Benefit and risks of local anesthetics in infants and children. Paediatr Drugs, 4(10), 649-672. https://doi.org/10.2165/00128072-200204100-00003

Ho, A. M.-H., Buck, R., Latmore, M., Levine, M., & Karmakar, M. K. (2021). Intercostal Nerve Block – Landmarks and Nerve Stimulator Technique. NYSORA. Retrieved 21 Dec. 2021 from https://www.nysora.com/regional-anesthesia-for-specific-surgical-procedures/thorax/intercostal-nerve-block/

Hutchens, D. J. (2018). Ear Anesthesia. Medscape Retrieved 20 Dec. 2021 from https://emedicine.medscape.com/article/82698-overview

Hwang, E. G., & Lee, Y. (2014). Effectiveness of intercostal nerve block for management of pain in rib fracture patients. J Exerc Rehabil, 10(4), 241-244. https://doi.org/10.12965/jer.140137

Ilfeld, B. M., Le, L. T., Meyer, R. S., Mariano, E. R., Vandenborne, K., Duncan, P. W., . . . Gearen, P. F. (2008). Ambulatory continuous femoral nerve blocks decrease time to discharge readiness after tri-compartment total knee arthroplasty: a randomized, triple-masked, placebo-controlled study. Anesthesiology, 108(4), 703-713. https://doi.org/10.1097/ALN.0b013e318167af46

Jeon, Y., & Kim, S. (2017). Treatment of great auricular neuralgia with real-time ultrasound-guided great auricular nerve block: A case report and review of the literature. Medicine (Baltimore), 96(12), e6325. https://doi.org/10.1097/md.0000000000006325

Kasibhatla, R. D., & Russon, K. (2009). Femoral nerve blocks. J Perioper Pract, 19(2), 65-69. https://doi.org/10.1177/175045890901900204

Kendall, J. M., Allen, P., Younge, P., Meek, S. M., & McCabe, S. E. (1997). Haematoma block or Bier's block for Colles' fracture reduction in the accident and emergency department--which is best? Journal of Accident & Emergency Medicine, 14(6), 352. https://doi.org/10.1136/emj.14.6.352

Kravchik, L., Ng, M., & VanHoy, T. B. (2021). Ear Nerve Block. In StatPearls. StatPearls Publishing. Copyright © 2021, StatPearls Publishing LLC.

Macario, A. (2021). Supratrochlear Nerve Block. Retrieved 17 Dec. 2021 from https://emedicine.medscape.com/article/1826449-overview

McCahon, R., & Bedforth, N. (2007). Peripheral nerve block at the elbow and wrist. Continuing Education in Anaesthesia Critical Care & Pain, 7(2), 42-44. https://doi.org/10.1093/bjaceaccp/mkm005

McGlone, R. (2017). Intravenous Regional Anaesthesia for Distal Forearm Fractures (Bier's Block). The Royal College of Emergency Medicine-Best Practice Guideline. Retrieved 22 Dec. 2021 from https://rcem.ac.uk/wp-content/uploads/2021/10/Biers_block_revised_Nov_2017.pdf

O'Reilly, N., Desmet, M., & Kearns, R. (2019). Fascia iliaca compartment block. BJA Educ, 19(6), 191-197. https://doi.org/10.1016/j.bjae.2019.03.001

RCEM. (2020b). Fascia Iliaca Block in the Emergency Department. Royal College of Emergency Medicine. Retrieved 17 Dec. 2021 from https://www.embeds.co.uk/wp-content/uploads/2020/10/Fascia_Iliaca_Block_in_the_Emergency_Department_Revised_July_2020_v2.pdf

Smith, M., Wolfram, W., & Rose, R. (1992). Toxicity--seizures in an infant caused by (or related to) oral viscous lidocaine use. J Emerg Med, 10(5), 587-590. https://doi.org/10.1016/0736-4679(92)90143-h

| 24 |

Resuscitative Hysterotomy

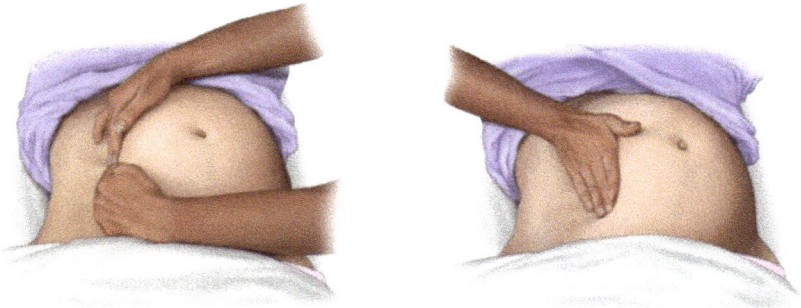

Overview

In 2015, the American Heart Association (AHA) published a statement on "Cardiac arrest in pregnancy", which is considered to be one of the most challenging clinical scenarios to manage in an emergency (Jeejeebhoy et al., 2015). Performing cardiopulmonary resuscitation (CPR) to a pregnant woman shares similar features with the general population, explicitly dealing with two patients in one resuscitative event. Furthermore, Cardiopulmonary resuscitation (CPR) in pregnancy is challenging given the physiological changes of pregnancy and the gravid uterus pushing onto the inferior vena cava leading to a decrease in venous return to the maternal heart. Therefore, in 2015, the American Journal of Obstetrics and Gynaecology revised the terminology from "perimortem caesarean delivery (PMCD)" and "perimortem caesarean section (PMCS)" to "resuscitative hysterotomy (RH)." This new nomenclature emphasises the significance of the procedure to a successful resuscitation during maternal cardiopulmonary arrest

(MCPA). Therefore, resuscitative hysterotomy is delivering a foetus from a pregnant patient through an incision in the abdomen during or after MCPA. This approach aims to immediately deliver the foetus to alleviate aortocaval compression, improve hemodynamics, and maximise maternal and neonatal survival.

The maternal collapse in pregnancy carries an incidence of around 1/36000 pregnancies (Beckett et al., 2017). Maternal mortality is described as maternal death during pregnancy and up to 42 days after delivery or termination of pregnancy if the cause of death is related to or aggravated by the pregnancy or its management (Jeejeebhoy et al., 2015).

According to the AHA recommendation, when a pregnant woman fails the initial CPR and manual displacement of the uterus, rapid hysterotomy might make resuscitation more effective and prevent permanent brain hypoxia in the mother (Tambawala et al., 2020). In addition, resuscitative hysterotomy and delivery of the foetus result in a higher return of spontaneous circulation (ROSC) and survival to hospital discharge in mothers.

To date, there is no consensus concerning the exact timing of the procedure and who should perform this procedure first among the obstetricians, surgeons, or emergency physicians. This generates further stress and uncertainty. As emergency physicians, the Royal College of Emergency medicine (RCEM) recommend that we comprehend the indications and improve the ability to perform the procedure efficiently, thus offering both the mother and neonate an increased chance of survival (Krywko et al., 2021). This chapter will guide the reader step by step with evaluating and managing resuscitative hysterotomy in the ED.

Objectives

- By the end of this module, you should be able to:
    - Recall the indications and contraindications for resuscitative hysterotomy.
    - Describe the technique of resuscitative hysterotomy.

○ Outline the complications of resuscitative hysterotomy.

Indications
- Maternal cardiac arrest for >4 minutes

and

- Gestation of >20 weeks (indicated by a fundus palpable above the umbilicus) (Emergency Care institute, 2020)
- *Classically accepted rule-of-thumb landmarks (Jeejeebhoy et al., 2015):*
  - ○ *Gestational age is 12 weeks if the uterus is palpable above the pubic symphysis*
  - ○ *Gestational age is 20 weeks if the uterus is palpable at the level of the umbilicus*
  - ○ *Gestational age is 36 weeks if the uterus is palpable at the level of the xiphisternum*

Contraindications
- Maternal cardiac arrest for >15 minutes
- Known gestation less than 24 weeks
- Return of spontaneous circulation (ROSC) after a short period of resuscitation

ACLS modifications for resuscitative hysterotomy
- Chest compressions 2-3 cm higher on the sternum
- Manually displace the uterus to the left*
- Avoid femoral lines
- Obtain IV access above the diaphragm

*To help reduce aortocaval compression, the recent recommendation is to keep the pregnant woman supine and apply leftwards pressure (rather than the old recommendation to have the patient in 30 degrees left lateral decubitus) *to promote high-quality chest compressions that may be challenging with the old 30-degree lateral decubitus recommendation (Helman, 2021)*

Equipment (caesarean section)
- Scalpel
- Scissors (blunt-ended)
- Retractors (or assistant's hand can retract)
- Clamps or haemostats (two for cord clamping, extra for bleeding vessels)
- Gauze swabs
- Large absorbable sutures and needle holder

Equipment (neonatal resuscitation)
- Dry linen
- Baby warmer (Resuscitaire)
- Neonatal bag valve mask, airway adjuncts and suction
- Cannula, umbilical venous line and resuscitation drugs

Pre-procedural care
- As a medical emergency, informed consent is not required
- Procedural hygiene
  - Standard precautions
  - Aseptic non-touch technique
  - PPE: sterile gloves and gown, surgical mask, protective eyewear/shield
- Staff needed:
  - Proceduralist and assistant
  - Maternal resuscitation team
  - Neonatal resuscitation team
- Medication
  - Oxytocin 10 units IV
  - Cephazolin 2g IV
  - Tranexamic acid 1g IV

ACLS Recommendations

Basic Life Support

Exactly as for non-pregnant patient (Jeejeebhoy et al., 2015).

- Place the patient in a supine position*
- No modification of Chest compressions
    - Rate: 100-120 per minute
    - Depth: at least 2 inches (5 cm)
    - Allow for full chest recoil between compressions
- Avoid interruptions as much as possible
- No modification of Ventilation
    - Use bag-ventilation
    - Compression to breath ratio: 30:2 before advanced airway

Left lateral decubitus (left lateral tilt) positioning is no longer advised during CPR because of the reduced efficacy of chest compressions

Advanced cardiorepiratory Life Support

Exactly as for non-pregnant patient (Jeejeebhoy et al., 2015).

- No modification of Ventilation
    - One breath every 6 seconds (10 BPM) with advanced airway
- No modification of medications
    - Use 1 mg Epinephrine of epinephrine every 3-5 minutes
- No modification to defibrillation
    - Use adhesive pads on the patient
- Place in anterolateral position
    - A Lateral pad should be placed under the breast tissue

- ○ Defibrillate for Ventricular fibrillation or Ventricular tachycardia
- Use usual Voltages
  - ○ Biphasic: 120-200 Joules
  - ○ Resume compressions after delivering a shock

Special Considerations during resuscitation

- Obtain access above the diaphragm to lessen the effect of aorto-caval compression on the administration of drugs
- Perform left uterine deviation (LUD) during resuscitation to decrease aortocaval compression
- Call for help early if a gravid patient suffers a cardiac arrest to prepare for the need for resuscitative hysterotomy and the resuscitation of the foetus early
- Palpate the size of the gravid uterus
- If above the height of the umbilicus, then the patient is most likely greater than 20 weeks gravid and a candidate for resuscitative hysterotomy
- Strongly consider performing resuscitative hysterotomy if the patient does not achieve ROSC by the **4-minute mark** and qualified staff to perform the procedure are present
- Aim to have the procedure done by the **5-minute mark**
- Consider performing resuscitative hysterotomy sooner if the maternal prognosis is a poor or prolonged period of pulselessness
- Resuscitative hysterotomy should be performed at the site of the resuscitation
- Do not delay procedure to prepare abdomen
- May pour iodine solution over abdomen prior to incision
- Do not delay the procedure for surgical equipment if a scalpel is available
- Continue performing LUD while performing RH

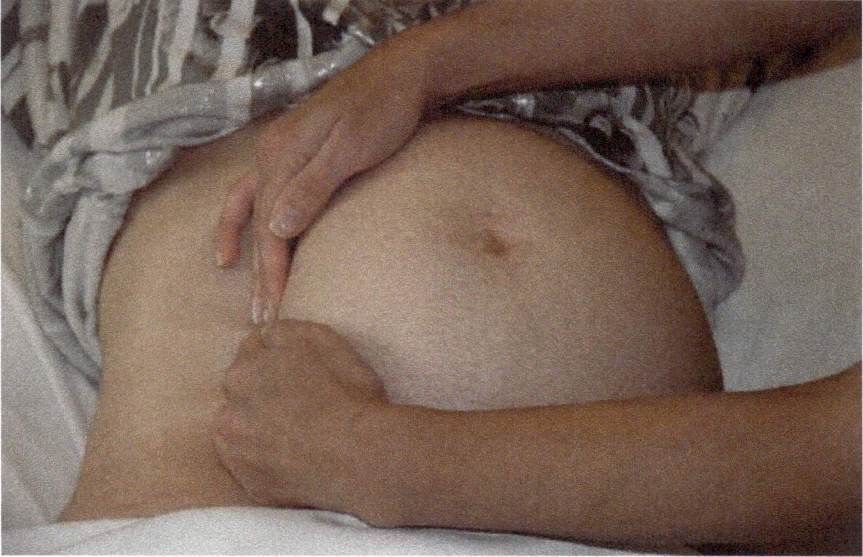

Fig.1.24.1. Manual left uterine displacement by the 2-handed technique from the left of the patient
(Jeejeebhoy et al., 2015)

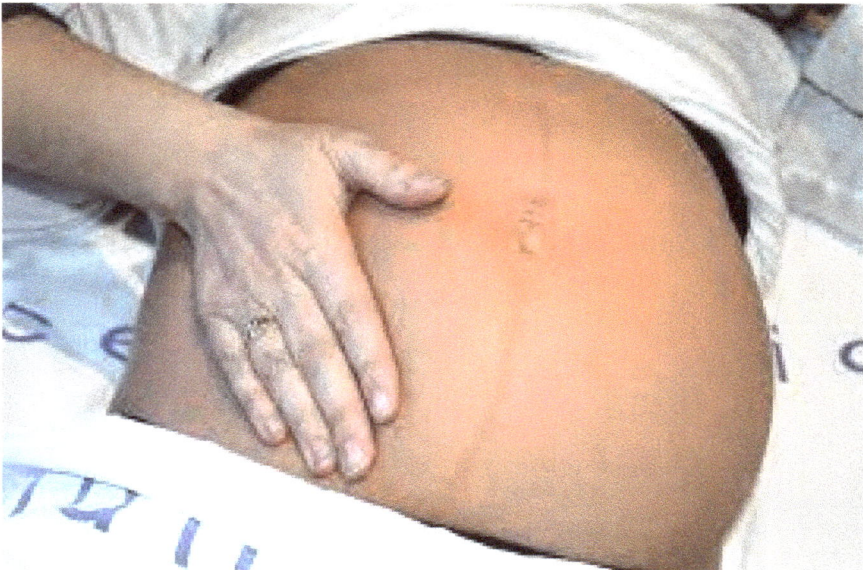

Fig.1.24.2. Manual left uterine displacement by the 1-handed technique from the right of the patient during adult resuscitation
Credit - Trauma Victoria

Procedure

- Continue with maternal resuscitation as per ACLS/ALS algorithm
- Incise vertically from the umbilicus to the symphysis pubis (approximately 20cm) through the skin, subcutaneous tissue and the fascial layer.
- Split the rectus muscles with your hand to reveal the peritoneum
- Incise the parietal peritoneum with scissors or a scalpel
- Ask the assistant to pull the abdominal wall laterally on both sides by hand to expose the uterus
- Make a midline incision starting at the lower uterus, avoiding the bladder inferiorly
- Outstretch the incision upwards towards the uterine fundus (1cm thick) with scissors
- Incise anteriorly until a gush of amniotic fluid (through placenta if encountered)
- With your dominant hand, uncover the presenting part and disengage from the pelvis (head, bottom or feet)
- Elevate the foetal body part through the incision while the assistant applies transabdominal pressure
- Use traction along with further transabdominal pressure to deliver the rest of the baby
- Clamp the umbilical cord twice and cut immediately between clamps
- Pass the baby to the neonatal resuscitation team
- The placenta is delivered next by using traction to the remaining cord or separating manually
- Clear the inside of the uterus of remaining debris using a large gauze swab
- Massage the uterine fundus to stimulate uterine contraction and lessen further blood loss
- Apply clamps to any actively bleeding uterine vessels and temporarily pack the uterus with large gauze swabs
- Give oxytocin (10 units by slow IV injection)

- Consider internal cardiac massage (compress heart against anterior chest wall) and aortic compression
- If ROSC, large absorbable sutures may be required to close the uterus

Post-procedure care
- If the maternal return of spontaneous circulation is achieved, provide:
- Analgesia, sedation, and intubation
- Oxytocin infusion at 10 units per hour
- Cephazolin 2g IV
- Tranexamic acid 1g IV, activate MTP, resuscitate with blood products if required
- Transfer mother to theatre for closure of the abdomen

Considerations
- The perceived time of maternal cardiac arrest may not be the time circulation ceases
- Consider the possibility of low-flow states with apparent pulseless electrical activity arrest while considering the procedure
- The primary purpose of resuscitative hysterotomy is to improve the chances of maternal survival
- The target is one minute total duration from initial incision until removal of the foetus

Complications
- Foetal injury
- Haemorrhage
- Neurovascular or visceral injury (bladder, bowel)

Further reading
AHA-Cardiac Arrest in Pregnancy-A Scientific Statement from the American Heart Association: https://www.ahajournals.org/doi/full/10.1161/CIR.0000000000000300

References

Beckett, V., Knight, M., & Sharpe, P. (2017). The CAPS Study: incidence, management and outcomes of cardiac arrest in pregnancy in the UK: a prospective, descriptive study. BJOG: An International Journal of Obstetrics & Gynaecology, 124(9), 1374-1381.

Emergency Care institute. (2020). Circulation - Hysterotomy (resuscitative). Emergency Care institute New South Wales. Retrieved 24 Dec. 2021 from https://www.aci.health.nsw.gov.au/networks/eci/clinical/procedures/procedures/575756

Helman, A. (2021). EM Cases: Perimortem C-section – The Resuscitative Hysterotomy. EMDocs. Retrieved 24 Dec. 2021 from http://www.emdocs.net/em-cases-perimortem-c-section-the-resuscitative-hysterotomy/

Jeejeebhoy, F. M., Zelop, C. M., Lipman, S., Carvalho, B., Joglar, J., Mhyre, J. M., . . . Callaway, C. W. (2015). Cardiac Arrest in Pregnancy. Circulation, 132(18), 1747-1773. https://doi.org/10.1161/CIR.0000000000000300

Krywko, D. M., Sheraton, M., & Presley, B. (2021). Perimortem Cesarean. Statpearls. Retrieved 28 Dec. 2021 from https://www.ncbi.nlm.nih.gov/books/NBK459265/

Tambawala, Z. Y., Cherawala, M., Maqbool, S., & Hamza, L. K. (2020). Resuscitative hysterotomy for maternal collapse in a triplet pregnancy. BMJ Case Reports, 13(7), e235328. https://doi.org/10.1136/bcr-2020-235328

| 25 |

Tracheostomy Tube Displaced

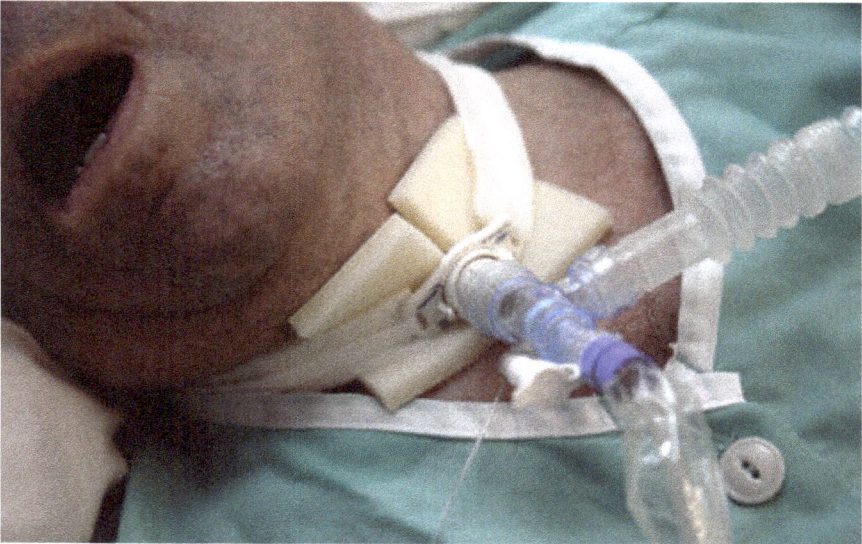

What is your first step once you confirm that the tracheostomy tube is displaced?

- Call for help
- Give/switch 100% oxygen
- Check capnography (ETCO2): if not on, put it on
- Call for difficult airway trolley

- Look if the chest is moving or not?

What will you do if the patient is breathing normally and the ETCO2 trace is normal?

- Suggests tracheostomy displacement is unlikely
- Consider other causes for deterioration (pneumothorax, bronchospasm)
- Assess breathing and circulation, follow ALS algorithm if necessary

What will you do if the patient is not breathing normally and the ETCO2 trace is not normal?

- Suggests a problem with tracheostomy:
  - Is tracheostomy blocked? – pass suction catheter via tracheostomy, ensure inner tube removed
  - Has cuff herniated over the end of tracheostomy? – deflate and reinflate cuff

What will you do if the patient is deteriorating?

- Deflate the tracheostomy cuff and remove the tracheostomy
- Cover tracheostomy with sterile gauze and occlusive dressing
- Ventilate with 100% O2 using bag and facemask with Guedel airway and two hands-on mask
- Consider LMA/I-gel/ Proseal LMA
- Intubate if you have the skills
- When senior help arrives consider:
  - GEB guided insertion of tracheostomy (extreme care if tracheostomy tract <7 days old)
  - RSI and oral reintubation.

2. Child Tracheostomy Tube Displaced

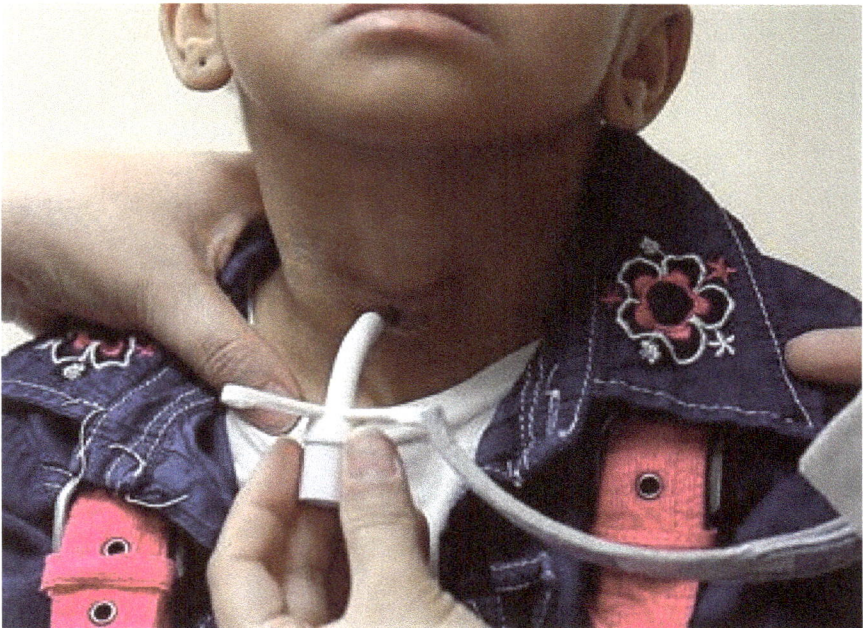

What will be your first Resuscitation steps in the event of finding an unresponsive tracheostomised child?

- Attempt to arouse the child while calling for help
- Attempt to suction the airway

What if there is difficulty suctioning or the tracheostomy tube is blocked?

- Change the tracheostomy tube immediately and attempt suctioning again

What If this fails?

- Consider inserting a smaller size tracheostomy tube

What If this fails?

- A tracheal suction tube is passed down the lumen of the smaller tube and an attempt is made to guide the tracheostomy tube over the suction tube

What If this fails?

- If still unsuccessful, a flexible endoscope with a tube first threaded over it may be used by experienced staff to insert the tracheostomy tube under direct vision
- Concurrently with the above steps, any other possible means of ventilating the child are employed i.e., bag & mask, endotracheal tube intubation etc.; the possibility of doing this depends on the underlying pathology
- Only experienced personnel should use tracheostomy dilators or an artery clip to dilate the tracheal stoma if it has started to close down
- Check whether the child is breathing after reinserting the tracheostomy tube; a self-inflating bag ventilation device may be required to provide rescue breaths

| 26 |

Tracheal Tube Displaced

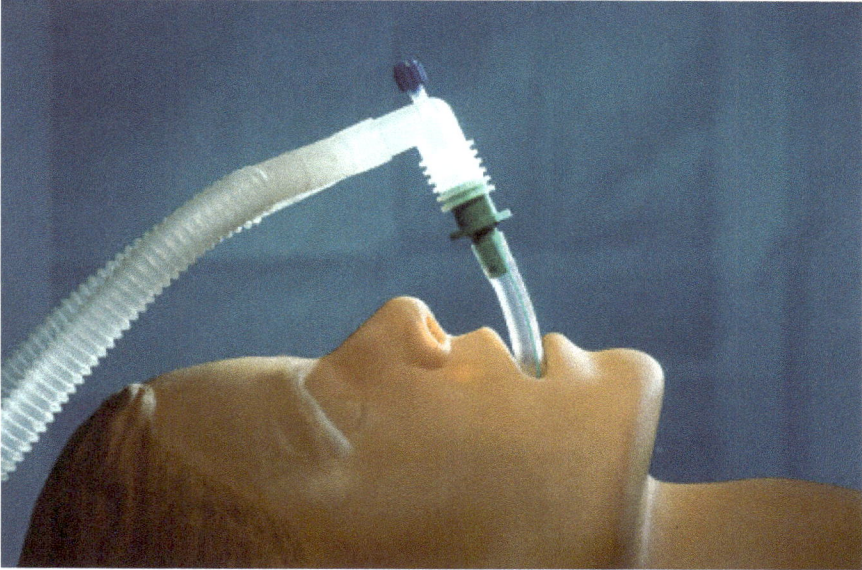

What is your first step once you confirm that the endotracheal tube is displaced?

- Give 100% oxygen
- Check capnography (ETCO2): if not on, put it on
- Call for difficult airway trolley
- Look if the chest is moving or not?

What if the patient is breathing normally and the ETCO2 trace is normal? What will you do?

- Suggests problem with tracheal tube unlikely
- Consider other causes for deterioration (pneumothorax, bronchospasm)
- Assess breathing and circulation, follow ALS algorithm if necessary

What if the patient is not breathing normally and the ETCO2 trace is not normal? What will you do?

- Suggests a problem with tracheal tube (TT):
    - Check TT markings at teeth- has TT been pushed in or partially fallen out?
    - Is TT blocked? – pass suction catheter
    - Is patient biting on TT? - give ATRACURIUM 50mg IV
    - Has cuff herniated over end of TT? - deflate and reinflate cuff

What will you do if the patient is deteriorating?

- Remove tracheal tube and call for senior anaesthetist
- Ventilate with 100% O2 using bag/mask with Guedel airway + two hands on mask
- Consider LMA/I-gel/ Proseal LMA
- Oral tracheal intubation if you have the skills

What if the patient is not deteriorating?

- 100% Oxygen and await senior anaesthetist
- Paralyse
- Consider passing bronchoscope via TT ± railroading TT into place
- If no doubt, laryngoscopy, and re-intubation

| 27 |

Thoracentesis

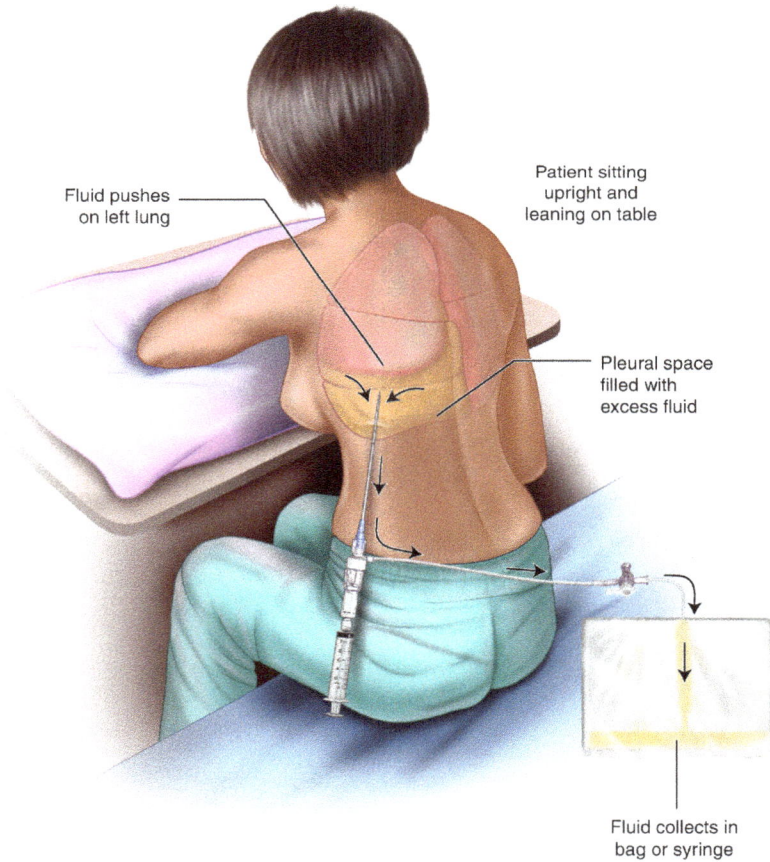

Fluid pushes on left lung

Patient sitting upright and leaning on table

Pleural space filled with excess fluid

Fluid collects in bag or syringe

Overview

Emergency practical procedures require the identification of surface anatomical landmarks to lessen the risk of injury to other structures (Ferrie et al., 2005). Thoracentesis (thoracocentesis) is a core procedural skill for Emergency physicians, critical care physicians, and physicians (Brauner, 2020). Thoracentesis is performed in whatever position the patient is the most comfortable (sternal, sitting, lateral recumbency) through the seventh intercostal space. If the patient is in sternal or sitting, the thoracentesis is performed at the junction between the dorsal and middle one-third for air and the junction middle and ventral one-third for fluid.

Objectives
- By the end of this chapter, you should be able to:
  - Outline the indications and contraindications for thoracentesis.
  - Learn the technique involved in performing thoracentesis.
  - Highlight landmark for safely performing thoracentesis.
  - Describe the complications of thoracentesis.

Bedside Ultrasonography
- Before the procedure, bedside ultrasonography can be used to determine the presence and size of pleural effusions and to look for loculations.
- During the procedure, bedside ultrasonography can be used in real time to facilitate anaesthesia and then guide needle placement.

Indications
- **Therapeutic thoracentesis** is performed to relieve dyspnoea, hypoxia, or otherwise compromised respiratory function due to a large pleural effusion.
- **Diagnostic thoracentesis** is performed to aid in the diagnosis and workup of:
  - Pleural effusions of unknown cause
  - Unilateral pleural effusions
  - Pleural effusions originally determined to be due to heart failure but persisting after 3 days of diuresis

Contraindications

- **Absolute:**
  - None
- **Relative:**
  - Coagulopathy
  - Thrombocytopenia
  - Small or loculated pleural effusion - these will increase the risk of missing the effusion and causing lung injury
  - Positive-pressure ventilation
  - Skin infection over the needle insertion site

Equipment

- Antiseptic solution with applicators, drapes, and gloves
- Thoracentesis needle and plastic catheter
- Local anaesthetic (e.g., 10 mL of 1% lidocaine),
- 25-gauge and 20- to 22-gauge needles,
- 10-mL syringe
- 3-way stopcock
- 30- to 50-mL syringe
- Wound dressing materials
- Bedside table for patient to lean on
- Appropriate containers for collection of fluid for laboratory tests
- Collection bags for removal of larger volumes during therapeutic thoracentesis
- Ultrasound machine

Consent

- Informed Consent: should be obtained from the patient or parent if minor.
- Provide a focused set of risks and complications.
- Discuss how these risks can be avoided or prevented (e.g., proper positioning, ensuring that the patient remains as still as possible during the procedure, adequate analgesia).

Patient Preparation

- Patient preparation includes adequate anaesthesia and proper positioning.

Anaesthesia

- In addition to local anaesthesia, mild sedation may also be considered.
- IV Midazolam or Lorazepam.
- The skin, subcutaneous tissue, rib periosteum, intercostal muscle, and parietal pleura should all be well infiltrated with local anaesthetic.

Positioning

- Alert and cooperative patients are most comfortable in a seated position inclining slightly forward and resting the head on the arms or hands or on a pillow laid on an adjustable bedside table.
- This position helps access the posterior axillary space, which is the most dependent part of the thorax.
- Unstable patients and those who are unable to sit up may lie supine for the procedure.

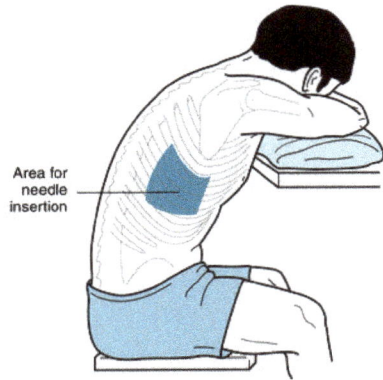

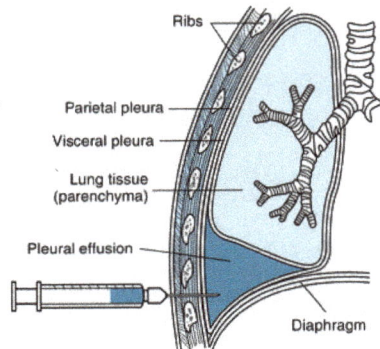

Fig.1.27.1. Positioning and landmark for thoracentesis
Credit - Nurse Key

Landmarks

- Traditionally, this is between the 7th and 9th rib spaces and between the posterior axillary line and the midline.

Considerations

- The use of bedside ultrasound is highly recommended, the US-guided approach is proven to reduce the risk of pneumothorax.
- Initially appreciate the height, width, and depth of the effusion by scanning the chest and observing the effusion through the intercostal spaces.
- Re-expansion pulmonary oedema is a rare but feared complication of thoracentesis. The cause is not fully understood but, it is recommended to limit the volume of pleural fluid removed to no more than 1–1.5 L.
- If available, pleural manometry can be considered to control intrapleural pressures from reaching more negative values.

Diagnostic Analysis of Pleural Fluid

- The following laboratory tests should be requested:
  - pH level
  - Gram stain, Culture, Cell count and Differential
  - Glucose level, protein levels, and lactic acid dehydrogenase (LDH) level
  - Cytology
  - Creatinine level if Urinothorax is suspected
  - Amylase level if oesophageal perforation or pancreatitis is suspected
  - Triglyceride levels if chylothorax is suspected (e.g., after coronary artery bypass graft [CABG], especially if the inferior mesenteric artery [IMA] was used; milky appearance is not sensitive

Complications

- Pneumothorax
- Re-expansion pulmonary oedema
- Haemothorax, hematoma
- Intra-abdominal organ injury
- Air embolism

- Empyema
- Damage to the intercostals or internal mammary vessels,
- Diaphragmatic injury
- Cough
- Pain
- Risk of Catheter fragment left in the pleural space.

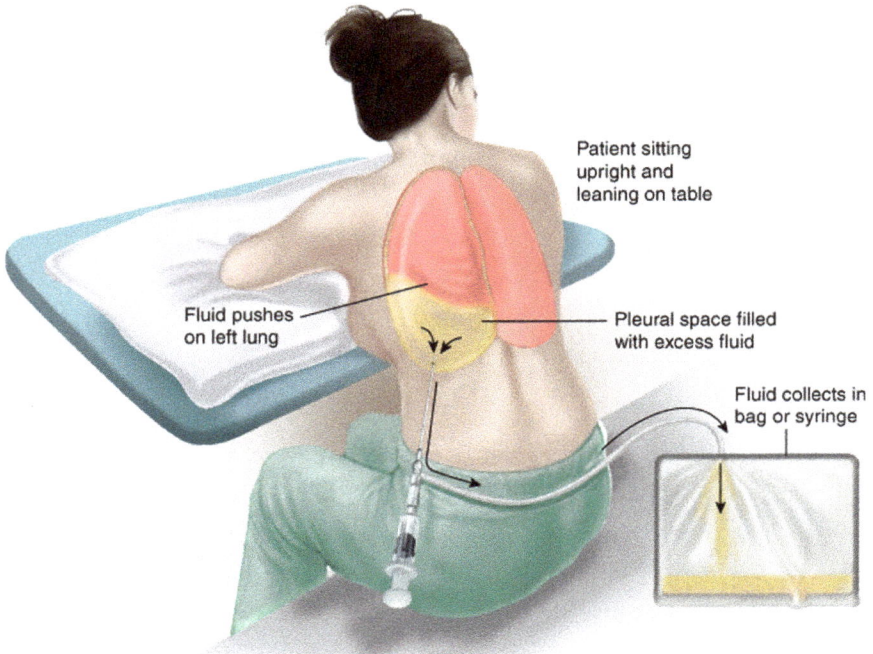

Patient sitting upright and leaning on table

Fluid pushes on left lung

Pleural space filled with excess fluid

Fluid collects in bag or syringe

Fig.1.25.2. Drainage of pleural fluid
Credit - Health Jade

Post-procedure care

- Analgesia
- Advise patients to inform if any shortness of breath or chest pain, coughing.
- It has been standard practice to obtain a chest x-ray after thoracentesis to rule out pneumothorax, document the extent of fluid removal, and view lung fields previously obscured by fluid, but evidence suggests that routine chest x-ray is not necessary for asymptomatic patients.

- A chest x-ray is needed for any of the following (Dezube, 2019):
- The patient is ventilated
- Air was aspirated
- The needle was passed more than once
- Symptoms or signs of pneumothorax develop

Further reading

Medscape- Thoracentesis: https://emedicine.medscape.com/article/80640-overview

Video from NEJM- Thoracentesis NEJM: https://www.youtube.com/watch?v=ivTyH09BcHg

References

Brauner, M. E. (2020). Thoracentesis. Medscape. Retrieved 21 Nov. 2021 from https://emedicine.medscape.com/article/80640-overview

Ferrie, E. P., Collum, N., & McGovern, S. (2005). The right place in the right space? Awareness of site for needle thoracocentesis. Emergency Medicine Journal, 22(11), 788. https://doi.org/10.1136/emj.2004.015107

Dezube, R. (2019). How To Do Thoracentesis. MSD Manual. Retrieved 24 Nov. 2021 from https://www.msdmanuals.com/professional/pulmonary-disorders/how-to-do-pulmonary-procedures/how-to-do-thoracentesis

| 28 |

Thoracostomy – Needle Decompression

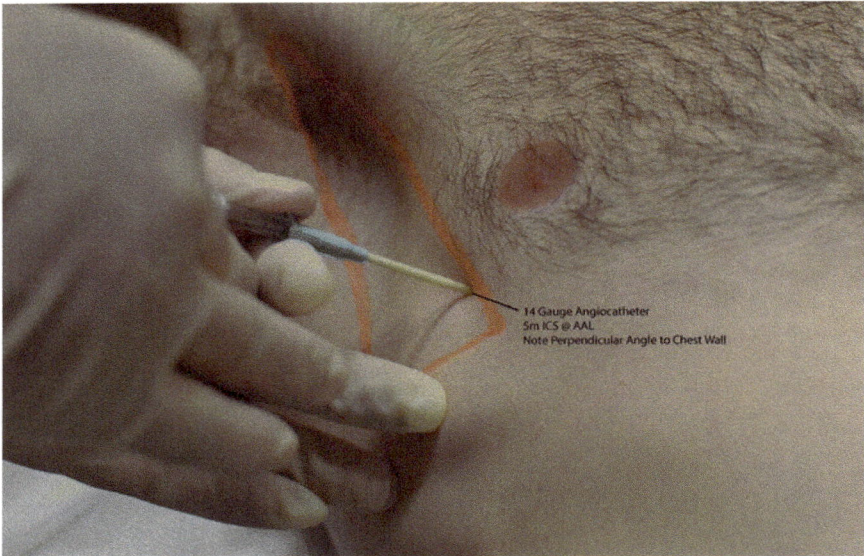

14 Gauge Angiocatheter
5m ICS @ AAL
Note Perpendicular Angle to Chest Wall

Overview

Tension Pneumothorax (TP) is one of the life-threatening complications of traumatic chest injury. Historically, the decompression of tension pneumothorax implied a direct insertion of a wide bore catheter (14-16 gauge) into the second intercostal space (ICS) in the midclavicular line (MCL). The chest tube insertion succeeded in the fifth ICS anterior to the mid-axillary line (MAL) (Elhariri et al., 2019). In 2018, the 10th Advanced Trauma life support (ATLS) edition revised that landmark to the fifth intercostal space anterior to the MAL. The evidence attests that the thickness of the chest wall is significantly less at the fifth intercostal space MAL when compared to 2nd ICS in MCL and that an 8cm length catheter has greater efficacy in comparison to 5cm catheter, as proved by radiographic measurements (Elhariri et al., 2019).

Objectives

- By the end of this chapter, you should be able to:
  - Outline the indications and contraindications for needle thoracostomy.
  - Learn the technique involved in performing needle thoracostomy.
  - Highlight landmark for safely performing needle thoracostomy.
  - Describe the complications of needle thoracostomy.

Indications

- Needle decompression thoracostomy is a procedure used in the emergent treatment of a tension pneumothorax.

Contraindications

- None
- This procedure is only done in response to an immediate threat to life superseding other considerations.

Equipment

- Large-bore needle/angiocatheter (min of 16 gauge)
- 10-mL syringe (optional)
- One-way valve (optional)
- Betadine (povidone-iodine) swab/chlorhexidine scrub
- Tape

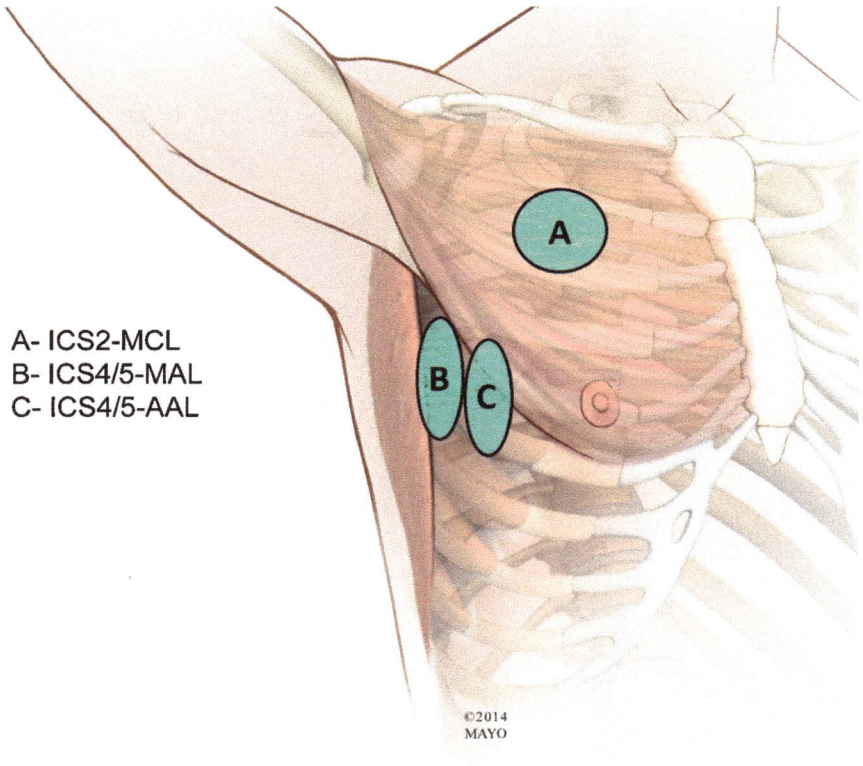

A- ICS2-MCL
B- ICS4/5-MAL
C- ICS4/5-AAL

©2014
MAYO

Fig.1.28.1. Landmark for needle thoracostomy

New ATLS Considerations

According to the 10th edition ATLS manual (Advanced Trauma Life Support® Tenth edition, 2018):

Tension pneumothorax can be managed initially by rapidly applying the finger decompression technique.

Due to the variable thickness of the chest wall, kinking of the catheter, and other technical or anatomic complications, needle decompression may not be successful. In this case, a finger thoracostomy is an alternative approach.

Chest wall thickness influences the likelihood of success with needle decompression.

Evidence suggests that a 5-cm over-the-needle catheter will reach the pleural space >50% of the time, whereas an 8-cm over-the-needle catheter will reach the pleural space >90% of the time.

Studies have also demonstrated that over-the-needle catheter placement in the field into the anterior chest wall by paramedics was too medial in 44% of patients.

Recent evidence supports placing the large, over-the-needle catheter at the fifth interspace, slightly anterior to the midaxillary line. However, even with an over-the-needle catheter of the appropriate size, the manoeuvre will not always be successful.

Successful needle decompression converts tension pneumothorax to a simple pneumothorax. However, there is a possibility of subsequent pneumothorax because of the manoeuvre, so continual reassessment of the patient is necessary.

Thoracostomy is mandatory after needle or finger decompression of the chest.

Complications
- Failure to resolve the tension pneumothorax.
- Obese or muscular patients may require a longer needle and catheter to reach the pleural space or, alternatively, may require proceeding immediately to tube thoracostomy.
- Iatrogenic pneumothorax.
- Laceration of intercostal artery or nerve.
- Rapid re-expansion may result in the development of pulmonary oedema.

Post procedure care
- Reassess the patient after insertion of the cannula.
- *Causes of needle decompression failure* (Jones & Hollingsworth, 2002; Leigh-Smith & Harris, 2005):
  - Inadequate length of the cannula
  - Obstruction (blood, tissue, kinking) (Leigh-Smith & Harris, 2005)

- ○ Missing a localised tension pneumothorax
- ○ Air leaks from the lung faster than it can drain through the cannula
- ○ Requirement for repeated needle decompression

Further reading

Pulmcast - needle decompression 2.0: something you never thought you had to relearn: http://pulmcast.com/discussion/2018/4/23/needle-decompression-20-something-you-never-thought-you-had-to-relearn

References

Advanced Trauma Life Support® Tenth edition. (2018). Student Course Manual. Chapter 4- Thoracic Trauma. In (pp. 66): American College of Surgeons.

Elhariri, S. Y., Mohamed, H., Burud, I. A., & Elhariri, A. (2019). Changing Trends in the Decompression of Tension Pneumothorax. Journal of Surgery and Research, 2, 261-2

Leigh-Smith, S., & Harris, T. (2005). Tension pneumothorax—time for a re-think? Emergency Medicine Journal, 22(1), 8. https://doi.org/10.1136/emj.2003.010421

Jones, R., & Hollingsworth, J. (2002). Tension pneumothoraces not responding to needle thoracocentesis. Emerg Med J, 19(2), 176-177. https://doi.org/10.1136/emj.19.2.176

| 29 |

Thoracostomy – Chest Drain

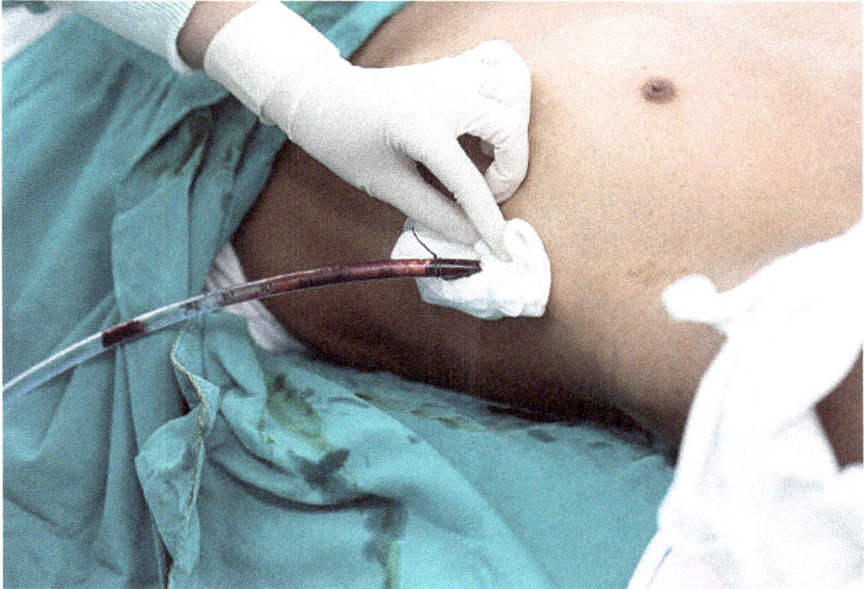

Overview

Thoracic injury is one of the causes of mortality after trauma. Countless victims of thoracic trauma die after reaching the hospital. However, many deaths could have been prevented with prompt diagnosis and treatment. Less than 10% of blunt chest injuries in thoracic trauma and only 15% to 30% of penetrating chest injuries require operative intervention (Advanced Trauma Life Support® Tenth edition, 2018). Tube thoracostomy is the insertion of a tube (chest tube) into the pleural cavity to drain air, blood, bile, pus, or other fluids (Mattox & Allen, 1986). Tube thoracostomy is an invasive procedure, and complications may result from lacking skills and training. These complications can be as technical or infective. Trocar technique is associated with a higher complication rate, and its usage is highly discouraged (Dural et al., 2010).

Objectives

- By the end of this chapter, you should be able to:
    - Outline the indications and contraindications for tube thoracostomy.
    - Learn the technique involved in performing tube thoracostomy.
    - Highlight landmark for safely performing tube thoracostomy.
    - Describe the complications of tube thoracostomy.

Indications

- Spontaneous pneumothorax (large and/or symptomatic)
- Tension pneumothorax (or suspected)
- Iatrogenic pneumothorax
- Penetrating chest injuries
- Hemopneumothorax in acute trauma
- Patient in extremis with evidence of thoracic trauma
- Empyema/Chylothorax/haemothorax/
- Post-thoracic surgery
- Bronchopleural fistula

Contraindications

- **Absolute**
    - Emergent thoracotomy
- **Relative**
    - Coagulopathy
    - Pulmonary bullae
    - Pulmonary, pleural, or thoracic adhesions
    - Loculated pleural effusion or empyema
    - Skin infection over the chest tube insertion site

Consent

- Informed Consent: should be obtained from the patient or parent if minor.
- Provide a focused set of risks and complications.
- Discuss how these risks can be avoided or prevented (e.g., proper positioning, ensuring that the patient remains as still as possible during the procedure, adequate analgesia).

Equipment

- Chest tube tray (that includes Kelly clamps x 2 and forceps x 1)
- Sterile gloves, gown, hair covering, drapes and towels
- Petroleum-based and regular gauze dressings and tape
- Cleansing solution such as 2% chlorhexidine solution
- Local anaesthetic such as 1% lidocaine
- 25- and 21-gauge needles
- 10-mL and 20-mL syringes
- 2 Haemostat or Kelly clamps
- Nonabsorbable, strong silk or nylon suture (e.g., 0 or 1-0)
- Scalpel (size 11 blade)
- Suction
- Water seal drainage apparatus and connecting tubing
- Chest tube (size is influenced by the reason for placement)
  - *Adults*:
    - 36 - 38 F for large pneumothorax or haemothorax
    - 24 - 32 F for simple/nontraumatic pneumothorax
  - *Paediatrics*:
    - Based on Broselow tape but ranges 12 - 28 F for children and 12 - 18 F for infants

Pre-procedure

- Aseptic technique: intrathoracic drains should be inserted with full aseptic precautions (washed hands, don gloves, and gown, antiseptic preparation for the insertion site and satisfactory sterile field) to prevent wound site infection or secondary empyema.

- Patient position: The patient should be positioned suitably; this will depend on the reason for insertion and the clinical state of the patient. Generally, the patient reclines 45° with their arm raised behind the head to reveal the axillary area or in a forward lean position. The procedure may also be performed with the patient lying on their side with the affected side uppermost. In trauma situations, emergency drain insertion is more likely to be performed whilst the patient is still in supine as part of the primary trauma survey.
- Premedication/local anaesthetic

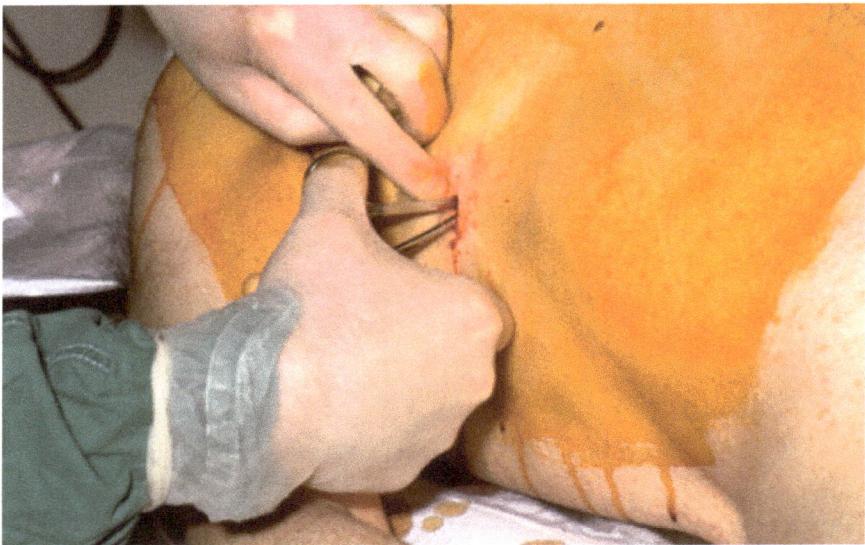

Fig.1.29.1. Chest drain insertion

Landmarks

- The 5th intercostal space anterior to the mid-axillary line for most situations.
- This area is commonly known as the "safe triangle".
- Any other placement should be discussed with a senior clinician (apical pneumothorax), placement of a chest tube in the 2nd intercostal space should be considered.
- A specific position may also be required for a loculated effusion.

Triangle of Safety

- The triangle of safety is an anatomical region in the axilla that forms a guide as to the safe position for intercostal catheter (ICC) placement.
- With the arm abducted, the apex is the axilla, and the triangle is formed by the:
- *Lateral border of the pectoralis major anteriorly*
- *Anterior border of the latissimus dorsi posteriorly*
- *Inferiorly, by a line superior to the horizontal level of the nipple and an apex below the axilla*

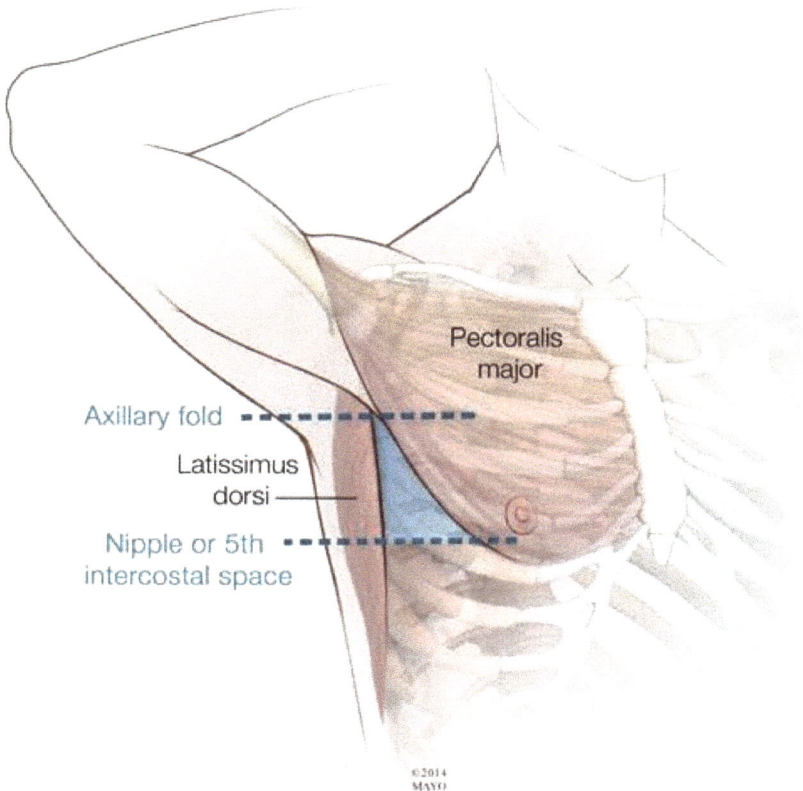

Pectoralis major

Axillary fold

Latissimus dorsi

Nipple or 5th intercostal space

©2014
MAYO

Fig.1.29.2. Safe triangle

Procedure

- Mark the insertion area.
- Clean the field with topical antiseptic
- Drape the area using sterile technique
- Identify the 6th rib and intercostal space
- Inject a local anaesthetic such as 1% lidocaine into the skin, sub-cutaneous tissue, rib periosteum (of the rib below the insertion site), and the parietal pleura.
- Roughly make a 1.5- to 2-cm skin incision, and then bluntly dissect the intercostal soft tissue down to the pleura by advancing a clasped haemostat or Kelly clamp and opening it.
- Locate the rib below the insertion site and move over the rib to identify the pleural space above the rib.

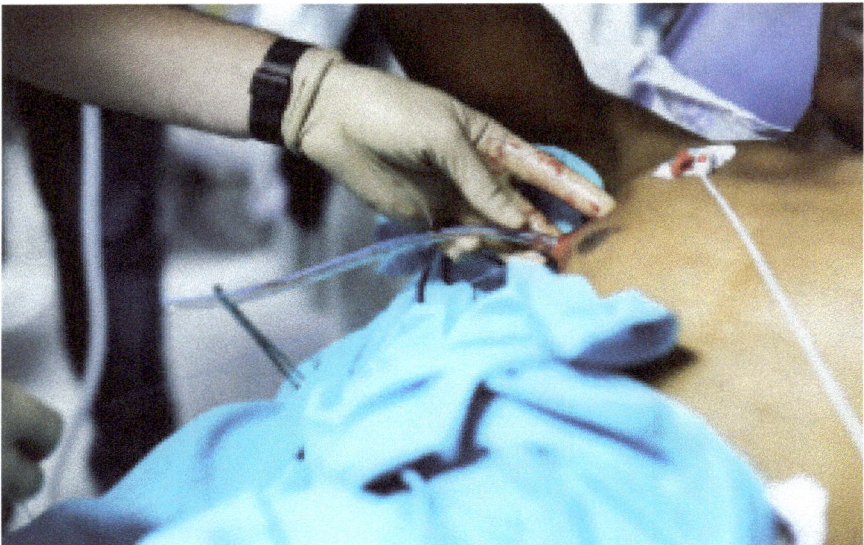

Fig.1.29.3. Chest drain insertion site. Image credit RCEMLearning

- Then penetrate the pleura with the clamped instrument and open in the same way.
- With the Kelly clamp still inside the chest cavity, insert your index finger into the hole to keep the track open and take out the Kelly clamp.

- Sweep the inside of the chest cavity to feel for adhesions and to ensure that you are in the intrathoracic cavity and not in the intraperitoneal cavity.
- Do not take your index finger out if you are in the right location.
- Clamp the chest tube on the outside end.
- Take the chest tube with the Kelly clamp and forceps still in place with your other hand and advance the tip of the chest tube along your index finger to ensure you enter the intrathoracic cavity.
- Once you have verified the chest tube in the right place, remove the Kelly clamp.
- Advance the tube further in a posterior direction and up towards the apex (superior aspect) of the lung until all the holes on the chest tube inside the chest cavity.
- Take out your index finger and now release the forceps attached to the end of the chest tube and connect the end of the chest tube quickly to an underwater seal.
- Suture the chest tube to the skin of the chest wall using one of the various suture methods available.
- Apply dressings.

Complications
- Improper placement for pneumothorax
- Tube dislodgment
- Pain, Bleeding, Infection,
- Damage to local structures,
- Empyema (chest drain introduces bacteria into the pleural space)
- Retained pneumothorax (may require second chest drain)
- Re-expansion pulmonary oedema
- Subcutaneous emphysema

Post procedure care

- Place drain on free drainage but monitor closely
- If the patient has a chronically collapsed lung and you drain more than 1-1.5l in the first 24 hours there is risk of re-expansion pulmonary oedema
- Analgesia
- Post procedure CXR
- Document procedure clearly and document length of drain inserted
- Respiratory review and advise on onward management
- Check the underwater seal oscillates during respiration
- Advise the patient to keep the underwater bottle upright and below the drain insertion site.
- Any changes to the chest drain/drainage system following initial insertion should be clearly documented.

Further reading

Life In the fast Lane- Emergency thoracocentesis: https://litfl.com/emergency-thoracocentesis/

References

Advanced Trauma Life Support® Tenth edition. (2018). Student Course Manual. Chapter 4- Thoracic Trauma. In (pp. 66): American College of Surgeons.

Dural, K., Gulbahar, G., Kocer, B., & Sakinci, U. (2010). A novel and safe technique in closed tube thoracostomy. Journal of Cardiothoracic Surgery, 5(1), 21. https://doi.org/10.1186/1749-8090-5-21

Mattox, K. L., & Allen, M. K. (1986). Systematic approach to pneumothorax, haemothorax, pneumomediastinum and subcutaneous emphysema. Injury, 17(5), 309-312. https://doi.org/10.1016/0020-1383(86)90152-x

| 30 |

Thoracostomy - Seldinger Technique

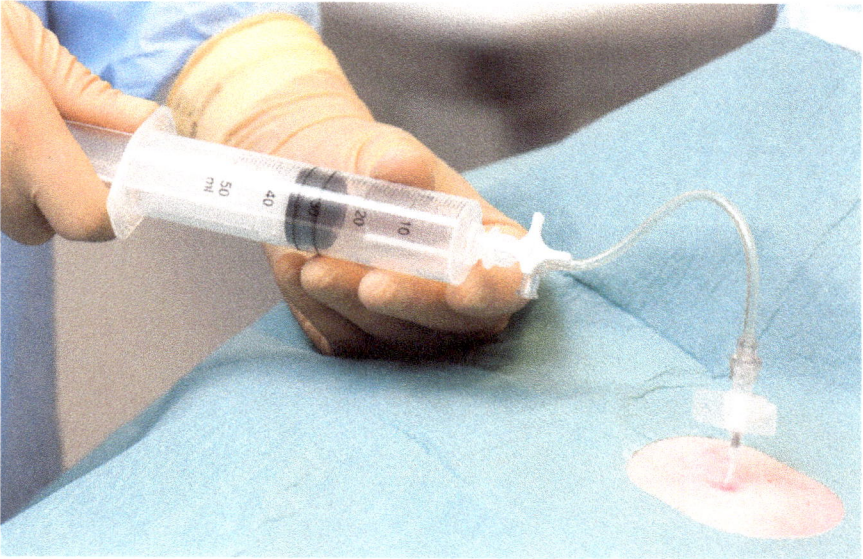

Overview

Despite the popular practice of tube thoracostomy, high-quality prospective data to guide postplacement management of chest drains are lacking, and the management of patients with thoracic drains has been driven mainly by anecdotal expertise and institutional protocols (Martin et al., 2013). Nevertheless, the Seldinger chest drain insertion technique has rapidly become the favoured method for most emergency departments. The procedure is believed to be less "invasive" than the trocar technique and, with practice, can be inserted quickly and safely. However, as with any procedure, it bears risks and as such appropriate preparation and technique are vital.

Objectives
- By the end of this chapter, you should be able to:
  - Outline the indications and contraindications for the Seldinger technique.
  - Learn the technique involved in performing Seldinger chest drain.
  - Highlight landmark for safely performing Seldinger chest drain.
  - Describe the complications of Seldinger chest drain.

Indications
- Angiography,
- Insertion of chest drains and central venous catheters,
- Insertion of PEG tubes using the push technique,
- Insertion of the leads for an artificial pacemaker or implantable cardioverter-defibrillator, and
- Numerous other interventional medical procedures.

Pre-procedure
- Time Out check has been completed
- Baseline observations including SpO2 are taken and recorded
- Supplemental oxygen is administered
- SpO2 continuous monitoring is in place
- The patient has received adequate analgesia
- The small-bore catheter kit is present.

Consent
- Written consent should be obtained whenever possible and documented in the patient's record

- The identity of the patient should be checked and the site for insertion of the chest drain confirmed by reviewing the clinical signs and the radiological information.

Aseptic technique

- All drains should be inserted with full aseptic precautions (washed hands, gloves, gown, antiseptic preparation for the insertion site and adequate sterile field) in order to avoid wound site infection or secondary empyema.

Procedure

- Ensure full aseptic conditions are maintained at all times; Perform surgical hand wash, don apron and sterile gloves
- Open pack keeping contents sterile, take additional equipment from assistant in a sterile fashion
- Clean the skin using Antiseptic skin preparation such as Chlorhexidine
- Apply sterile drape
- Make a small incision (3-5 mm) in the skin where the drain is to be inserted
- Using the needle and syringe in the pack gently insert (avoiding excess force) towards the upper border of the chosen rib aspirating continuously until air in the syringe confirms the position of the needle in the pleural cavity
- *Best Practice Statement:* Air or fluid must be aspirated before wire is inserted (stop and get help or arrange USS guidance if you cannot achieve this). Both the needle and dilator should be inserted without force
- **Rationale:** Confirm correct position and minimise risk of damage to underlying structures
- Hold the needle steady and remove the syringe. Feed the wire gently through the needle into the pleural cavity (at any stage in the procedure one hand should always be holding the wire)

- Remove the needle leaving the guidewire in place, make sure that the wire does not shear.
- Feed the first dilator down over the wire and into the pleural cavity. Repeat the process for the second dilator if present.
- Remove the dilator leaving the wire in place. Estimate the depth of insertion on the scale on the drain from the apex to the skin. Feed the 12F chest drain over the wire until it is in the pleural cavity to desired depth. Remove the wire making sure that the chest drain stays in position *DO NOT LET GO OF THE DRAIN NOW*.
- Attach the end of the drain onto the underwater seal system and make sure that the chest drain bottle is placed below the patient. Check that the water in the chest drain is bubbling or swinging, if in doubt ask the patient to cough gently. An adhesive dry dressing such as MEPORE is normally all that is required to secure the drain to the skin
- Remove the drape and Dispose of all waste and sharps appropriately

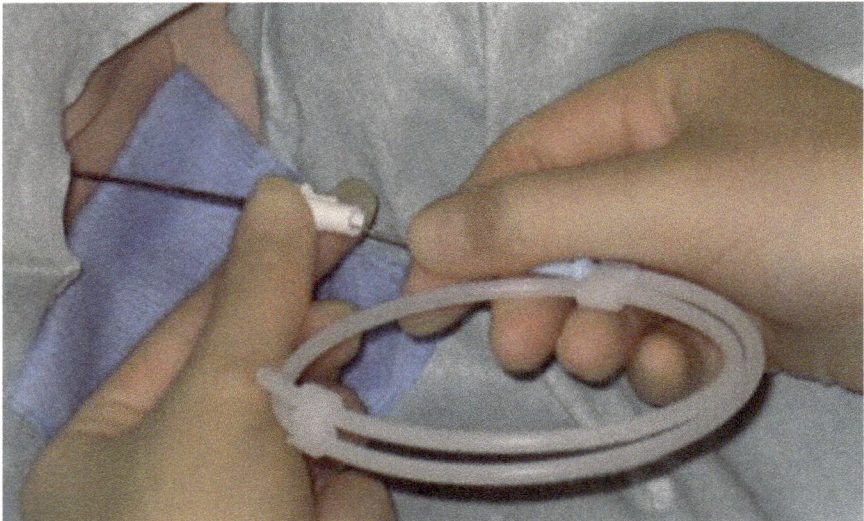

Fig.1.30.1. Seldinger chest drain - guidewire insertion
Credit - NHS Scotland

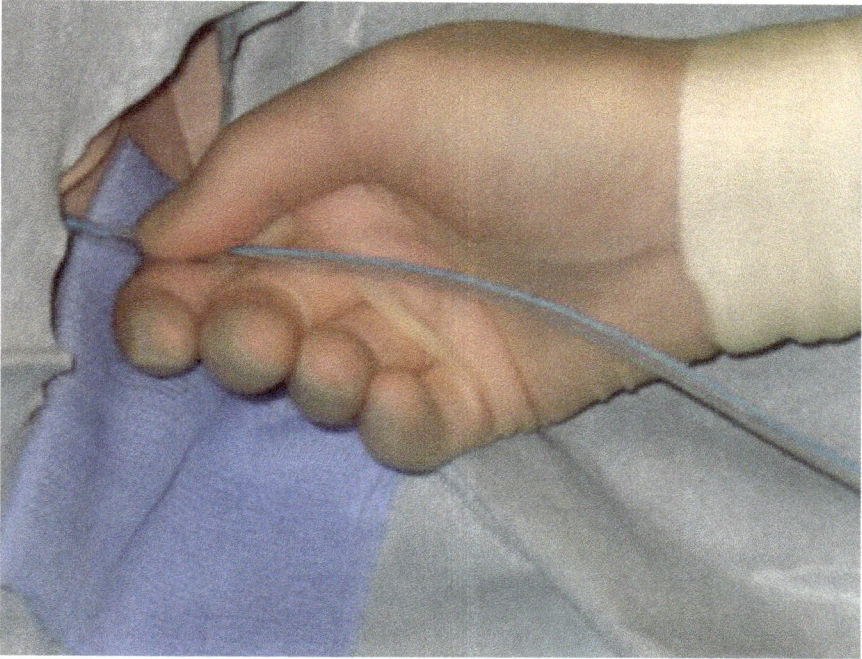

Fig.1.30.2. Seldinger chest drain insertion
Credit - NHS Scotland

Post-Procedure

- Place drain on free drainage but monitor closely
- If the patient has a chronically collapsed lung and you drain more than 1-1.5l in the first 24 hours there is risk of re-expansion pulmonary oedema
- Analgesia
- Post procedure CXR
- Document procedure clearly and document length of drain inserted
- Respiratory review and advise on onward management
- Check the underwater seal oscillates during respiration
- Advise the patient to keep the underwater bottle upright and below the drain insertion site.
- Any changes to the chest drain following initial insertion should be clearly documented.

In the event of failure
- Stop procedure and seek senior help
- Re-review imaging and patient with a senior colleague to ensure presence of fluid
- Consider further imaging or chest drain insertion in radiology

Complications
- Haemorrhage: Puncture of the intercostal artery (Maskell et al., 2010).
- Organ perforation
- Infection: non-aseptic technique.
- Inadequate "stay" suture allowing the chest tube to fall out.
- Tube blockage
- Pneumothorax if the procedure is for an effusion.

Further reading
Whittington NHS-Pleural Procedures Guideline for Adult Patients: Chest Drain Insertion and Pleural Aspiration for Pleural Fluid: https://www.whittington.nhs.uk/document.ashx?id=6071

References
Martin, M., Schall, C. T., Anderson, C., Kopari, N., Davis, A. T., Stevens, P., . . . Mosher, B. D. (2013). Results of a clinical practice algorithm for the management of thoracostomy tubes placed for traumatic mechanism. SpringerPlus, 2(1), 642. https://doi.org/10.1186/2193-1801-2-642

Maskell, N. A., Medford, A., & Gleeson, F. V. (2010). Seldinger chest drain insertion: simpler but not necessarily safer. Thorax, 65(1), 5. https://doi.org/10.1136/thx.2009.117200

| 31 |

Thoracotomy - Emergency

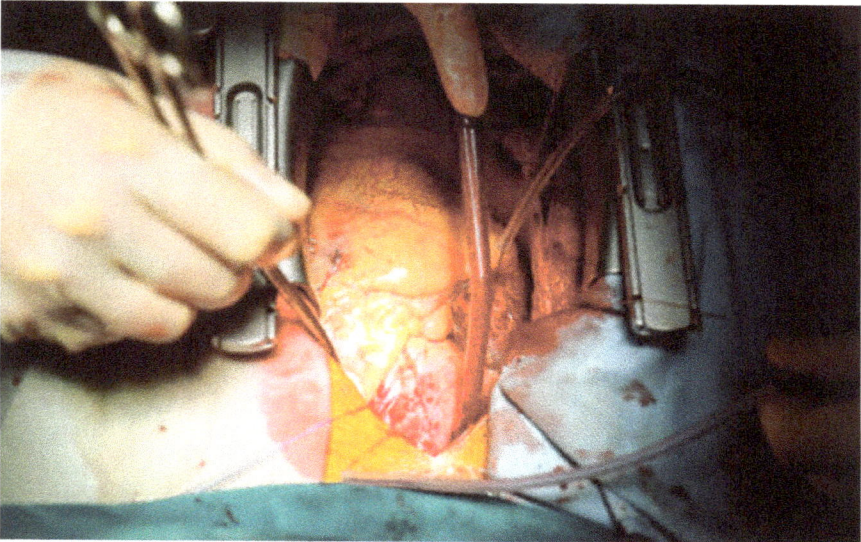

Overview

Emergency thoracotomy might be indicated following a cardiac arrest after penetrating chest trauma (Wise et al., 2005). A successful outcome is possible if the patient has a cardiac tamponade and the definitive intervention is performed within 10 minutes of loss of cardiac output (Asensio et al., 1998). Survival rates are low; however, this is because it is a life-saving measure aimed at temporising a critical patient until a definitive repair can be achieved in the operating room (Weare & Gnugnoli, 2021).

Objectives

- By the end of this chapter, you should be able to:

○ Describe the indications for emergency room thoracotomy.

○ Name the equipment, personnel, preparation, and technique in regard to emergency room thoracotomy.

○ Review the expected outcomes of emergency room thoracotomy.

Indications

- Penetrating chest trauma with recent or imminent loss of vital signs
- Consider in blunt trauma with pericardial tamponade or exsanguination where aortic occlusion may provide proximal control

Contraindications

- Prolonged cessation of vital signs
- Injury profile obviously incompatible with life
- Absence of surgical services to whom care can be transferred

Materials & Medications

- Betadine (povidone-iodine) for rapid skin preparation
- Size10 Scalpel
- Mayo or long Metzenbaum scissors
- Finochietto retractor (rib spreader)
- Long DeBakey or other tissue forceps (2)
- Satinsky vascular clamp and/or straight vascular clamp
- Long needle holders (2)
- Lebsche knife or sternal osteotome with hammer
- Lap sponges or gauze pads

Preparation

- An emergency room thoracotomy offers limited time for preparation when required.
- Preparation should be completed before the procedure is needed.

- An emergency department provider should be aware of the closest location of equipment to be used when needed.
- All staff and materials should be assembled and available before commencing the procedure.
- Antibiotics are justified before any cardiothoracic surgery; however, resuscitative thoracentesis should not be delayed waiting for antibiotics. Universal precautions should be followed with gowns, gloves, and eye protection for any staff involved in the resuscitative efforts (Wise et al., 2005).

Procedure summary
- Full aseptic technique (Nickson, 2020).
- Scalpel through the skin and intercostal muscles to the mid-axillary line.
- Insert heavy-duty scissors into thoracostomy incisions.
- Cut through the sternum.
- Lift up (clamshell)
- Relieve tamponade (longitudinal incision through pericardium)
- Repair cardiac wounds (non-absorbable sutures, 3.0)
- Stop massive lung or hilar bleeding with a finger (partial or intermittent occlusion may be performed to avoid right heart failure)
- Identify aortic injuries (repair with 3.0 non-absorbable sutures or use finger)
- Consider aortic cross-clamping at the level of diaphragm (limits spinal cord ischaemia)

Complications
- Injury to care providers, by means of scalpel, needlestick, or sharp foreign body, is the principal concern.
- Post-emergency department thoracotomy infections are rare, even given the less-than-optimal sterile conditions.
- Damage to lung parenchyma during the initial incision is common and often leads to air leak in survivors.

- Neglect of the mammary arteries, often divided during emergent thoracotomy and not briskly bleeding in the shock state, will result in intrathoracic haemorrhage if not tied off.

Further reading

RebelEM- If You're Going to do the Thoracotomy...do a Clamshell: https://rebelem.com/if-youre-going-to-do-the-thoracotomydo-a-clamshell/

Medscape- Emergency Bedside Thoracotomy: https://emedicine.medscape.com/article/82584-overview

References

Asensio, J. A., Murray, J., Demetriades, D., Berne, J., Cornwell, E., Velmahos, G., . . . Berne, T. V. (1998). Penetrating cardiac injuries: a prospective study of variables predicting outcomes. J Am Coll Surg, 186(1), 24-34. https://doi.org/10.1016/s1072-7515(97)00144-0

Nickson, C. (2020). Resuscitative Thoracotomy. Life in the fast Lane. Retrieved 2 Dec. 2021 from https://litfl.com/resuscitative-thoracotomy/

Weare, S., & Gnugnoli, D. M. (2021). Emergency Room Thoracotomy. StatPearls. Retrieved 2 Dec. 2021 from https://www.ncbi.nlm.nih.gov/books/NBK560863/

Wise, D., Davies, G., Coats, T., Lockey, D., Hyde, J., & Good, A. (2005). Emergency thoracotomy: "how to do it". Emergency Medicine Journal, 22(1), 22. https://doi.org/10.1136/emj.2003.012963

PART TWO: POINT OF CARE ULTRASOUND "POCUS" IN EMERGENCY MEDICINE

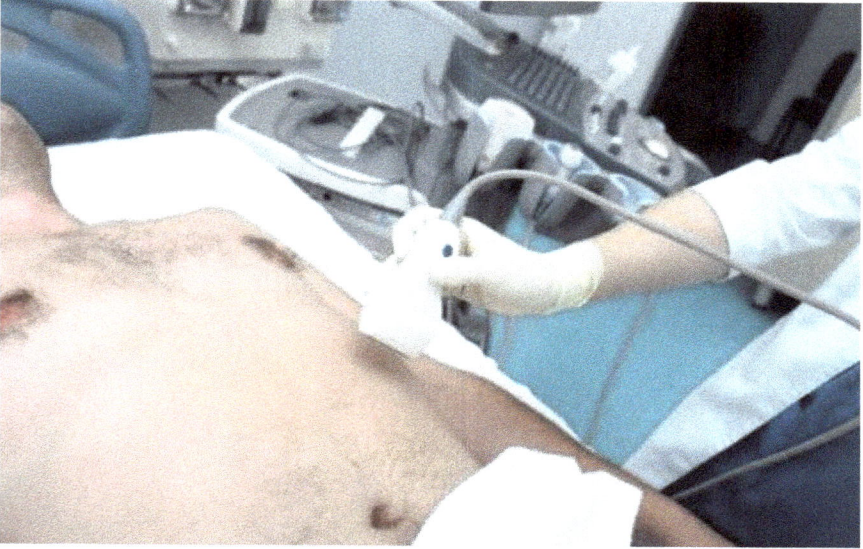

| 32 |

Ultrasound Physics

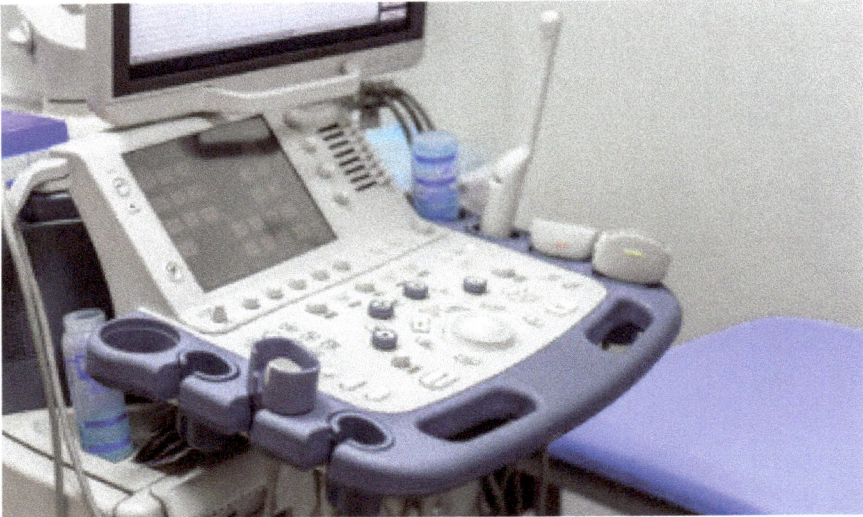

Fig.2.32.1. Basic components of US scan

1. Basic components of an ultrasound system

- Transducer probe - a probe that sends and receives the sound waves
- Central processing unit (CPU) - computer that does all the calculations and contains the electrical power supplies for itself and the transducer probe
- Transducer pulse controls - changes the amplitude, frequency and duration of the pulses emitted from the transducer probe
- Display - displays the image from the ultrasound data processed by the CPU
- Keyboard/cursor - inputs data and takes measurements from the display

- Disk storage device (hard, floppy, CD) - stores the acquired images
- Printer - prints the image from the displayed data

2. Generation and detection of ultrasound
- According to Au & Zwank (Au & Zwank, 2020):
    - **Sound** is a series of pressure waves propagating through a medium
    - One **cycle** of the acoustic wave is composed of a complete positive and negative pressure change
    - The **wavelength** is the distance crossed during one cycle
    - The **frequency** of the wave is measured in cycles per second or Hertz (cycles/s, Hz)

Ultrasound is sound owning a frequency above 2000 MHz, the upper limit for human hearing. The essential part of the US machine remains the transducer probe, it generates the sound waves and receives the echoes. therefore, it is known as the mouth and ears of the ultrasound machine. By generating and receiving sound waves, the transducer probe operates the piezoelectric (pressure electricity) effect (Freudenrich, 2001).

The piezoelectric effect: is the capacity of certain materials to generate an electric charge in response to applied mechanical stress. With ultrasound, it is the reversible process of transformation of electrical energy to mechanical energy and back to electrical energy. Hence, the probe function as both a transmitter and receiver of ultrasound (Freudenrich, 2001).

Transducer probes are made in various shapes and sizes. The shape defines its field of view, and the frequency of emitted sound waves determines how deep the sound waves penetrate and the resolution of the image.

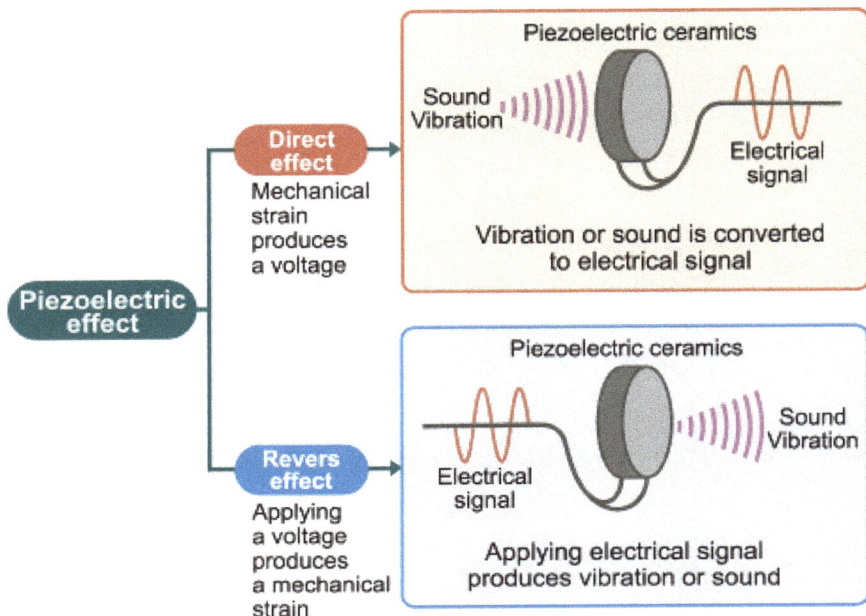

Fig.2.32.2. The piezoelectric effect

Attenuation effect:

This means that the amplitude and intensity of ultrasound waves decrease as they travel through tissue.

This energy is required to overpower the internal friction intrinsic to any material.

Given a fixed propagation space, attenuation impacts high-frequency ultrasound waves to a more significant degree than lower-frequency waves.

- **Causes of attenuation:**
  - Divergence
  - Deflection

Reflection: This means that the remaining energy is either transmitted to deeper tissues or reflected in the probe. The amount of reflection relies on the ability of the sound wave to traverse through tissues and the interface between various tissues.

Scattering: hits small irregular objects and go in a different direction, i.e., blood cells

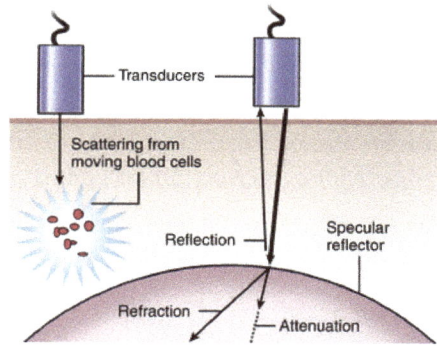

Fig.2.32.3. Ultrasound-Tissue Interaction
Credit - Thoracic Key

Refraction: the sound is bent as it goes through a specular reflector, i.e., straw suspended in a glass of water

3. The Pulse-Echo Principle - Echolocation

The acoustic energy out of the beam is deflected by reflection, refraction, and scattering which also reduces the intensity. The main reason for attenuation in the body is absorption, in which energy is transferred from the sound beam to the tissue and ultimately is degraded into heat. The amount of absorption depends on the frequency of the ultrasound beam. For most tissues within the body, the relationship is linear.

Acoustic Impedance: The resistance to the propagation of ultrasound waves through tissues. Each tissue type has a unique acoustic impedance. Acoustic impedance is the product of the density and speed of sound in the tissue. The greater the difference in acoustic impedance between two materials, the stronger will be the echo arising from their interface.

Ultrasound gel: because of the significant acoustic impedance mismatch between air and skin, nearly all the ultrasound beams will be reflected. The use of a gel ensures an air-free sound path and allow penetration of the ultrasound beam into the body.

1. A-MODE

A-Mode or **Amplitude Modulation** is the ultrasonographic modality that provides simple displays that are plotted as a series of peaks, the height of which represents the depth of the echoing structure from the transducer. It is indicated for ophthalmology studies to detect findings in the optic

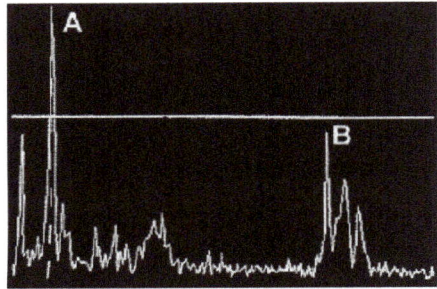

Fig.2.32.4. A Mode

nerve. A-Mode consists of an x and y-axis, the depth is represented by an X and the amplitude by a Y.

2. B-MODE

B-Mode or Brightness Modulation, the most common form of ultrasound imaging, is the production of a 2D map of B-Mode data. Unlike the A-Mode, the B-Mode is generated from the brightness without vertical spikes. Thus, the brightness relies upon the amplitude or intensity of the echo. There is no y-axis on B-Mode, the echo intensity or am-

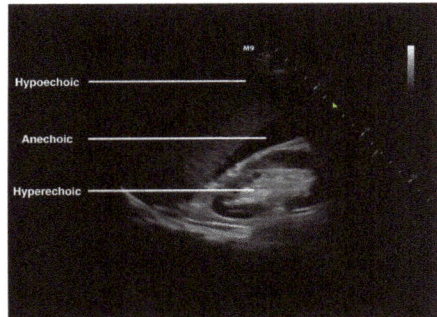

Fig.2.32.5. B-Mode image of free fluid in the right upper quadrant (Au & Zwank, 2020)

plitude is represented by the Z-axis and the depth by the X-axis. B-Mode will exhibit an image of large and small dots respectively representing strong and weak echoes. It is two-dimensional real-time

B-mode scanning that forms the basis for emergency medicine scans, such as FAST and AAA.

3. M-MODE

M-Mode or Motion Mode or Time Motion or TM-Mode is a form of ultrasound imaging carrying a high clinical utility in the emergency department. It is the display of a one-dimensional image used for analysing moving body parts commonly in cardiac and foetal cardiac imaging. Basically, the M-mode takes a single line of the B-mode image and exhibits modifications within this over time. The single sound beam

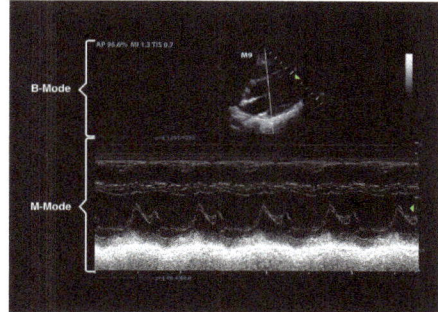

Fig.2.32.6. M-Mode (lower portion of the image) combined with B-Mode image. In this still image the M-mode captures the movement of a particular part of the heart) (Au & Zwank, 2020)

is transmitted, and the reflected echoes are displayed as dots of varying intensities thus forming lines across the screen.

4. Doppler modes

Doppler modes analyse the characteristics of direction and speed of tissue motion and blood flow and present it in audible, colour or spectral displays. It uses the "Doppler shift" phenomenon which is a change in frequency from the sent to the returning sound wave. These shifts are induced by sound waves reaching moving particles. The change of frequency/amount of shift correlates

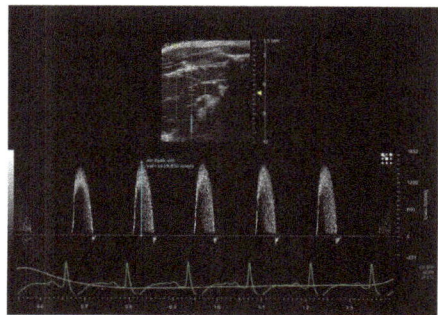

Fig.2.32.7. Doppler mode ultrasound

with the velocity and direction of particle motion (Au & Zwank, 2020).

5. Colour Doppler ultrasound

Colour Doppler ultrasound is also called colour-flow ultrasound. It is utilised to show blood flow or tissue motion in a selected two-dimensional area. Direction and velocity of tissue motion and blood flow are colour coded and superimposed on the corresponding B-mode image. Typically, red depicts movement towards the transducer, while blue depicts movement away from the transducer (Au & Zwank, 2020).

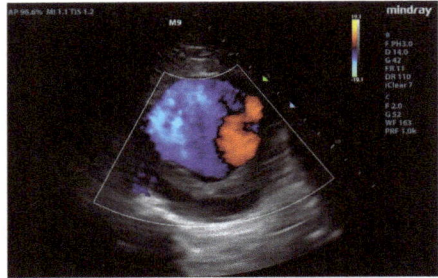

Fig.2.32.8. Colour doppler showing turbulent blood flow in a large abdominal aortic aneurysm (Au & Zwank, 2020).

5. Probes and acoustic 'beams'

Ultrasound probes are made in various types and sizes and the emergency physician should be familiar with three different types of probes.

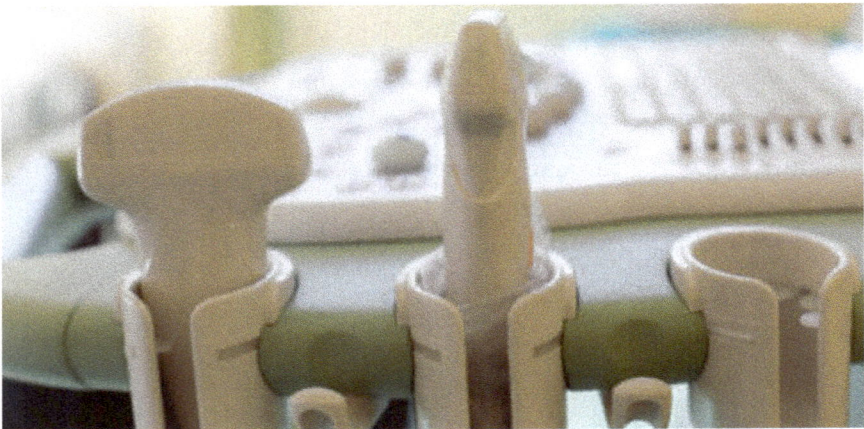

Fig.2.32.9. Ultrasound probes

Linear Probe

A linear probe uses high-frequency ultrasound to create high-resolution images of structures near the body surface. As most are of a higher frequency, the depth is limited.

This probe is ideal for vascular imaging and central line placement.

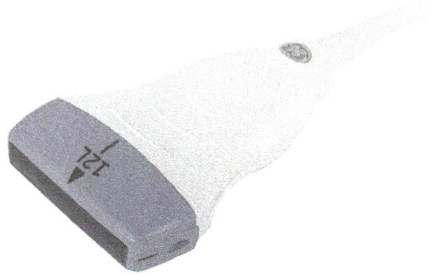

Fig.2.32.10. Ultrasound linear probe

Curvilinear probe

A curvilinear probe utilises lower frequency ultrasound allowing deep penetration and a wide depth of field. This makes it an ideal probe for the imaging of intra-abdominal structures.

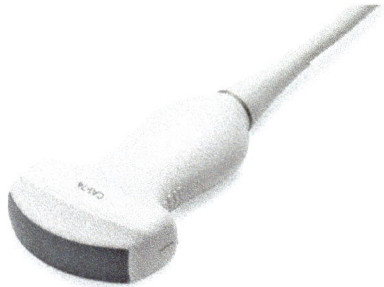

Fig.2.32.11. Ultrasound curvilinear probe

Phased Array Probe

Phased array probes provide a large depth of field with a small footprint allowing the ultrasound to view deep structures through a small acoustic window. This makes it the ideal probe for viewing structure in the chest as the ultrasound waves are beamed between the ribs.

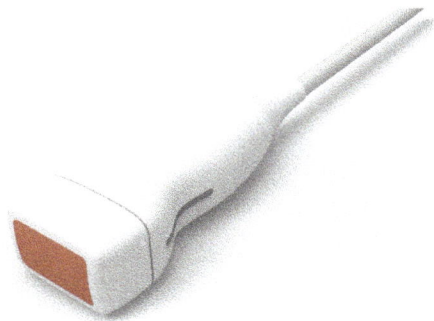

Fig.2.32.12. Ultrasound phased array probe

6. Gain, Focus, and Mode of Scanning

Gain

The gain function compensates for attenuation, changing the gain will change the amount of white, black, and grey on the monitor. Increasing the gain will amplify the received signal (not the send signal). The image will therefore become brighter. An excessive increase in gain will add "noise" to the image. Therefore, outlining different "shades" of grey will not be possible as all reflectors above a certain brightness will have the same (maximal) grayscale value. A very low gain will not display tissue with a low reflector intensity. It is also possible to adjust gain in specific depths of the image (far or near field) with the aid of time compensation gain (TGC) knobs. Some scanners have a function whereby gain (and the dynamic range) is automatically adjusted throughout the image in "real-time" to compensate for attenuation. Modern US machines have useful "nerve", "angio" or "general" modes.

Focus

The "focus" function helps to enhance the visualisation of the targeted structure. This function is seldom required for superficial structures if the depth is correctly set.

Callipers

Callipers are an important feature of ultrasound machines that allows measurements of the distance of specific structures of interest. Modern US machines let callipers be placed and then moved via a mouse or rollerball, numerically providing a measure on the screen. In general, front to back measures of circular structures are better (e.g., vessels) as edge artefacts may lead to a loss of definition at the edges.

Scanning planes

Scanning planes are utilised to show the direction that which the ultrasound beam penetrates the body and the piece of anatomy being visualised from that direction. There are 3 standards described scan planes: Coronal, Sagittal and Transverse. Scanning planes provide two-dimensional ultrasound images. Body structures are generally viewed longitudinally and axially.

- Longitudinal views show a structure's length and depth.
- Axial views show width and depth.

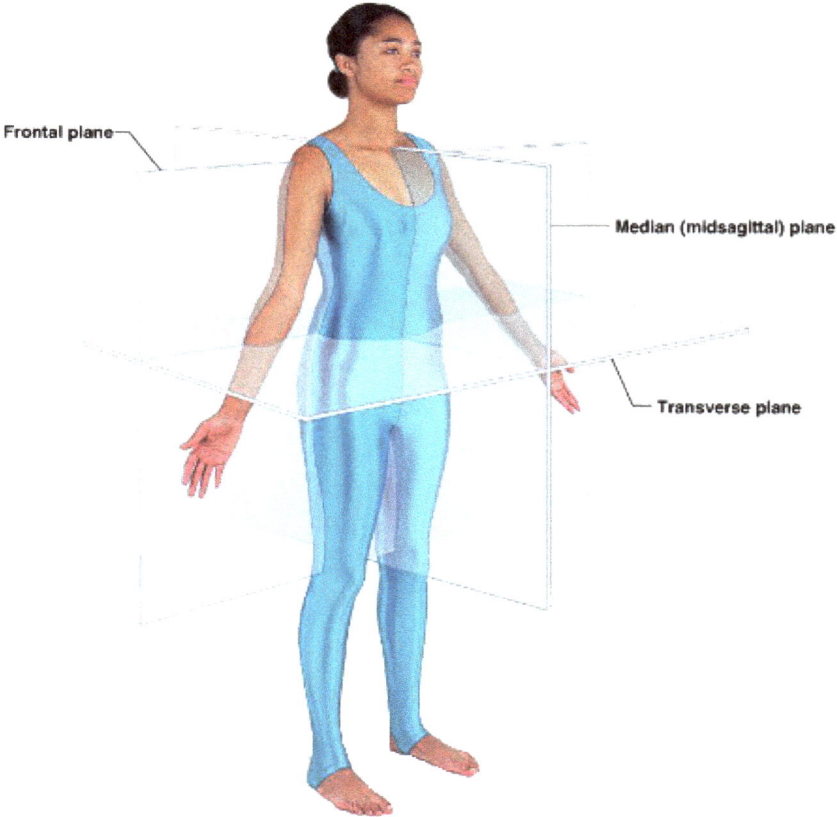

Fig.2.30.13. Ultrasound scanning planes

Do not confuse scanning planes with views. e.g., "transverse" is not a view, it is a scanning plane.

Depth settings

The depth buttons adjust the displayed image field in one-centimetre gradation increments. Increasing the depth lowers the image resolution. High depth penetration is indispensable to achieve an overview of the anatomy but goes hand in hand with slower image acquisition because an echo signal must be sent/received for each additional image line.

Probe orientation

Every probe has an orientation notch that is a small marker or grooved line on one side of the probe. The probe is held with the thumb side of your hand near the orientation notch or groove.

1. Longitudinal plane

For longitudinal orientation, the probe is held so that the orientation notch is pointing towards the patient's head. The patient's head will be to the left of the image and their legs will be to the right. Longitudinal US images are taken parallel to the vessel thus, the artery will appear like a horizontal pipe.

2. Transverse plane

For transverse orientation, the probe is held so that the notch is directed towards the patient's right side. This will orient the screen to the related plane. The artery appears like a cross-sectional circle, thus, any plaque bulging out into the lumen can be easily noticed. Transverse views are also valuable for uncovering a vessel's location.

Probe manipulation

Holding the ultrasound probe and correct movement is crucial to acquiring optimal ultrasound images. Traditionally, there are 4 basic movements to be performed when scanning with ultrasound: Slide, Rock, Tilt (Fan), Rotate. A fifth cardinal movement to be considered is Compression.

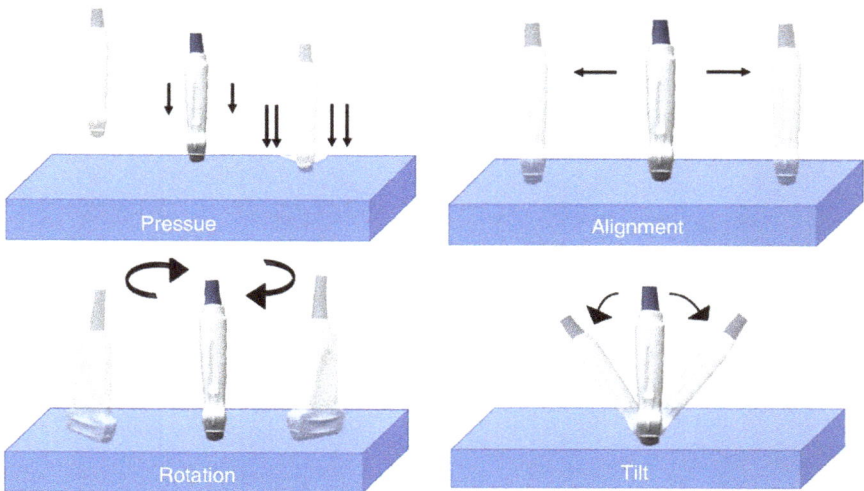

Fig.2.30.14. Different ultrasound probe manipulation

1. Alignment (Sliding)

By sliding, the entire probe is moving in an exact direction to uncover a better imaging window. The principal purpose of this technique is to identify and optimally position the structure of interest on the screen for needle advancement. This is usually used to find the best window, move to different areas of the body, or follow a specific structure (such as a vessel).

2. Rocking

Rocking refers to motion in the same plane as the field of view. It enables focusing in the area of interest or extending the field of view in one direction or the other.

3. Tilt

Tilting the ultrasound probe, typically known as "Fanning", implicates moving the transducer from side to side along the short axis of the probe. It allows the visualization of multiple cross-sectional images of a structure of interest.

4. Rotation

Rotating the ultrasound probe means twisting the transducer in a clockwise or counterclockwise direction along its central axis. This is mostly utilised to switch between the long and short axis of a specific structure such as a vessel, the heart, the kidney, etc.

Rotating the probe 90° from the initial position, the view of the structure can change from its short axis to its long axis, and vice versa.

5. Pressure

Compression with the ultrasound probe involves placing downward pressure on the probe to assess the compressibility of a structure or organ of interest. It is commonly used to differentiate between artery versus vein, assess deep vein thrombosis, and evaluate for appendicitis (non-compressible). This technique affects the echogenicity of the tissue and shortens the distance to the structure of interest. Applying the correct pressure can considerably enhance the image quality. Excessive pressure can induce discomfort to the patient and may significantly underestimate the depth of the relatively deep structure.

Further reading

Fikri M Abu-Zidan, Ashraf F Hefny, and Peter Corr - Clinical ultrasound physics: https://www.ncbi.nlm.nih.gov/pmc/articles/PMC3214508

ERS - Basic Ultrasound Physics: https://www.ers-education.org/lr-media/2016/pdf/298677.pdf

References

Au, A., & Zwank, M. (2020). Ultrasound Physics and Technical Facts for the Beginner. Sonoguide. https://www.acep.org/sonoguide/basic/ultrasound-physics-and-technical-facts-for-the-beginner/

Freudenrich, C. (2001). How Ultrasound Works. Retrieved 21 Dec. 2021 from https://science.howstuffworks.com/ultrasound2.htm

| 33 |

e-FAST Examination

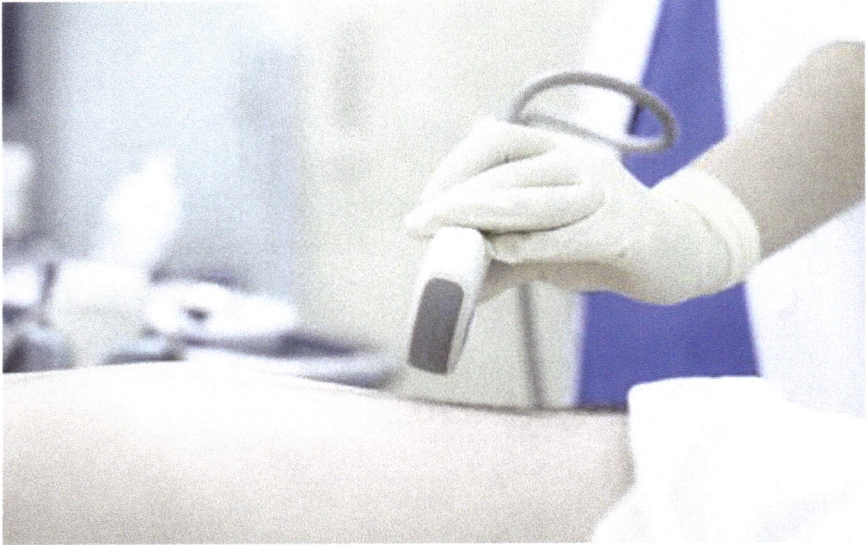

Overview

Trauma is understood to be a significant cause of mortality and morbidity across the globe. Daily, more than 15000 deaths from injuries are registered, and for every death, thousands of injured individuals will survive with persistent sequelae (Mock C, 2004). More than 80% of traumatic injuries are blunt, with most deaths secondary to hypovolaemic shock (Bloom & Gibbons, 2021). Blunt abdominal trauma (BAT) is one of the main presentations to the emergency department (ED) (Jang, 2017). Intraperitoneal bleeds happen in 12% of blunt trauma (Bloom & Gibbons, 2021). Historically, Diagnostic peritoneal lavage (DPL) was indicated to pick which patients required exploratory laparotomy, but the procedure is challenging in pregnant patients, not adequate for serial examination, and leads to a high rate of negative laparotomies (Jansen & Logie, 2005). Furthermore, abdominal computed tomography (CT), carrying a greater specificity than DPL for intra-abdominal injuries in BAT, is not indicated in haemodynamically compromised patients. CT scan is expensive, requires removing patients from the clinical location, and is relatively contraindicated in pregnant patients (Griffin & Pullinger, 2007).

Focused assessment with sonography for trauma (FAST), recommended by international panel consensus and incorporated into the advanced trauma life support (ATLS) course, is an essential and valuable diagnostic alternative to DPL and CT that can usually enable a timely diagnosis for patients with BAT (Bahner et al., 2008; Jang, 2017). FAST aims to identify free fluid, which necessarily suggests blood in acute trauma settings, in three possible body spaces (pericardial, pleural, and peritoneal spaces). The four target areas of scanning include the pericardial view, right upper quadrant (RUQ) view, left upper quadrant (LUQ) view and pelvic view. FAST has a significant role in triage and directing the diagnosis and management of trauma patients. Ollerton et al. discovered that the management was adjusted in 32.8% of patients after FAST. In addition, diagnostic peritoneal lavage (DPL) has decreased from 9% to 1%, while CT utilisation has decreased from 47% to 34% (Ollerton et al., 2006). E-FAST (Extended Focused Assessment with Sonography in Trauma) is a bedside ultrasonographic protocol designed to detect peritoneal fluid, pericardial fluid, pneumothorax, and haemothorax in a trauma patient (Habrat, 2021).

Objectives

- By the end of this chapter, you should be able to:
  - Outline the indications and contraindications for a Focused Assessment with Sonography for Trauma (FAST) exam.
  - Describe the limitations of a Focused Assessment with Sonography for Trauma (FAST) exam.

- Understand the advantages and disadvantages of FAST over the CT scan
- Describe how to perform a Focused Assessment with Sonography for Trauma (FAST) exam.

Indications

- Indications for the eFAST exams include:
  - Blunt abdominal trauma
  - Penetrating abdominal trauma
  - Thoracic trauma
  - Evaluation of injury, hypotension, and/or shock of unknown aetiology in a trauma patient to determine the need for interventions
  - Evaluation of unexplained hypotension or shock in the non-trauma patient
  - To identify rupture of an ectopic pregnancy

Contraindications

- **Absolute contraindications**
  - Clear need for time-sensitive definitive care: eFAST should not delay resuscitative efforts for patients in extremis.
- **Relative contraindications**
  - None

Equipment

- Bedside ultrasound machine
- Low-frequency (e.g., 2 to 5 MHz) probe (transducer), either curvilinear or phased-array*
- High-frequency (e.g., 5 to 10 MHz) linear probe, for examining the pleura
- Ultrasound gel (non-sterile) or, often, water-based surgical lubricant
- Glove, to cover probe tip (providing barrier protection)

- A phased array probe is often preferred for E-FAST because its small footprint can more readily be placed between the ribs.

Advantage of FAST

The benefits of the FAST examination include the following:

- Decreases the time to diagnosis for acute abdominal injury in BAT
- Helps accurately diagnose hemoperitoneum
- Helps assess the degree of hemoperitoneum in BAT
- It is non-invasive
- Can be integrated into the primary or secondary survey and can be performed quickly, without removing patients from the clinical arena
- Can be repeated for serial examinations
- Is safe in pregnant patients and children, as it requires less radiation than CT
- Leads to fewer DPLs; in the proper clinical setting, can lead to fewer CT scans (patients admitted to the trauma service and to receive serial abdominal examinations)

The Standard FAST views

Ten spaces can be viewed via 4 windows in a FAST examination; other views may be included and other structures evaluated. The windows and what is evaluated include:

1. **Right Upper Quadrant (RUQ):**
   - Morrison's Pouch (hepatorenal recess),
   - Liver tip (right paracolic gutter) and
   - Lower right thorax
2. **Left Upper Quadrant (LUQ):**
   - Subphrenic space,
   - Splenorenal recess,
   - Spleen tip (left paracolic gutter) and

    ◦ Lower left thorax.

3. **Pelvic:**

    ◦ Rectovesical pouch (male patients) or,

    ◦ In female patients, rectouterine / pouch of Douglas.

4. **Cardiac (most often subxiphoid, but other views may be obtained):**

    ◦ Pericardium and

    ◦ Heart chambers, especially the right ventricle

5. **Additional views may include:**

    ◦ Additional cardiac views (apical, parasternal long and short axis)

    ◦ Inferior vena cava / Cavo-atrial junction – to help assess volume status

    ◦ Pleural line views, which may be performed in one or more areas of each side of the chest – to evaluate for pneumothorax (as part of the extended FAST, or eFAST)

1. The Right Upper Quadrant (RUQ) View

The RUQ is the area to scan first, as free fluid will usually be viewed in this area earlier than in other areas.

Technique

- With the indicator marker on the US probe pointing towards the patient's head,
- Place the transducer in the mid-axillary line at approximately the level of the 10th rib or slightly inferior to the xiphoid if it's difficult to see the ribs
- This may display the liver, the right kidney, or both.
- Only the kidney is visualised:
  - Slide the probe cephalad along the mid-axillary line one rib space at a time until the liver is seen.
- Only the liver is seen:

○ Slide the probe caudad one rib space at a time until you find the kidney.

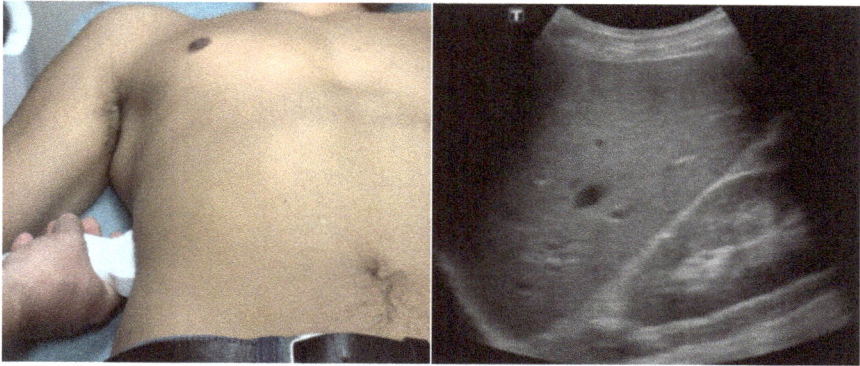

Fig.2.33.1. Right Upper quadrant probe placement and Ultrasonographic view of the liver-kidney interface (Morrison's pouch)

- Cannot see the kidney:
  ○ You may be too far anterior.
  ○ Slide your probe posterior and repeat the caudad/cephalad exploration.
- Cannot find either the liver or the kidney:
  ○ Ensure your machine is turned on, the depth is correct, the gain is up...
- Can visualise the liver and kidney interface:
  ○ Adjust the probe to centre the hepatorenal space on the screen,
  ○ Tilt the probe in all directions to fully evaluate the area.
- I have shadows:
  ○ you can first try rotating the probe around its axis
  ○ pointing the US probe indicator marker more posteriorly
  ○ If this is not successful, you can have the patient take a breath in and out to help acquire the image.
  ○ This is often necessary to work around rib shadows.
- **Normal view**
  ○ The liver and kidney are tightly juxtaposed, with a hyper-echoic line separating them.

- **Positive view**
  - The presence of free fluid at the hepatorenal space (Morrison's pouch), the paracolic gutter past the tip of the liver and the right subphrenic recess.

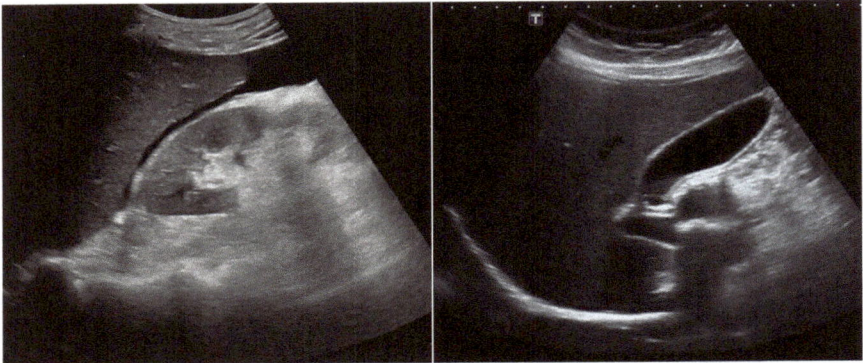

Fig.2.33.2. FAST-free fluid seen in the Morrison's pouch and Ultrasonographic view of the gallbladder

- **False Negatives**
  - Unskilled sonographer
  - Limited to a single view
  - Thus, a negative FAST exam does not rule injuries out
- **False Positives**
  - Mistaking the gallbladder for free fluid if scanned too anteriorly.
  - Renal cysts can also look like free fluid
  - The IVC can also be mistaken for free fluid if scanned too posterior.

2. The Left Upper Quadrant (LUQ) View

- The LUQ is the area to scan next.
- The spleen is located more posterior and superior to the liver. Therefore, the probe is to be slightly higher, i.e. toward the axilla, than the RUQ view.

- With the indicator marker on the probe pointing towards the patient's head
- Place the transducer in the posterior axillary line at the level of the 8th rib
- This may reveal the spleen, the left kidney, or both.
- The spleen being smaller than the liver, it can be challenging to visualize immediately
- Slide the probe along the chest wall cephalad/caudad until you have a good view of the spleen.
- Only the kidney is seen:
  - Use that as a base and explore cephalad to that.

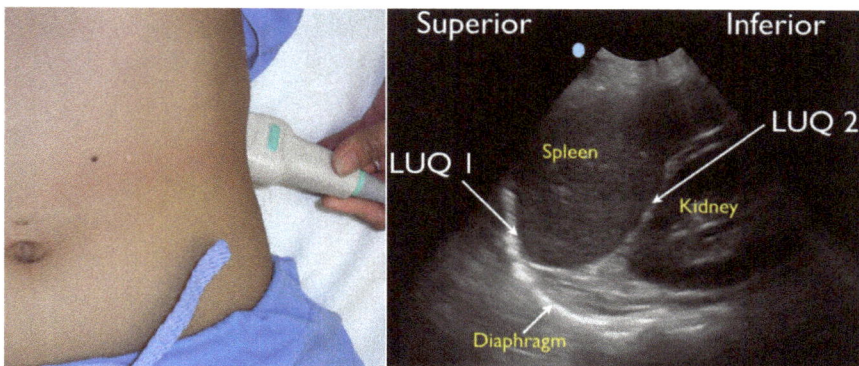

Fig.2.33.3. LUQ probe placement and Normal left upper quadrant FAST view showing spleno-diaphragmatic space (LUQ1) and spleno-renal space (LUQ2).

- Cannot see the spleen
  - Move more posterior and try again.
- Can visualise the spleen and kidney interface:
  - Tilt the probe in all directions to fully evaluate the area.
  - Rotating the probe so the indicator marker points a little posterior, utilizing the diaphragm to push things around, and using a respiratory variation to get ribs out of the way are almost always necessary.
- **Normal View**
  - The spleen and kidney are tightly juxtaposed, with a hyperechoic line separating them.

○ The diaphragm is the echogenic line just cephalad to the spleen.

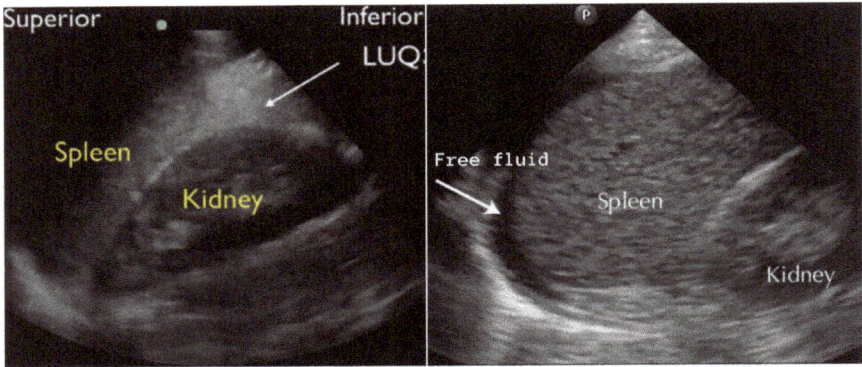

Fig.2.33.4. Normal left upper quadrant view of FAST showing left paracolic gutter (LUQ3) and Positive left upper quadrant view (free fluid between spleen and diaphragm).

- **Positive view**
  ○ The presence of fluid can appear in the splenorenal recess and the subphrenic space.
- **False Negatives**
  ○ Failure to correctly evaluate the splenorenal recess
  ○ Fluid in the subphrenic space is harder to image than the splenorenal recess.

3. The Pericardial View

- The pericardium is easily visualised using the sub-xiphisternal or parasternal views
- Adjust the settings to limit the view to the area being examined.
- Patient body habitus can limit the subxiphoid window.
- Pericardial collections are visualised posteriorly at first.
- For the pericardial view, try the subxiphoid approach first.
- Alternatively, the parasternal view may be better.
- The probe is placed just below the xiphoid process in the transverse orientation.

- Increase the depth to view the entire pericardium.
- The liver is used as an acoustic window to improve the image.
- Generally, a shallow probe angle of lesser than 15 degrees is essential to see the entire cardiac silhouette (Bloom & Gibbons, 2021).
- An overhand grip is ideal to achieve this angle of approach.
- Have the patient inhale deeply or try parasternal windows to assess for pathologic pericardial fluid.

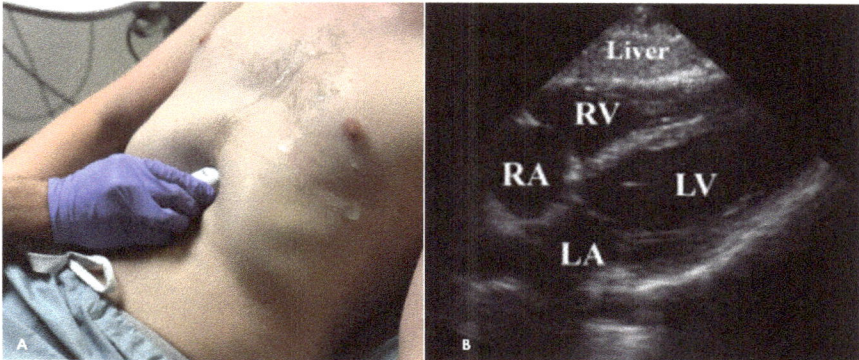

Fig.2.33.5. (A) Subxiphoid probe placement and normal subxiphoid ultrasonic view

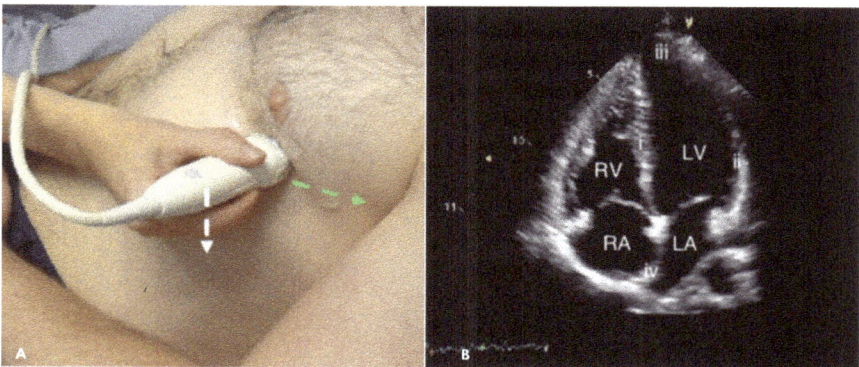

Fig.2.33.6. (A) Cardiac probe placement and (B) normal apical 4 chamber views.

4. The Pelvic Views

- The pelvic cavity is a more difficult area to scan and takes experience. A small amount of fluid in the pouch of Douglas, in the female pelvis, may be normal following ovulation. ***Do not assume free fluid is blood.***
- The marker on the probe should always be orientated towards the patient's head, or to their right (except in the long axis parasternal view).
- Find the pubic symphysis and place the transversely oriented probe immediately cephalad to it.

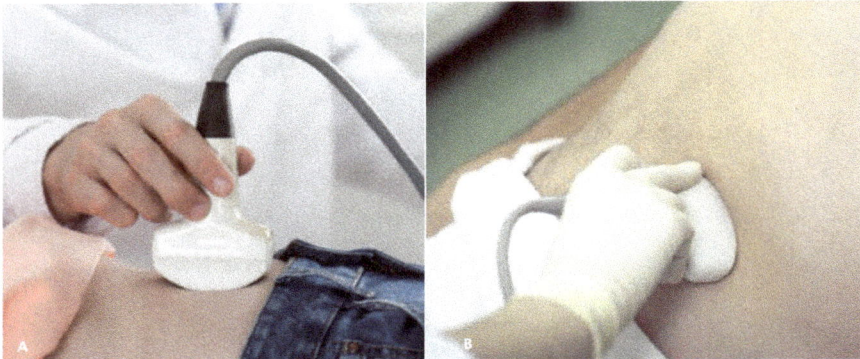

Fig.2.33.7. (A)Sagittal pelvic view of the FAST exam using the curved array transducer and (B) Transverse pelvic view of the FAST examination using the phased array transducer

- Preferably, the bladder should be full. However, if the bladder is decompressed aim the probe caudally.
- Increase the depth to visualise posterior to the bladder where free fluid collects.
- Sweep caudally and cephalad to obtain full views of the rectovesical space in males and the rectouterine and vesico-uterine pouches in females. These pouches are the most dependent recesses of the intraperitoneal cavity.

- Rotate the probe 90 degrees clockwise into the sagittal orientation to best visualise the pouch of Douglas and vesico-uterine pouch in females.

5. e-FAST with Lung Views

Examine for pneumothorax:

- **Lung sliding**
  - ○ Absence: pneumothorax
  - ○ Presence: normal lung
- **M mode tracing**
  - ○ Stratosphere/Barcode sign: pneumothorax
  - ○ Seashore sign: normal lung

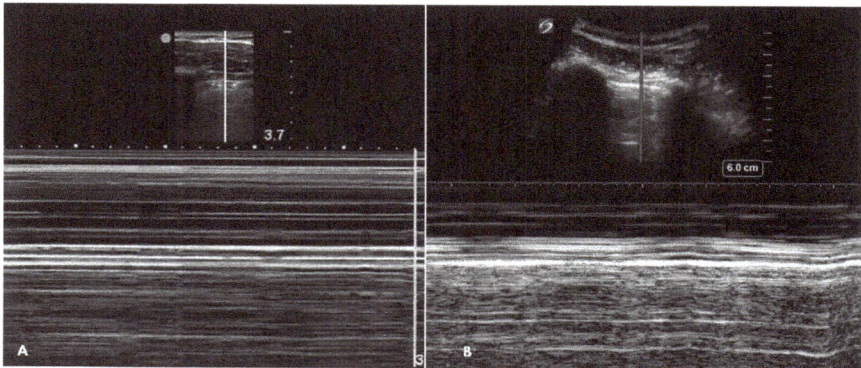

Fig.2.33.8. (A) Barcode sign suggestive of a pneumothorax and (B) Seashore sign confirming a normal lung.

Complications

- Overreliance on ultrasound to rule out abdominal injury: FAST examinations do not detect retroperitoneal bleeding, solid organ injury, contained subcapsular hematomas, and bowel injuries.
- Not scanning through the object in question could lead to false-negative results.

Further reading

Radiopaedia - Focussed Assessment with Sonography for Trauma (FAST) scan: https://radiopaedia.org/articles/focussed-assessment-with-sonography-for-trauma-fast-scan?lang=gb

References

Bloom, B. A., & Gibbons, R. C. (2021). Focused Assessment with Sonography for Trauma. StatPearls. Retrieved 25 Dec. 2021 from https://www.ncbi.nlm.nih.gov/books/NBK470479/

Griffin, X. L., & Pullinger, R. (2007). Are diagnostic peritoneal lavage or focused abdominal sonography for trauma safe screening investigations for hemodynamically stable patients after blunt abdominal trauma? A review of the literature. J Trauma, 62(3), 779-784. https://doi.org/10.1097/01.ta.0000250493.58701.ad

Habrat, D. (2021). How To Do E-Fast Examination. MSD Manual. Retrieved 25 Dec. 2021 from https://www.msdmanuals.com/en-gb/professional/critical-care-medicine/how-to-do-other-emergency-medicine-procedures/how-to-do-e-fast-examination

Jang, T. (2017). Focused Assessment with Sonography in Trauma (FAST). Medscape. Retrieved 25 Dec. 2021 from https://emedicine.medscape.com/article/104363-overview

Jansen, J. O., & Logie, J. R. (2005). Diagnostic peritoneal lavage - an obituary. Br J Surg, 92(5), 517-518. https://doi.org/10.1002/bjs.5003

Mock C, L. J., Goosen J, Joshipura M, Peden M. (2004). Guidelines for essential trauma care. In. Geneva: World Health Organization

Ollerton, J. E., Sugrue, M., Balogh, Z., D'Amours, S. K., Giles, A., & Wyllie, P. (2006). Prospective study to evaluate the influence of FAST on trauma patient management. J Trauma, 60(4), 785-791. https://doi.org/10.1097/01.ta.0000214583.21492.e8

| 34 |

Ultrasound of the Abdominal Aorta & IVC

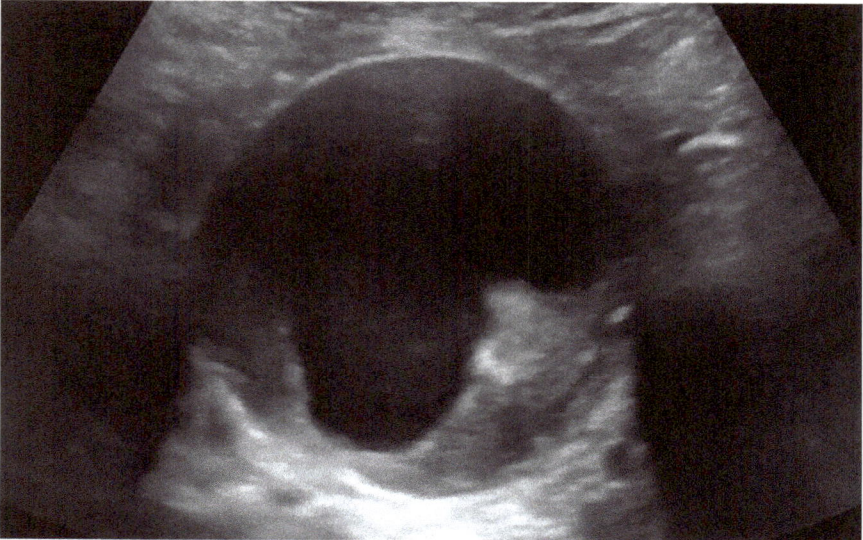

Overview

Adult patients commonly present to the emergency department (ED) with abdominal, back, and flank pain; In such cases, the emergency physician should always consider abdominal aortic aneurysm (AAA) in the differential diagnosis. Patients at most significant risk for AAA are men older than 65 years and have peripheral atherosclerotic vascular disease (Rahimi, 2021).

Several studies document that a well-trained emergency physician can competently and accurately identify an abdominal aortic aneurysm using bedside ultrasonography.

Aneurysms are focal dilations in an artery, with at least a 50% increase over the vessel's average diameter. Thus, enlargement of the diameter of the abdominal aorta to 3 cm or more fits the definition (Rahimi, 2021).

The recent increased use of ultrasound has contributed to the early diagnosis of AAA. Bengtsson et al.'s study from Malmo, Sweden, observed a prevalence of 4.3% in men and 2.1% in women detected on ultrasound (Bengtsson et al., 1991). The incidence of AAA ranges from 0.5% to 3%, increases after age 60 and peaks in the seventh and eighth decades of life (Shaw et al., 2021). Furthermore, AAAs are uncommon in Asian, African American, and Hispanic individuals, while the white male possesses the highest risk of developing AAAs (Zommorodi et al., 2018). A survey conducted by Kent et al. unveiled a prevalence of 1.4% or 1.1 million AAAs in those studied aged 50 to 84 (Kent et al., 2010). AAA's recognised risk factors include advancing age, male gender, smoking, and family history.

Often, it is challenging to define the limits or relations of the aneurysm in the emergency setting. Therefore, the ED sonographer will concentrate on the single issue of *whether it is aneurysmal or not*. Furthermore, ultrasound is not accurate in determining the presence of a leak from the aneurysm. Hence, In the ED setting, we concentrate on *whether aneurysmal change is present or not*.

Objectives

- By the end of this module, you should be able to:
  - ○ Describe normal ultrasound anatomy of the abdominal great vessels, including the aorta, inferior vena cava, its branches, as well as its relationship with surrounding structures
  - ○ Select the appropriate transducer and optimise image capture by adjusting function keys
  - ○ Able to determine if the aneurysm is present or not and if present, whether there is any change or not

Indications

A scan should always be carried out when a AAA is suspected. Features of a suspected abdominal aortic aneurysm include:

- Patients older than 50 years with the classic presentation of abdominal, back, or flank pain, a pulsatile abdominal mass, and hypotension should have a bedside aortic ultrasound examination.
- Renal colic in an older patient
- Any patient with unexplained hypotension, dizziness, or syncope should have a bedside aortic ultrasound.
- Patients presenting in cardiac arrest may have a ruptured AAA.
- Patients with pulseless electrical activity may be in a state of severe hypotension that could be reversed if the cause is rapidly identified and aggressively treated.

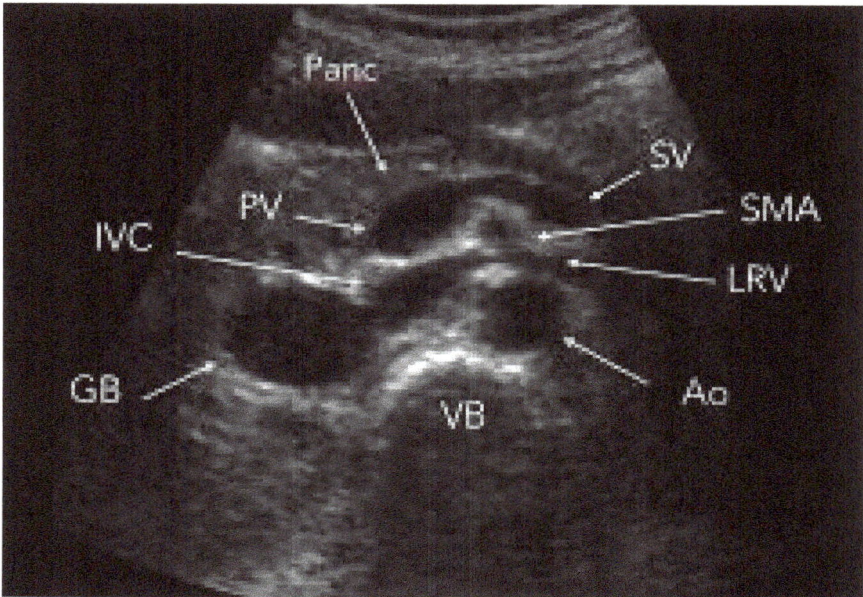

Fig.2.34.1. Abdominal Aorta bedside ultrasound. SV = Splenic Vein, SMA = Sup Mesenteric Artery, LRV = L Renal Vein, Ao = Aorta, VB = Vertebral Body, GB = Gallbladder, PV = Portal Vein. Note that the pancreas lies just anterior to the PV at this level.

Anatomical considerations

- Features of the IVC & Aorta
    - ○ The inferior vena cava (IVC) and aorta are both seen in most cases, as in this ultrasound scan. It is possible for a novice to confuse the two.
    - ○ The aorta is situated anterior to the vertebral bodies and left of the midline, whereas the IVC lies to the right of the midline.
    - ○ The aorta tapers and tends to be tortuous and move to the left.
    - ○ It can be calcified anteriorly which can make the ultrasound view more difficult.

The main features of the IVC	The main features of the aorta
• Right side • Thin-walled • Compressible • Transmitted pulse (double bounce) • Almond-shaped • Shape varies	• Left side • Thick-walled • Will not compress • Pulsatile • Round • Constant shape • Superior mesenteric artery demonstrated

Branches of the Abdominal Aorta

- Note the branches of the coeliac axis and their relationship to the superior mesenteric artery (SMA).
- The coeliac axis is 1-2 cm below the diaphragm,
- The SMA is 2 cm below the coeliac axis,
- The IMA is 4 cm above the bifurcation,

- The aorta bifurcates at, or immediately below, the umbilicus (L4),
- The maximum external diameter (measured from outer wall to outer wall) at different levels will vary, e.g., 3cm at the epigastrium, 1.5cm at the bifurcation.

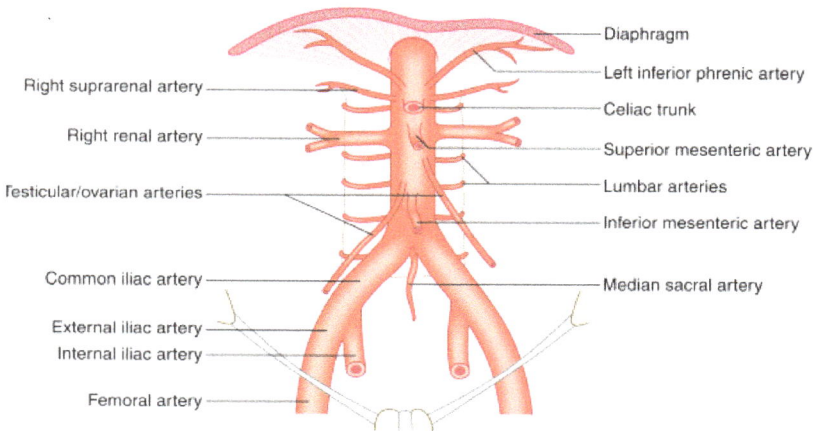

Fig.2.34.2. Normal anatomy of the aorta, including major branch vessels
Credit - Radiology key

Types of Aneurysms

- **Saccular aneurysms** appear like a small blister or bleb on the side of the aorta and are asymmetrical.
- **Fusiform aneurysms** are the type most seen in the abdominal aorta. Most fusiform aneurysms are true aneurysms. The weakness is often along an extended section of the aorta

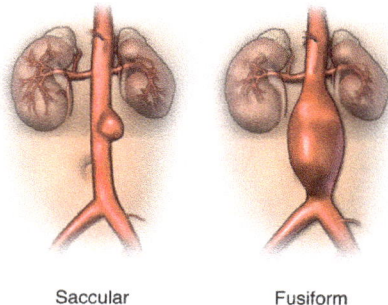

Saccular   Fusiform

Fig.2.34.3. Types of abdominal aortic aneurysm

and involves the entire circumference of the aorta. The weakened portion appears as a roughly symmetrical bulge, as shown in the image.

- They may be **pseudoaneurysms** caused by trauma, such as a car accident, or by a penetrating aortic ulcer.

AAA Ultrasound Procedure

- **Probe Selection:**
  - Curvilinear
  - Phased array Patient
- **Patient positioning:**
  - Place the patient in the supine position.
  - When bowel gas or adipose tissue prevents adequate visualisation, the patient can be placed in the lateral decubitus position.
  - Consider bending the patient's knees to decrease tension on the rectus muscles (ACEP Now, 2010).

Technique for scanning the abdominal aorta

1. Transverse View

Place probe in the subxiphoid region – transverse orientation, probe indicator oriented toward patient's right. Identify the vertebral shadow, which is a hyper-echoic rim with a posterior shadow, that appears like an upside-down "U" or "horseshoe sign". The aorta will be found anterior to the vertebral body and appear circular and pulsatile. The aorta in relation to the inferior vena cava (IVC) will appear on the right side of the screen, as it is oriented on the left side of the patient's body. Without removing the probe from the skin, continue to scan in the transverse orientation by sliding the probe towards the umbilicus. A complete exam of the abdominal aorta entails visualisation of the proximal, mid, and distal aorta. The normal diameter of the aorta is 3 cm.

The proximal and mid-aorta can also be evaluated in a longitudinal orientation.

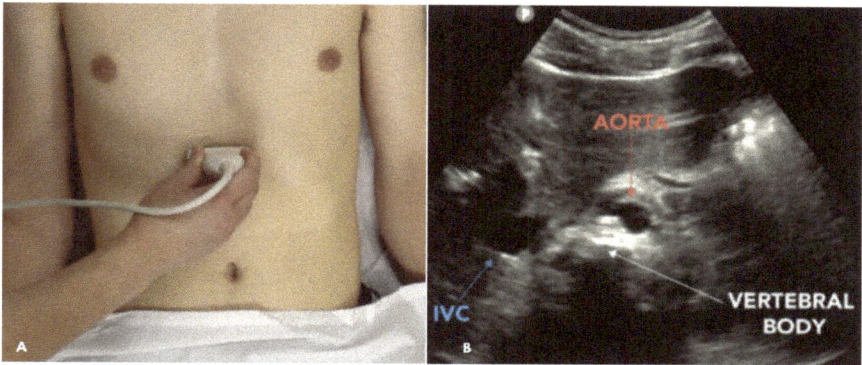

Fig.2.34.4. (A) Ultrasound aorta -Transverse probe placement and (B) Short axis view of the proximal aorta
Credit - POCUS 101

Proximal abdominal aorta (below the diaphragm)

The celiac trunk is the 1st major branch of the abdominal aorta. Look for the **"seagull sign"** – the wings are the hepatic (screen left) and splenic (screen right) arteries. The left gastric artery, the third component of the celiac trunk is usually not visualised on ultrasound.

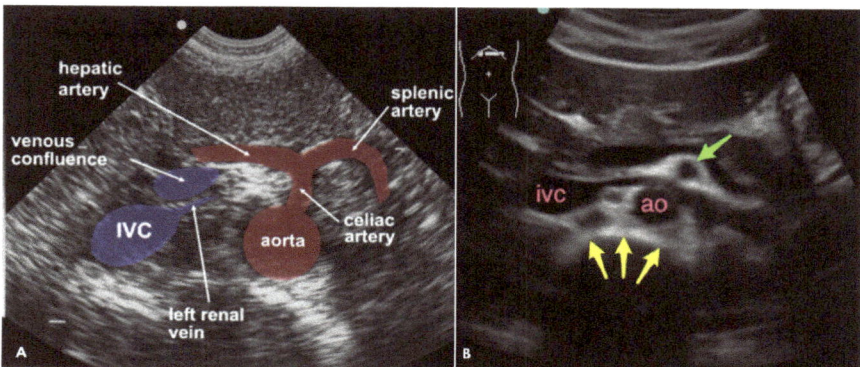

Fig.2.34.5. (A) Normal proximal transverse aorta. Note the anechoic circle of the aorta, the teardrop-shaped IVC, and the inverted "U" of the spine shadow. The celiac trunk bifurcating into hepatic and splenic arteries can be seen superficial to the aorta and (B) Mantle clock appearance of the SMA

Mid abdominal aorta (near the level of the renal arteries)

The superior mesenteric artery (SMA) is the second major branch of the abdominal aorta. The splenic vein passes anterior, and the left renal vein runs posterior to the SMA. The SMA view has been called the "**mantle clock**" sign given its resemblance to one.

Distal (Above and at the Iliac Bifurcation)

The aorta will bifurcate at the level of the umbilicus into the common iliac arteries. Slowly fan up and down to view the distal aorta branch off into the two branches of the iliac arteries.

2. Longitudinal View

Turning the transducer clockwise 90 degrees allows for the longitudinal view of the aorta to appear. The patient's head will be to the left of the screen, and the feet to the right. The celiac trunk (proximal aorta) and the SMA (mid-aorta) can be seen exiting the aorta, with the SMA running parallel to the aorta distally.

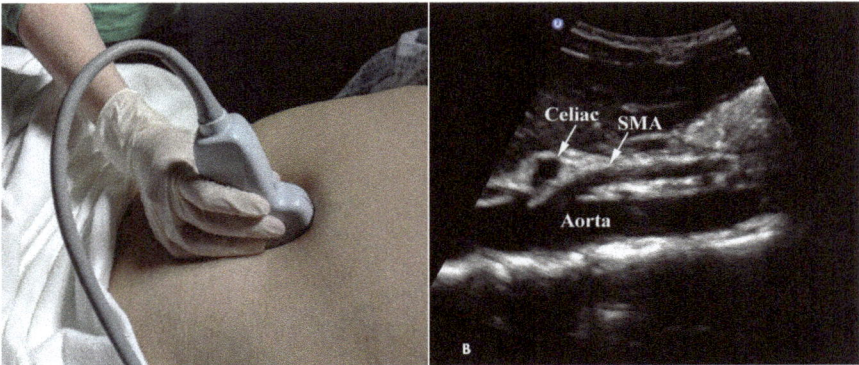

Fig.2.34.6. (A) Ultrasound aorta- Longitudinal probe placement and (B) The SMA is readily seen, together with the lumbar vertebral bodies and discs in the background.

3. IVC View (Longitudinal View)

Then, move the probe slightly over to the right to view the inferior vena cava (IVC) in the longitudinal section. Viewing the IVC as it passes through the diaphragm can give an indication of the load on the right side of the heart.

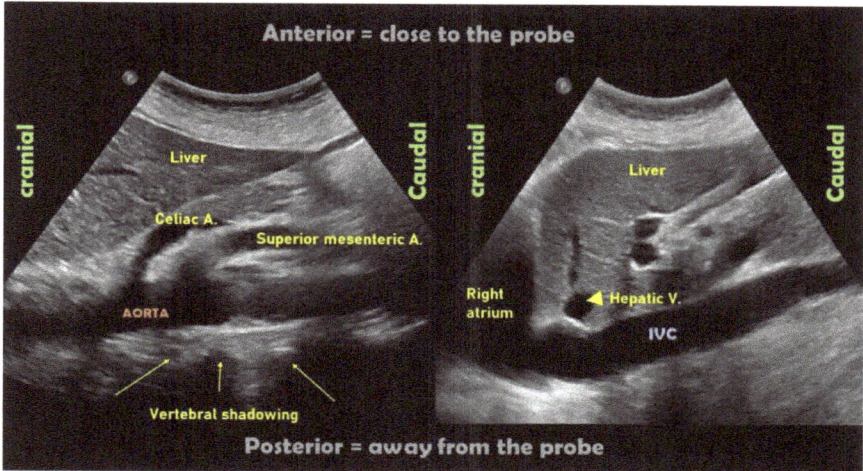

Fig.2.34.7. Aorta vs IVC. Note that: Aorta has anterior branches and is in front of the vertebral column; IVC joins the right atrium and the hepatic vein joins the IVC.
Credit - Renal fellow

IVC view interpretation:

- **The patient is not ventilated:**
  - IVC diameter (IVCD) is >2,5cm with minimal collapse, this suggests an increased right atrial pressure (RAP) seeing in Cor Pulmonale and fluid overload.
  - IVC diameter (IVCD) of <1,5cm with complete collapse is suggestive of being underfilled.
- **The patient is ventilated:**
  - The correlation between the IVCD and RAP is less reliable. Any diameter > 1,2cm appear to have no predictive value of RAP, whereas diameters below 1,2cm may.
  - An IVCD that is seen to vary throughout the respiratory cycle has been associated with fluid responsiveness, whereas minimally varying IVCD has been associated with less fluid responsiveness.

4. Anteroposterior Diameter of the Aorta

Lastly, evaluate the anteroposterior diameter of the aorta. The measurements should be from outer wall to outer wall of the vessel. Any clot or false lumen should be ignored when measuring. The apparent luminal diameter of the aorta should be estimated in both transverse and sagittal orientations. The surrounding soft tissue does not need to be included in the measurement.

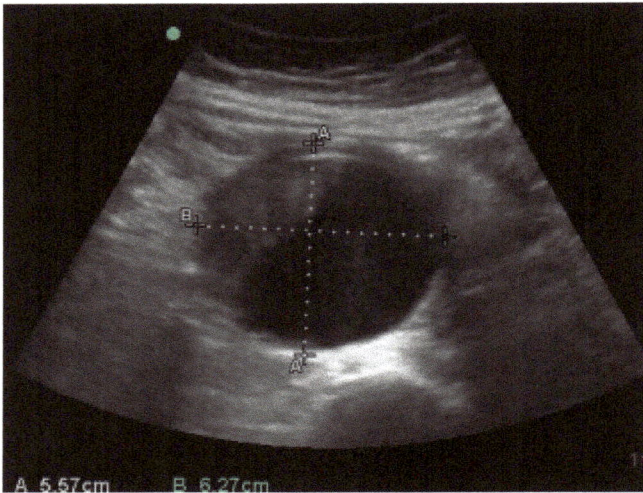

Fig.2.34.8. Correct measurement of an aneurysmal abdominal aorta, considering the luminal thrombus in both the AP and lateral measurements.

If the patient has AAA, measurements should consider the true lumen, including the area with plaque/clot rather than just the patent inner channel where there is blood flow. Any segment with a 3cm or more diameter should be considered aneurysmal. It is essential to obtain an accurate outer-layer-to-outer-layer measurement of the aorta in a plane perpendicular to the long axis of the vessel." This "outer to outer" recommendation is intended to ensure that the sonographer includes any plaque and/or thrombus in the measurement as described above. It is careful not to include large amounts of adjacent soft tissue within the callipers as it may lead to wildly exaggerated measurements of completely normal aortas.

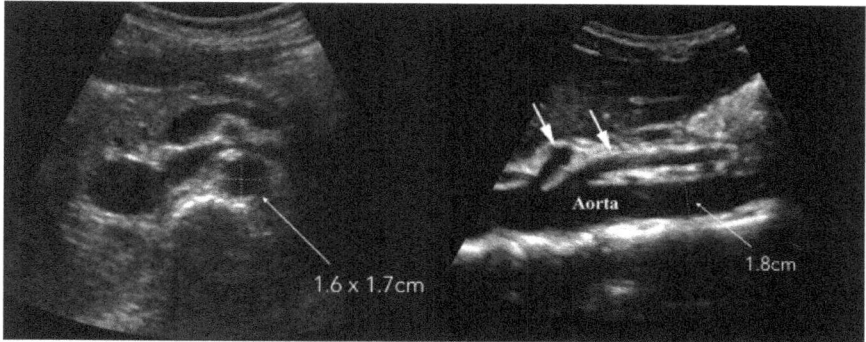

Fig.2.34.9. Correct AP and lateral measurements in a transverse view (left) and correct AP measurement in a sagittal view in a normal aorta.

The bottom line is that if there is an AAA, include any thrombus and plaque. If the aorta is entirely normal, it is impossible to differentiate the separate layers of the vessel, measure the apparent diameter as shown below, and the whole outer-to-outer thing is irrelevant.

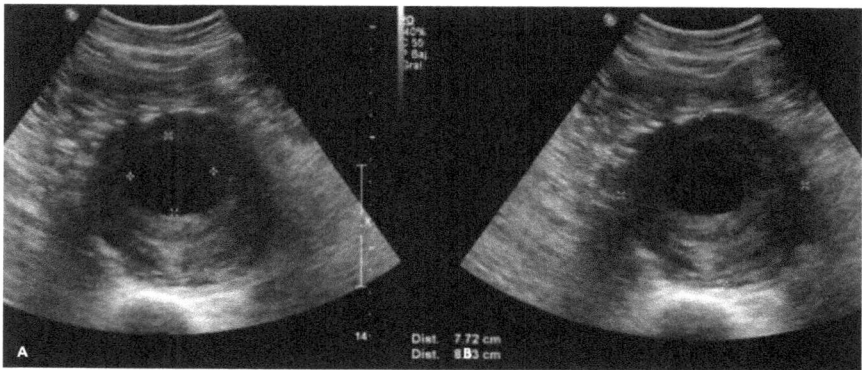

Fig.2.34.10. Left: Measurement of only the patent inner channel of an AAA. Right shows the correct measurement of the AAA.

Further reading

Cardioserv - Abdominal Ultrasound for Echocardiographers: Aorta and IVC: https://www.cardioserv.net/aorta-and-ivc-ultrasound/

References

ACEP Now. (2010). Bedside Ultrasound of the Abdominal Aorta. ACEP Now. https://www.acepnow.com/article/bedside-ultrasound-abdominal-aorta/3/?singlepage=1

Bengtsson, H., Bergqvist, D., Ekberg, O., & Janzon, L. (1991). A population based screening of abdominal aortic aneurysms (AAA). Eur J Vasc Surg, 5(1), 53-57. https://doi.org/10.1016/s0950-821x(05)80927-2

Kent, K. C., Zwolak, R. M., Egorova, N. N., Riles, T. S., Manganaro, A., Moskowitz, A. J., . . . Greco, G. (2010). Analysis of risk factors for abdominal aortic aneurysm in a cohort of more than 3 million individuals. J Vasc Surg, 52(3), 539-548. https://doi.org/10.1016/j.jvs.2010.05.090

Rahimi, S. (2021). Abdominal Aortic Aneurysm Workup. Medscape. Retrieved 06 Nov. 2021 from https://emedicine.medscape.com/article/1979501-workup

Shaw, P., Loree, J., & Gibbons, R. (2021). Abdominal Aortic Aneurysm. Statpearls. Retrieved 15 Nov. 2021 from https://www.ncbi.nlm.nih.gov/books/NBK470237/

Zommorodi, S., Leander, K., Roy, J., Steuer, J., & Hultgren, R. (2018). Understanding abdominal aortic aneurysm epidemiology: socioeconomic position affects outcome. J Epidemiol Community Health, 72(10), 904-910. https://doi.org/10.1136/jech-2018-210644

| 35 |

Ultrasound Guided Vascular Access

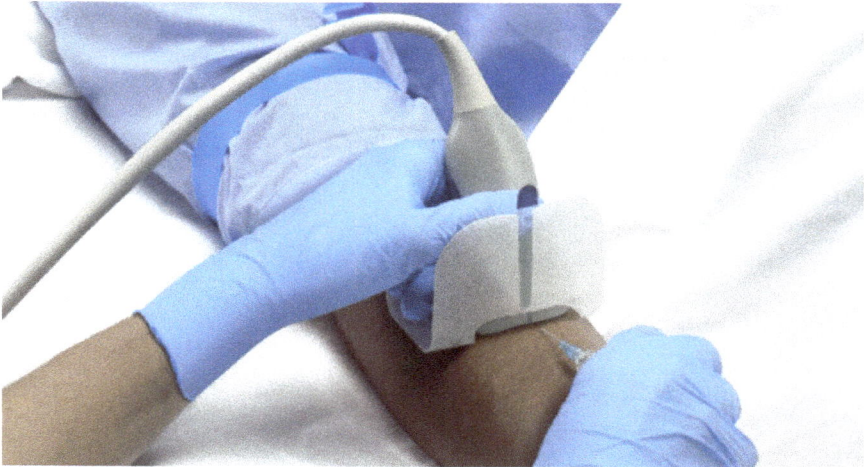

Overview

Venous and arterial cannulations are standard practices in critically ill patients worldwide. Establishing venous access is a crucial skill for the emergency physician but, this can sometimes be challenging. Although vascular accesses are generally performed using the anatomical landmark technique, this approach is not exempt from failures and complications.

The use of ultrasound to guide catheter placement is recommended to minimise complications, improve first-pass success, lessen the number of attempts, and enhance patient satisfaction (Troianos et al., 2012). Ultrasound guidance is indicated for central and peripheral venous catheters (Pittiruti et al., 2009).

Despite known advantages, ultrasound is less frequently used in the ED for other vascular applications, probably because these are technically challenging and demand additional experience (Reusz & Csomos, 2015). This module will master the reader's approach in guiding the needle into a vein, optimising the acquisition of the image, selecting the suitable vessel, using the correct infection prevention method and the best way of securing the device to cannulate the patient in the emergency department successfully.

Technique and Ultrasonographic Vascular Anatomy

Probe selection

Vascular structures being superficial, a linear array transducer (7–10MHz) is typically recommended to identify the vessels (Blanco, 2016).

2D vs 3D views

Two-dimensional imaging is mainly used, both in the short and long axis of the vessels. Occasionally, colour and spectral Doppler can be used. Three-dimensional ultrasound is barely used and is not recommended in practice for vascular cannulation (Blanco, 2016).

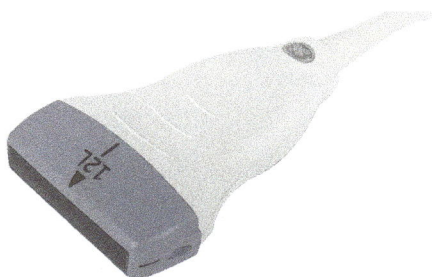

Fig.2.35.1. Linear probe

Probe orientation

- **Short-axis views:**
  - The probe indicator is pointed toward the operator's left side.

        ◦ The left side of the screen matches the operator's left side.
- **Long-axis views:**
  - ◦ The probe is rotated 90° clockwise from the latter position.
  - ◦ The left side of the screen matches the probe end located furthest from the operator.

Probe manipulation

Resting the medial edge and/or the transducer operator's fingers on the patient is the most acceptable method to control the transducer from unintentionally slipping (Blanco, 2016).

Depth, gain and focus

Depth, gain, and focal zones are the most important machine parameters that practitioners always need to optimize to carry out the best possible evaluation on the vessels (Blanco, 2016).

Preferably, tissue harmonic imaging must be switched off, especially for further needle recognition.

Artery vs Vein

- **Short-axis views:**
  - ◦ The veins are more oval than round, have an anechoic content, their walls are thin, they are fully compressible and, lastly, they are not pulsatile.
  - ◦ The arteries are round, also have an anechoic content, have a thicker wall in comparison with veins, are poorly compressible and, lastly, they have pulsatility.
- **Long-axis views:**
  - ◦ The vessels appear tubular.
  - ◦ Valves can sometimes be observed in the veins, with the corresponding normal opening and closing movements.

- Arteries lack valves.
- In some cases, when a proximal tourniquet is applied in the veins, stagnant blood, also called rouleaux, can be observed as internal mobile echoes within the vein, fully cleared when compressed with the transducer (Blanco, 2016).

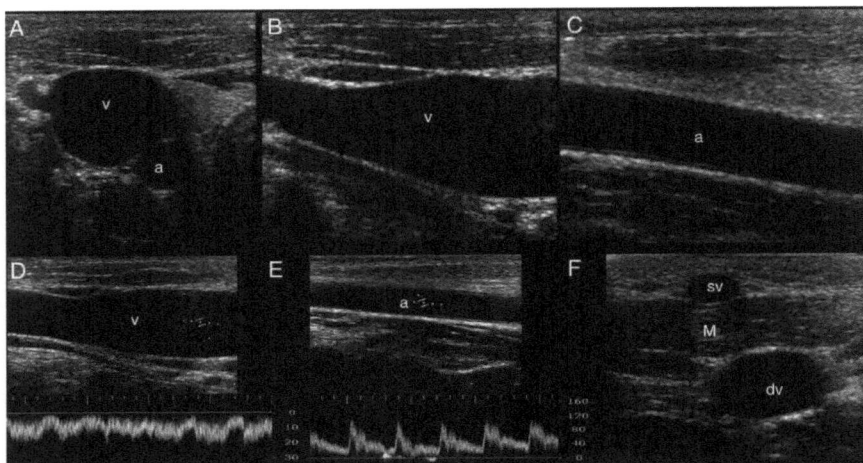

Fig.2.35.2. Vascular ultrasound. Long and short-axis views

- **Colour and spectral Doppler:**
  - Veins have a phasic flow (having augmentation with distal compression),
  - Superficial veins are found above the deep fascia and muscle, and they are not accompanied by arteries (Blanco, 2016).
  - Deep veins are located below the deep fascia and are always accompanied by arteries (and nerves) in the neurovascular bundle.
  - Arterial flow is pulsatile.

Ultrasound mapping before cannulation

After recognising the vascular structures, the next step is selecting an adequate vessel to be successfully cannulated. Ultrasonographic criteria for an optimal selection of a target vessel (Blanco, 2016):

- As superficial as possible
- Guaranteeing a safe pathway (far away from key structures, such as the pleura)
- Patent vessels (rule out a thrombosed vein or artery)
- Absence of atheromatous plaques in the selected site (arteries)
- Absence of valves in the selected site (veins)
- Central veins: anteroposterior diameter≥7mm
- Peripheral veins: anteroposterior diameter≥4mm; skin to vessel distance: <=16mm (longer catheters 8–20cm can still be used if the vessel has an appropriate size but the skin to vessel distance is >16mm)

Central Venous Accesses

- **Deep veins providing access to the superior vena cava:**
  - Internal jugular vein (IJV) - accompanied by the common carotid artery (CCA) in the neck),
  - Subclavian and axillary veins (accompanied by the corresponding subclavian and axillary arteries).
- **Deep veins providing access to the inferior vena cava:**
  - Common femoral vein (CFV)-accompanied by the common femoral artery (CFA) in the groin provide access to the inferior vena cava.

Internal Jugular Vein

Before proceeding, ensure sterile preparations and assessment of the IJ vein to evaluate the anatomy and patency and determine the size and location of access. The operator is positioned at the head of the bed, with the ultrasound screen facing the operator. Place the patient in the

Trendelenburg position to maximise the IJ vein size and minimise the possibility of air embolism (Bellazzini et al., 2009). If a patient is co-operative, attempt Valsalva or humming manoeuvres to increase the IJ vein size (Lewin et al., 2007). Minimise head rotation. In a transverse or short-axis view, the probe indicator should be oriented to the operator's left, corresponding to the left of the patient and the left side of the screen as it is viewed. Choose the correct site where the IJ vein is lateral to the carotid artery, as close as possible to the skin's surface.

Anterior approach: Insert the needle at the triangle's apex created by the sternal and clavicular heads of the sternocleidomastoid muscle. A posterior approach may also be used. Note the distance from the skin surface to the centre of the vessel, accounting for the angle of the needle pass to determine how far from the probe the needle should enter the skin. If it is impossible to avoid IJ vein and carotid artery overlap, an angle of approach should be chosen so that if the needle penetrates the IJ vein posteriorly, it will not enter the carotid artery (Blaivas & Adhikari, 2009). Once a backflow is noticed, place the probe aside on the sterile field to continue with the procedure. Advance the guidewire and correct positioning may be assisted by ultrasound visualisation (Moak et al., 2011).

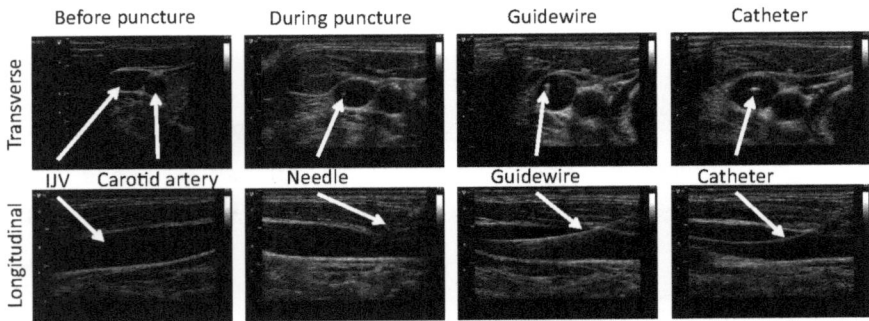

Fig. 2.35.3. Transverse and longitudinal ultrasonographic views during catheter placement of internal jugular vein (IJV). Note that in the longitudinal view, the carotid artery is not visualised simultaneously with the jugular vein.

Once the catheter is secured, perform a post-procedure assessment using ultrasound by visualising the heart's right atrium with a saline flush to determine central venous placement. Lung sliding may also be assessed using ultrasound to help demonstrate the absence of pneumothorax (Vezzani et al., 2010).

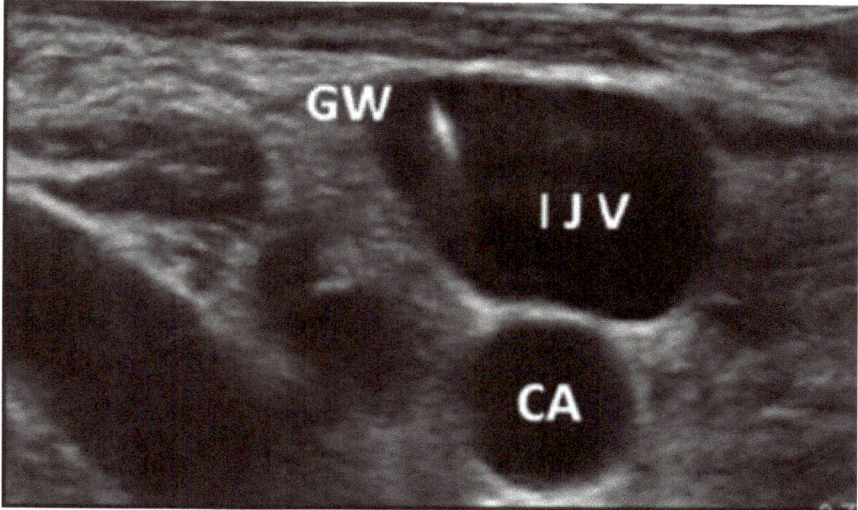

Fig.2.35.4. Short axis views of the internal jugular vein and surrounding

Subclavian & Axillary Veins

From an anatomical point of view, the subclavian vein is located under the clavicle (e.g., infraclavicular region); the axillary vein is in continuum with the subclavian vein, lateral to the outer border of the first rib at the teres major muscle (AIUM Practice Guidelines, 2012). The subclavian vein is accessed from a supraclavicular or an infraclavicular approach (the latter is the most common technique) (Rezayat et al., 2016). The main problem when cannulating this vein is the presence of the clavicle bone, which interferes with the probe positioning and fundamentally with the optimal view of this vessel.

In that respect, many practitioners who gain confidence with subclavian vein cannulation move more laterally and puncture the skin at the midclavicular point (Blanco, 2016). This probably means performing skin puncture over the axillary vein, but the subclavian or axillary vein may be punctured depending on the distance between the skin and the vein puncture sites. Uncertainties related to the utility of the subclavian vein cannulation are likely to be derived from the ambiguity implied by whether studies of US-guided access in this area refer to direct subclavian vein access or subclavian vein access via the axillary vein. As previously mentioned, the long axis (in-plane) technique is preferred when cannulating these veins since it is associated with high success rates and fewer complications.

The Trendelenburg position does not seem to improve venous distention of this vessel because it is in a relatively fixed position within the surrounding tissues. However, it reduces the risks of air embolism and thus, it is always recommended. In addition, evaluating the lung sliding before and after cannulating these vessels is recommended since it quickly detects the presence of pneumothorax (Blanco, 2016).

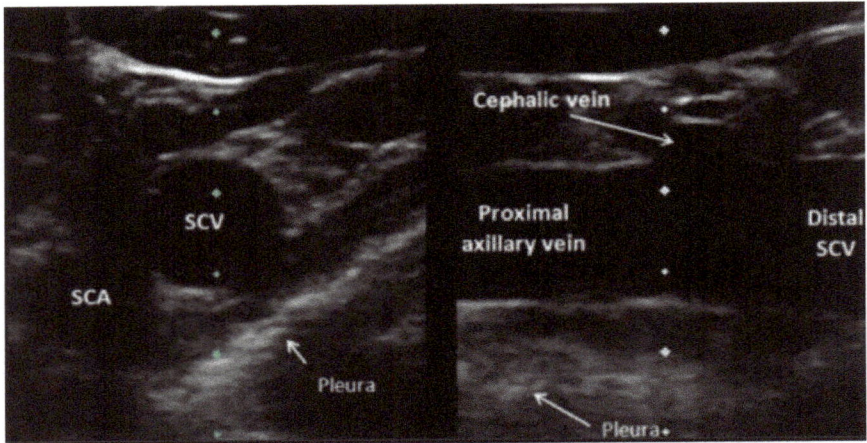

Fig.2.35.5. Short axis view of the subclavian vein using ultrasound vascular access

Common Femoral Vein (CFV)

CFV is in the femoral triangle below the inguinal ligament and medial to the common femoral artery (CFA) and femoral nerve in the neurovascular bundle. It originates from the junction of the deep femoral vein and femoral vein and receives the great saphenous vein. While

CFV is usually cannulated using the anatomical landmark technique because of the relatively constant location of the vein related to the artery at a safe entry point closer to the inguinal ligament (2–4cm); however, US guidance has demonstrated an 85% reduction in the rate of catheterization failure and an 86% reduction in arterial puncture rates (Blanco, 2016). Thus, US-guided femoral cannulation is recommended over the landmark technique and can be especially helpful in some circumstances, such as in obese patients, when arterial pulses are weak (e.g., the patient is in shock) or when there are anatomical alterations.

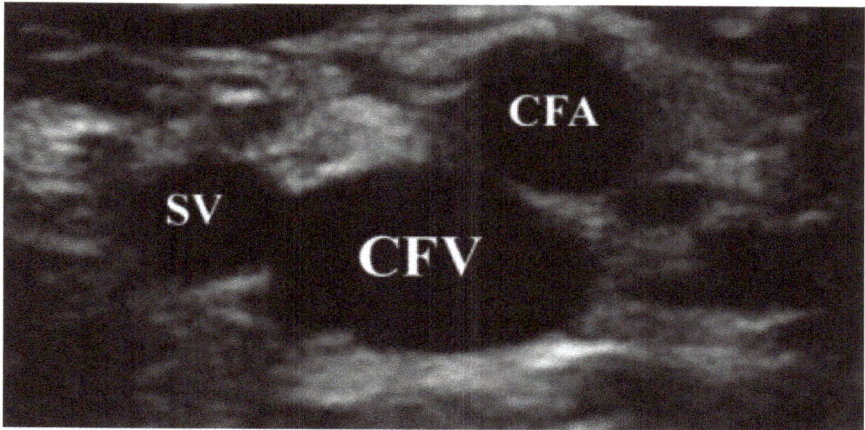

Fig.2.35.6. Mickey Mouse Sign. CFA: Common Femoral Artery, SV: Saphenous Vein and CFV: Common Femoral Vein

This vein is easily recognised medial to the CFA and receives the great saphenous vein. These structures are called the **"Mickey Mouse" sign** in the short axis. CFV is more distended when the hip has a slight external rotation and in the reverse Trendelenburg position. The vein receives the great saphenous vein in the long axis, and its bifurcation is distal to the CFA bifurcation (Blanco, 2016).

Peripheral Veins

Peripheral venous catheters are usually placed using the anatomical landmark technique. However, some patients are difficult or impossible to cannulate, for example, because they are obese, dehydrated, intravenous drug users or have prior multiple vein catheterizations. Therefore, US-guided peripheral venous cannulation can be first considered in this subgroup of patients. Superficial veins suited for US-guided cannulation are commonly found in the arms.

Two main veins are recognized: a lateral one, located in both the upper arm and the forearm, called the cephalic vein, which finally drains into the axillary vein; and a medial vein, called the basilic vein, which after running in the forearm and reaching the upper arm, it becomes deeper and joins the humeral veins and other tributaries to conform the axillary vein.

Tributaries of both main veins are also visible, including the connection between the cephalic and the basilic vein (median cubital vein) at the elbow. Basilic and cephalic veins also provide access to the superior vena cava through placing a peripherally inserted central catheter (PICC). Another peripheral vein able to be US-guided cannulated is the external jugular vein in the neck. Finally, peripheral deep veins for US-guided cannulation are the paired humeral veins located at both sides of the humeral artery (Blanco, 2016).

Radial Artery

Radial artery emerges from the bifurcation of the brachial artery at the elbow crease and is found in the lateral side of the distal forearm near the wrist, where it becomes more superficial and easier to palpate. Accordingly, this artery is usually well recognised by US and accessed from its distal ventral and more superficial segment. This vessel is accompanied by the paired radial veins located at both sides of the artery. Applying a tourniquet distal to the cannulation site has been shown to improve the arterial dimensions, and thus this manoeuvre can be considered in practice when the artery is too small.

Additionally, the radial artery can be recognised and cannulated using US in its dorsal segment, found in the anatomical snuffbox. This can be considered as a valid alternative when the more proximal radial artery cannot be accessed.

Finally, the permeability of the palmar arch must be assessed before cannulating this artery. This can be performed using the modified Allen test, plethysmographic Allen test or modified duplex Allen test (Barbeau et al., 2004).

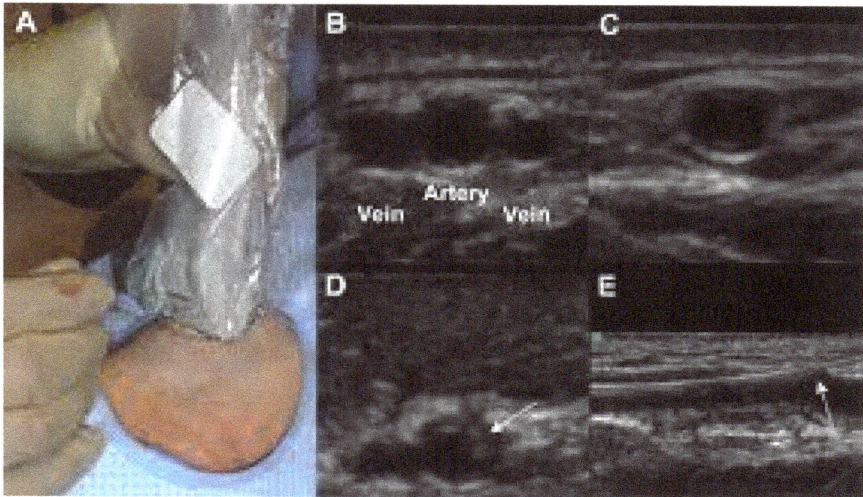

Fig.2.35.7. Real-Time Ultrasound Guidance Facilitates Trans-radial Access
Credit - JACC: Cardiovascular Interventions

The last one is done by placing the transducer in the anatomical snuffbox and identifying the radial artery flow by colour and spectral Doppler. After spectral waveforms are obtained, the radial artery is compressed proximal to the site of insonation. Normally, reversal of flow confirms patency of the deep palmar arch. Otherwise, an inadequate deep palmar arch is suspected, and thus, this artery is best avoided for cannulation.

Femoral Artery

As previously described, CFA is in the femoral triangle, lateral to the CFV and medial to the femoral nerve in the neurovascular bundle. 20% of the patients have a CFA bifurcation above the inferior border of the femoral head. Too high punctures may lead to retroperitoneal haemorrhage, while punctures below the femoral head may lead to pseudoaneurysm formation.

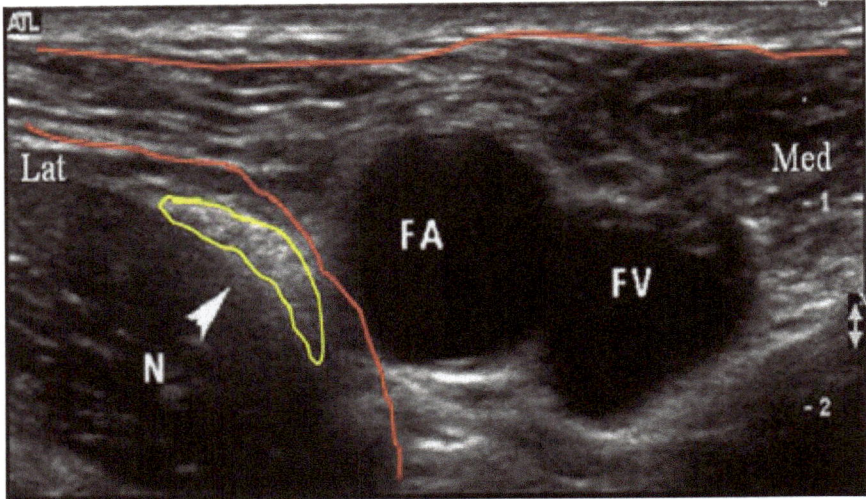

Fig.2.35.8. US of femoral anatomy. FA femoral artery, FV femoral Vein

Also, too low punctures may damage the superficial and the deep femoral arteries, an important complication that may lead to significant haemorrhage since these arteries are difficult to compress in thigh soft tissues. There is some overlapping between the CFA and CFV in 65% of the patients; therefore, an arteriovenous fistula formation can occur if an inadvertent posterior wall perforation occurs. In a recent meta-analysis including 719 patients with US-guided femoral arterial cannulation performed, a 44% reduced overall complication rate was noted compared to the landmark technique.

Furthermore, a 42% improvement in first-pass success was demonstrated. Thus, US-guided cannulation can be recommended as a first-line tool to place a femoral artery catheter safely.

Further reading

ESEM Ultrasound - Basic US Course: Ultrasound guided vascular Access: https://www.youtube.com/watch?v=hpdbxpiVDvo

Jason T Nomura - Ultrasound Guided Peripheral Access: https://www.youtube.com/watch?v=6jMo4c_WShs

References

AIUM Practice Guidelines. (2012). AIUM Practice Guideline for the use of Ultrasound to Guide Vascular Access Procedures. AIUM Practice Guidelines. Retrieved 27 Dec. 2021 from https://www.aana.com/docs/default-source/practice-aana-com-web-documents-(all)/use-of-ultrasound-to-guide-vascular-access-procedures.pdf?sfvrsn=acfc48b1_2

Barbeau, G. R., Arsenault, F., Dugas, L., Simard, S., & Larivière, M. M. (2004). Evaluation of the ulnopalmar arterial arches with pulse oximetry and plethysmography: comparison with the Allen's test in 1010 patients. Am Heart J, 147(3), 489-493. https://doi.org/10.1016/j.ahj.2003.10.038

Bellazzini, M. A., Rankin, P. M., Gangnon, R. E., & Bjoernsen, L. P. (2009). Ultrasound validation of maneuvers to increase internal jugular vein cross-sectional area and decrease compressibility. Am J Emerg Med, 27(4), 454-459. https://doi.org/10.1016/j.ajem.2008.03.034

Blaivas, M., & Adhikari, S. (2009). An unseen danger: frequency of posterior vessel wall penetration by needles during attempts to place internal jugular vein central catheters using ultrasound guidance. Crit Care Med, 37(8), 2345-2349; quiz 2359. https://doi.org/10.1097/CCM.0b013e3181a067d4

Blanco, P. (2016). Ultrasound-guided vascular cannulation in critical care patients: A practical review. medicina intensiva, 40(9), 560-571 https://doi.org/10.1016/j.medine.2016.07.002

Lewin, M. R., Stein, J., Wang, R., Lee, M. M., Kernberg, M., Boukhman, M., . . . Lewiss, R. E. (2007). Humming is as effective as Valsalva's maneuver and Trendelenburg's position for ultrasonographic visualization of the jugular venous system and common femoral veins. Ann Emerg Med, 50(1), 73-77. https://doi.org/10.1016/j.annemergmed.2007.01.024

Moak, J. H., Lyons, M. S., Wright, S. W., & Lindsell, C. J. (2011). Needle and guidewire visualization in ultrasound-guided internal jugular vein cannulation. Am J Emerg Med, 29(4), 432-436. https://doi.org/10.1016/j.ajem.2010.01.004

Pittiruti, M., Hamilton, H., Biffi, R., MacFie, J., & Pertkiewicz, M. (2009). ESPEN Guidelines on Parenteral Nutrition: central venous catheters (access, care, diagnosis and therapy of complications). Clin Nutr, 28(4), 365-377. https://doi.org/10.1016/j.clnu.2009.03.015

Reusz, G., & Csomos, A. (2015). The role of ultrasound guidance for vascular access. Curr Opin Anaesthesiol, 28(6), 710-716. https://doi.org/10.1097/aco.0000000000000245

Rezayat, T., Stowell, J. R., Kendall, J. L., Turner, E., Fox, J. C., & Barjaktarevic, I. (2016). Ultrasound-Guided Cannulation: Time to Bring Subclavian Central Lines Back. West J Emerg Med, 17(2), 216-221. https://doi.org/10.5811/westjem.2016.1.29462

Troianos, C. A., Hartman, G. S., Glas, K. E., Skubas, N. J., Eberhardt, R. T., Walker, J. D., & Reeves, S. T. (2012). Special articles: guidelines for performing ultrasound guided vascular cannulation: recommendations of the American Society of Echocardiography and the Society Of Cardiovascular Anesthesiologists. Anesth Analg, 114(1), 46-72. https://doi.org/10.1213/ANE.0b013e3182407cd8

Vezzani, A., Brusasco, C., Palermo, S., Launo, C., Mergoni, M., & Corradi, F. (2010). Ultrasound localization of central vein catheter and detection of postprocedural pneumothorax: an alternative to chest radiography. Crit Care Med, 38(2), 533-538. https://doi.org/10.1097/CCM.0b013e3181c0328f

| 36 |

Ultrasound Guided Femoral Nerve Block

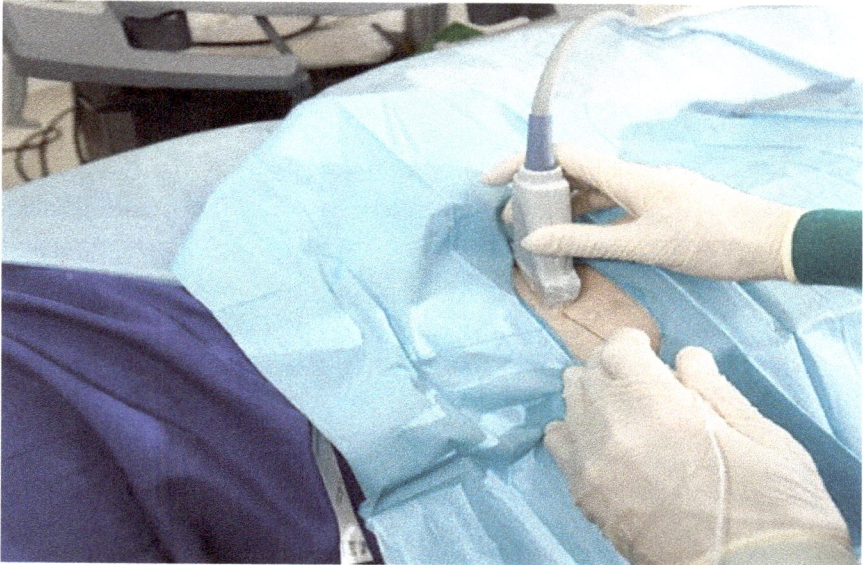

Overview

The femoral nerve is one of the major branches of the lumbar plexus. It is invariably lateral to the femoral artery, deep to the fascia iliaca and superficial to the iliopsoas muscle (USRA, 2020). Limb blocks can assist with practical and lengthy analgesia for major lower limb trauma (Neck of femur fracture) and surgery. Therefore, precise needle placement and drug delivery are the keys to success with nerve blocks (Munirama & McLeod, 2013). The use of ultrasound has enabled more rapid block onset (Perlas et al., 2008) and lengthy block duration (Oberndorfer et al., 2007) with the added advantages of a decrease in drug dosage and a lowering in the incidence of local anaesthetic toxicity (Latzke et al., 2010).

The ultrasound-guided technique of the femoral nerve blockade offers the advantage to the emergency physician to monitor the spread of local anaesthetic, the progress of the needle and make reasonable adjustments to achieve the expected disposition of the local anaesthetic. Furthermore, US also may decrease the risk of femoral artery puncture (Atchabahian et al., 2020). This module will provide you with the necessary knowledge and skills to enhance your ability to safely perform an ultrasound-guided femoral nerve block in the emergency department.

Indications

- A femoral nerve block with or without a perineural infusion to provide continuous pain relief after fractures of the femoral shaft.
- It may also provide a useful analgesic adjunct for femoral neck fractures.
- It is also indicated for knee replacement surgery, and skin grafts from the anterior thigh.

Equipment

The equipment needed for a femoral nerve block includes the following (Atchabahian et al., 2020):

- Ultrasound machine with linear transducer (8–18 MHz), sterile sleeve, and gel
- Standard nerve block tray
- One 20-mL syringe containing local anaesthetic
- A 50- to 100-mm, 22-gauge, short-bevel, insulated stimulating needle
- Peripheral nerve stimulator
- Injection pressure monitor
- Sterile gloves

Ultrasound Anatomy

Position the patient supine with the leg in the neutral position. Expose the groin and mark the inguinal crease. After skin and transducer preparation, place a transducer with the appropriate frequency range (10-12 MHz) along the inguinal crease. Suppose the femoral artery and nerve are deep (> 4 cm, use a 7 MHZ transducer). Optimize machine imaging capability; appropriate select depth of field (usually within 1-3 cm), focus range and gain (USRA, 2020). The ultrasound machine should be positioned on the opposite side so that the clinician's line of sight, needle, and screen is in a straight line (Munirama & McLeod, 2013). Medial to lateral sliding motions of the transducer aid visualisation of the pulsatile femoral artery. Visible structures are the fascia iliaca, femoral artery, and immediately below and lateral, the femoral nerve in a wedge-shaped space.

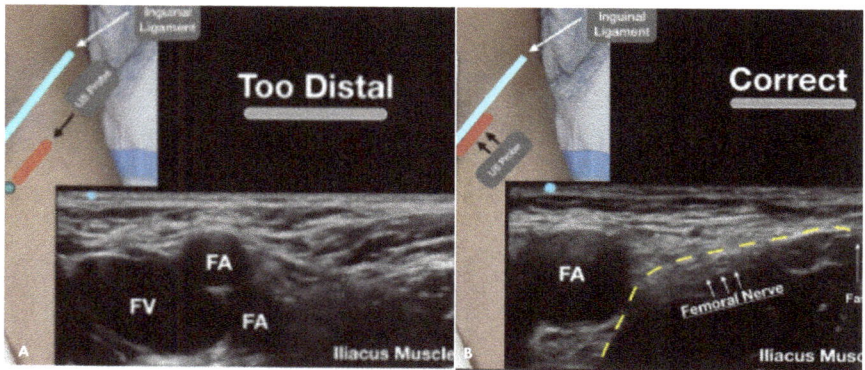

Fig.2.36.1. Ultrasound anatomy of the femoral nerve. Left-too distal, Right- correct probe position. FA = femoral artery, FN = femoral nerve, FV = femoral vein.
Credit - ACEPNow

The vein may not be visible until the transducer pressure on the skin is loosened. Deep to the femoral vessels is the iliopsoas muscle bulk. The femoral nerve is usually located within a triangular hyperechoic region, lateral to the femoral artery and superficial to the iliopsoas muscle. The femoral nerve may be quite thin and flat in this region as the nerve fans out into multiple branches. The fascia iliaca (a hyperechoic line) is superficial to the femoral nerve and its branches. Inguinal lymph nodes also appear hyperechoic and may confound with the nerve in the short axis view. To differentiate the inguinal lymph nodes to the nerve, scan proximally and distally in this region. A *nerve* is a continuous structure that can be traced while a lymph node is not and can be seen only in a discrete location (USRA, 2020).

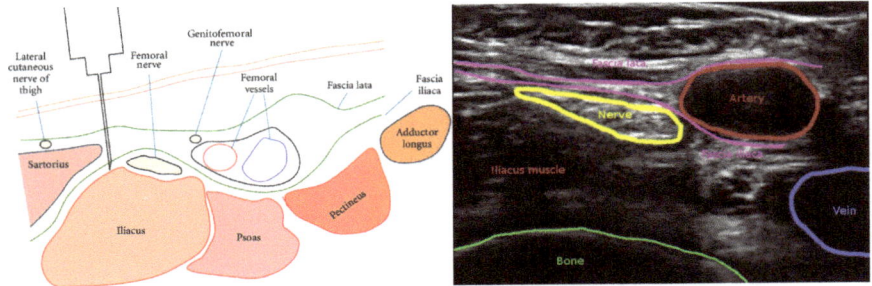

Fig.2.36.2. Ultrasound anatomy of the femoral nerve

Upon identifying the femoral nerve, make a 1cm skin wheal with the local anaesthetic away from the lateral border of the transducer. Insert the needle in-plane, lateral to medial orientation, and move toward the femoral nerve. If nerve stimulation is employed (0.5 mA, 0.1 msec), a motor response of the quadriceps muscle group will be noticed during the progression of the needle through the fascia iliaca and contact of the needle tip with the femoral nerve. Once the needle tip is adjacent (above, below, or lateral) to the nerve, after careful aspiration, 1–2 mL of local anaesthetic is injected to verify the correct needle placement (Atchabahian et al., 2020). The right injection

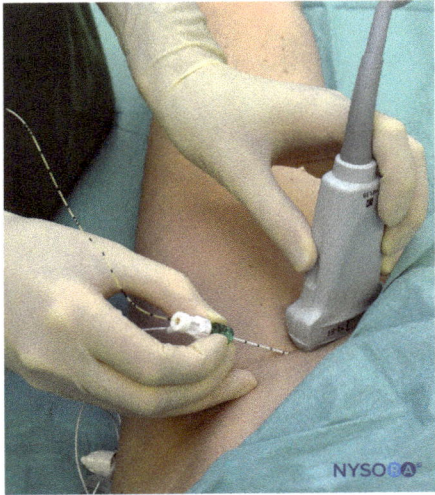

Fig. 2.36.3. Transducer position and needle insertion using an in-plane technique to nerve block the femoral nerve at the femoral crease
Credit - Nysora

will drive the femoral nerve away from the injection. Additional needle repositions and injections are done only when necessary.

Anatomic variations have been described with aberrant positions of the femoral nerve. In an adult patient, 10–15 mL of local anaesthetic is sufficient for an adequate nerve block.

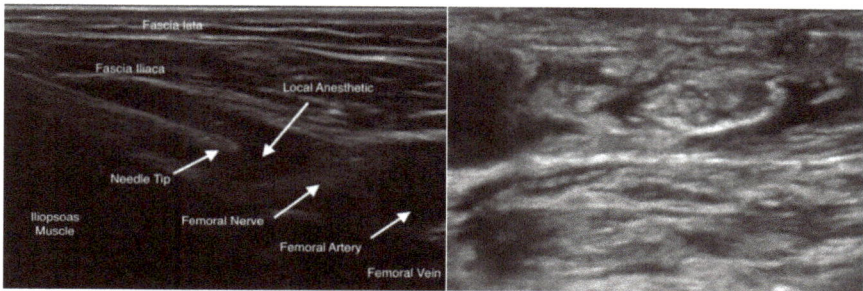

Fig.2.36.4. (A) In-plane needle approach showing the needle in contact with the femoral nerve. Arrowhead = femoral nerve. FA = femoral artery. FV = femoral vein. LA = local anaesthetic and (B) Femoral nerve with doughnut sign outlined after the injection of local anaesthetic.
Credit - WFSA

Further reading

NYSORA- Ultrasound-guided femoral nerve block: https://www.youtube.com/watch?v=tMy978ZwaDU&t=1s

References

Atchabahian, A., Leunen, I., Vandepitte, C., & Lopez, A. M. (2020). Ultrasound-Guided Femoral Nerve Block. Nysora. Retrieved 27 Dec. 2021 from https://www.nysora.com/techniques/lower-extremity/ultrasound-guided-femoral-nerve-block/

Latzke, D., Marhofer, P., Zeitlinger, M., Machata, A., Neumann, F., Lackner, E., & Kettner, S. C. (2010). Minimal local anaesthetic volumes for sciatic nerve block: evaluation of ED 99 in volunteers. Br J Anaesth, 104(2), 239-244. https://doi.org/10.1093/bja/aep368

Munirama, S., & McLeod, G. (2013). Ultrasound-guided femoral and sciatic nerve blocks. Continuing Education in Anaesthesia Critical Care & Pain, 13(4), 136-140. https://doi.org/10.1093/bjaceaccp/mkt005

Oberndorfer, U., Marhofer, P., Bösenberg, A., Willschke, H., Felfernig, M., Weintraud, M., . . . Kettner, S. C. (2007). Ultrasonographic guidance for sciatic and femoral nerve blocks in children. Br J Anaesth, 98(6), 797-801. https://doi.org/10.1093/bja/aem092

Perlas, A., Brull, R., Chan, V. W., McCartney, C. J., Nuica, A., & Abbas, S. (2008). Ultrasound guidance improves the success of sciatic nerve block at the popliteal fossa. Reg Anesth Pain Med, 33(3), 259-265. https://doi.org/10.1016/j.rapm.2007.10.010

USRA. (2020). Femoral Nerve Block. USRA. Retrieved 27 Dec. 2021 from http://www.usra.ca/regional-anesthesia/specific-blocks/lower-limb/femoralnerveblock.php

| 37 |

Deep Vein Thrombosis Ultrasound

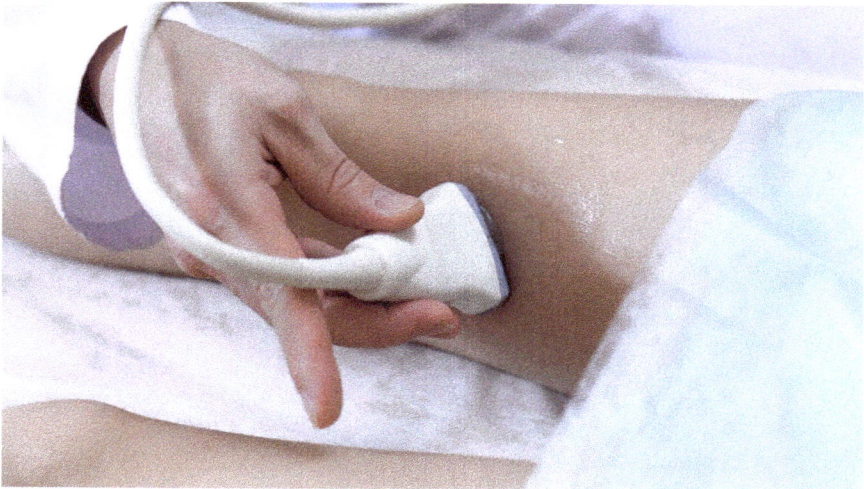

Overview

A lower limb Deep Vein Thrombosis (DVT) might have a significant consequence if gone unnoticed or untreated by the emergency physician because a dislodged clot may lead to a pulmonary embolism and hemodynamic instability (Ahn & Dinh, 2021). Although DVTs generally occur in the lower limbs, they are not uncommon in the upper limb and neck veins (Gaillard & Knipe, 2021).

Venous ultrasound is the standard imaging modality to diagnose DVT (Needleman et al., 2018). In the emergency department, Point of Care Compression Ultrasound is a fast and non-invasive diagnostic approach to assess DVT with very high sensitivity and specificity if conducted by a skilled operator (Burnside et al., 2008).

Objectives

- By the end of this module, you should be able to:
    - Describe the indications and contraindications for a Point of Care Compression Ultrasound for DVT
    - Recall steps needed for a Point of Care Compression Ultrasound for DVT
    - Assess for DVT using Compression, Clot Visualisation, and Colour Doppler Augmentation.
    - Identify DVT Ultrasound False Positives.

Indications

- Any suspicion of DVT (Ahn & Dinh, 2021):
    - Unilateral lower extremity associated with leg pain, tenderness, swelling and erythema
    - Positive Homans' Sign (pain on calf compression during the physical exam)

Contraindications

- Theoretically, a clot may dislodge with compression with a risk of pulmonary embolism (rare) (Lockhart et al., 2005).

Preparation

- The patient is in the supine position
- Leg externally rotated and Knee bent (*Frog Leg position*)

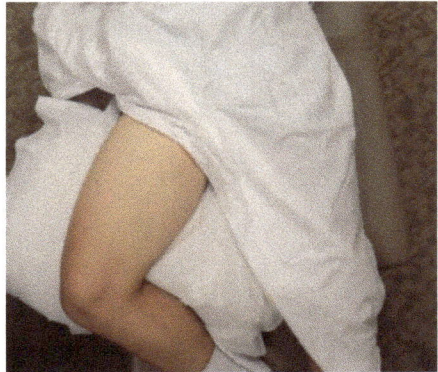

Fig.2.37.1. Frog Leg Position

- Place a pillow under the patient's knee to increase comfort
- Transducer: Linear Ultrasound Probe
- Pre-set: Venous

- Ultrasound Machine Placement: usually on the patient's right side so you can scan with your right hand and manipulate ultrasound controls with your left hand (Ahn & Dinh, 2021).

DVT Ultrasound Anatomy

- The venous anatomy of the lower extremity (Ahn & Dinh, 2021):
  - Common Femoral Vein (CFV)
  - Great Saphenous Vein
  - Bifurcation of CFV into Femoral Vein (formerly called Superficial Femoral Vein) and Deep Femoral Vein
  - Popliteal Vein
  - Trifurcation of the Popliteal Vein
    - Anterior Tibial Vein
    - Posterior Tibial Vein
    - Peroneal Vein

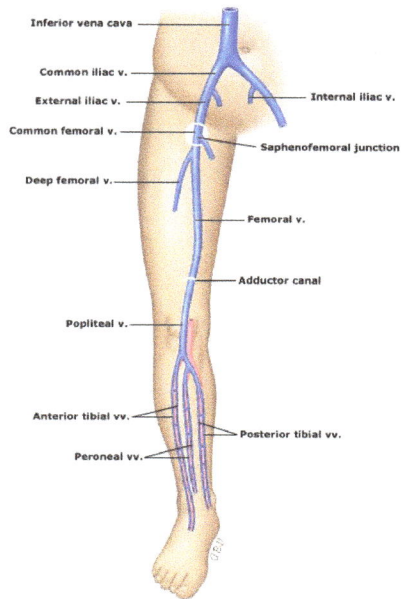

Fig.2.37.2. Tributaries of the Common Femoral Vein
Credit - Uptodate

The **Common Femoral Vein (CFV) is** *the most proximal vessel giving off the great saphenous vein, the deep femoral vein, and a **femoral vein**. The femoral vein enters the adductor canal and passes posterior to the knee to become the **popliteal vein**. The popliteal vein gives rise to three other deep veins: the **anterior tibial vein**, the **posterior tibial vein**, and the **peroneal vein** (Zitek et al., 2016).*

DVT Ultrasound Protocol

- **2-Point Lower Extremity DVT Ultrasound:** This tests the compressibility of the common femoral vein (CFV) and the popliteal vein (PV).
- **3-Point Lower Extremity DVT Ultrasound:** This tests the compressibility of the CFV, superficial femoral vein (SFV), and PV, as well as detects isolated SFV thrombosis of lower extremity DVT.
- **Whole Leg/Complete Lower Extremity DVT Ultrasound:** This scans the leg using compression, colour Doppler, and pulse wave Doppler from the common femoral vein to the ankle while evaluating the calf veins.

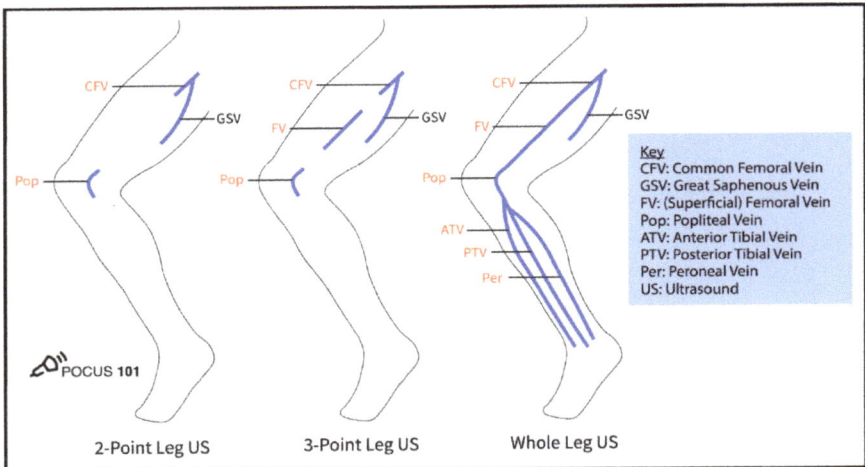

Key
CFV: Common Femoral Vein
GSV: Great Saphenous Vein
FV: (Superficial) Femoral Vein
Pop: Popliteal Vein
ATV: Anterior Tibial Vein
PTV: Posterior Tibial Vein
Per: Peroneal Vein
US: Ultrasound

2-Point Leg US   3-Point Leg US   Whole Leg US

Fig.2.37.3. Different DVT Ultrasound protocols (Ahn & Dinh, 2021)

Vein Compression approach

- The ability to correctly compress a vein during a DVT ultrasound is of great importance to minimise false positives for DVTs. Apply pressure until the pulsatile artery compresses slightly:
  - *The adjacent vein compresses fully, DVT is ruled out.*
  - *The vein does not filly compress, a clot in the area is likely.*

Step 1: Common Femoral Vein Scan

- Place the transducer along the inguinal ligament midway between the pubic symphysis and the anterior superior iliac spine (ASIS).
- Then perpendicularly direct the probe to the skin with the indicator towards the patient's right for a transverse view.
- Locate the common femoral vein and artery (CFV is medial to the CFA).
- A firm pressure should be applied to barely compress the artery
- Normally, this should compress the vein entirely.

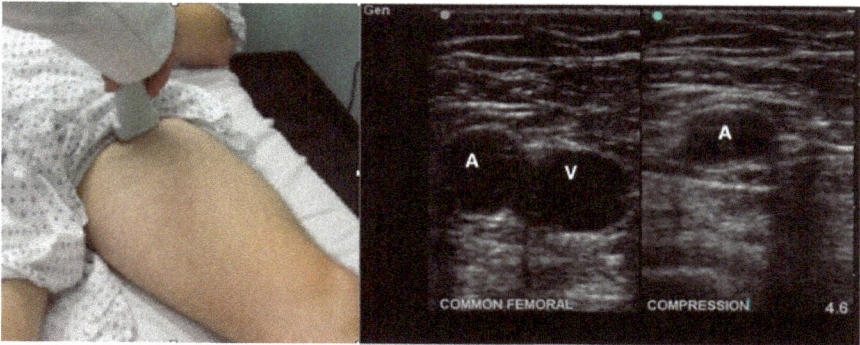

Fig.2.37.4. Transducer location to evaluate the femoral vein and normal ultrasound images showing common femoral artery (A) and fully compressible vein (V)
Credit - AliEMcards

Step 2: Great Saphenous Vein Scan

- The transducer is slid 1-2 cm down to uncover the location where the great saphenous vein branches off the CFV.
- Keep moving the transducer distally, the artery will typically bifurcate first and then the vein.
- At the level of the junction of the CFV with the Great Saphenous Vein, compress the CFV.

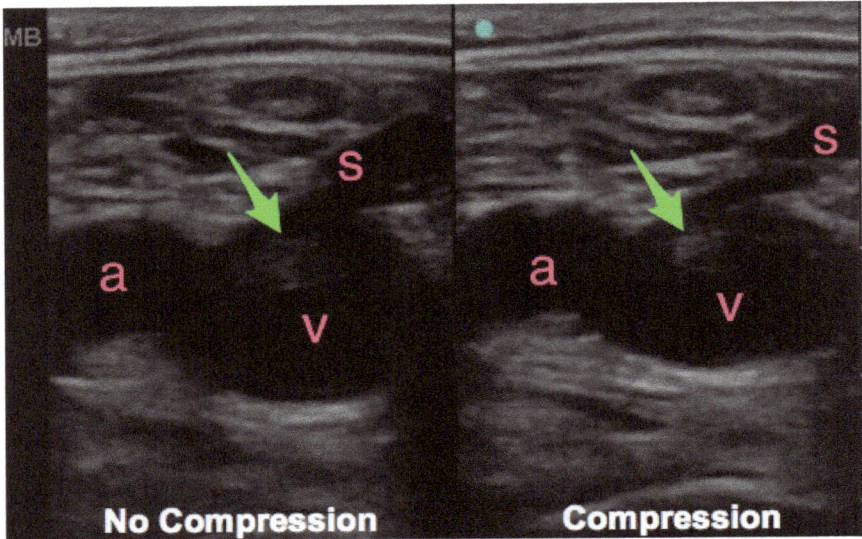

Fig.2.37.5. Positive DVT study showing thrombus in the femoral vein (v), adjacent to the femoral artery (a) and involving the greater saphenous vein (s). The image on the right demonstrates that the vein does not collapse with compression.

Step 3: Superficial Femoral Vein Scan

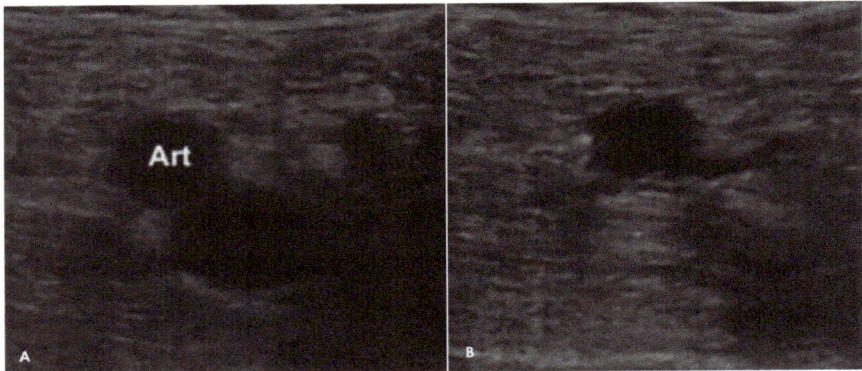

Fig.2.37.6. Normal femoral vein at baseline and acute DVT at 1-week follow-up. A and B, Ultrasound images of a normal femoral vein without (A) and with (B) compression. The artery (Art) is anterior to the vein. After compression, the vein is completely collapsed, indicating normal compressibility
(Needleman et al., 2018)

- The transducer is slid 1-2 cm down to uncover the location where the CFV branches into the deep femoral vein and (superficial) femoral vein.
- At this level, the deep femoral vein will plunge deep into the thigh while the (superficial) femoral vein remains adjacent to the femoral artery.
- Then compress the (superficial) femoral vein just distal to the bifurcation.

Step 4: Popliteal Vein Scan

- Place the linear transducer in transverse position in the popliteal fossa.
- Locate the popliteal artery and vein and assess for compressibility of the vein.

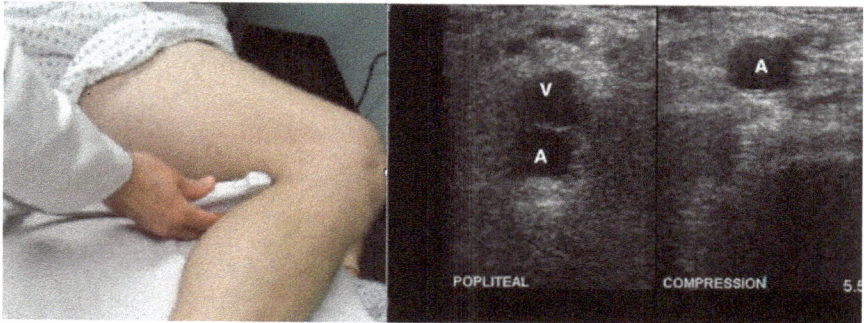

Fig.2.37.7. Transducer location to evaluate the popliteal vein and normal ultrasound images showing popliteal artery (A) and fully compressible vein (V).
Credit - AliEMcards

Step 5: Trifurcation of the Popliteal Vein Scan

- To fully evaluate the popliteal region, slide distally following the popliteal vein to allow for visualisation of the proximal portion of the anterior and posterior tibial veins, and the peroneal vein. At this trifurcation, assess for compressibility of all three veins.
- This junction signals the end of the examination.

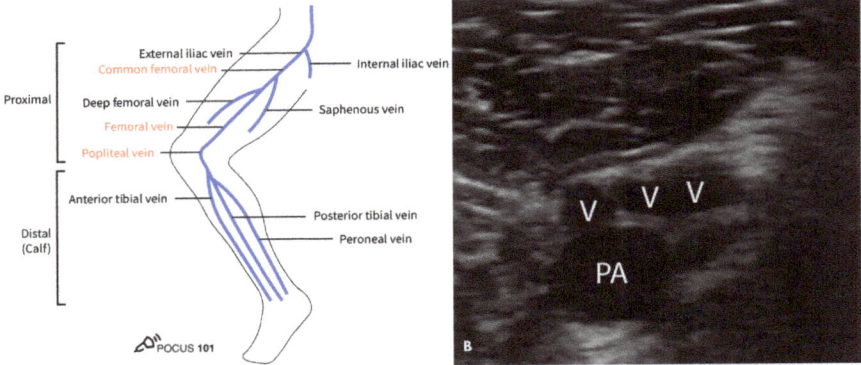

Fig.2.37.8. Popliteal Vein Trifurcation
Credit - POCUS 101

Pathological DVT Ultrasound

- Three ways to detect DVT (Ahn & Dinh, 2021):
    - Direct clot visualisation
    - Non-compressibility of the vein
    - Augmentation with Colour Doppler.

Direct clot Visualisation

Acute thrombi are difficult to visualise as they are anechoic or hypoechoic and often located near the edges of the lumen. An echogenic mass may be seen inside the vessel if the transducer lies over the mass.

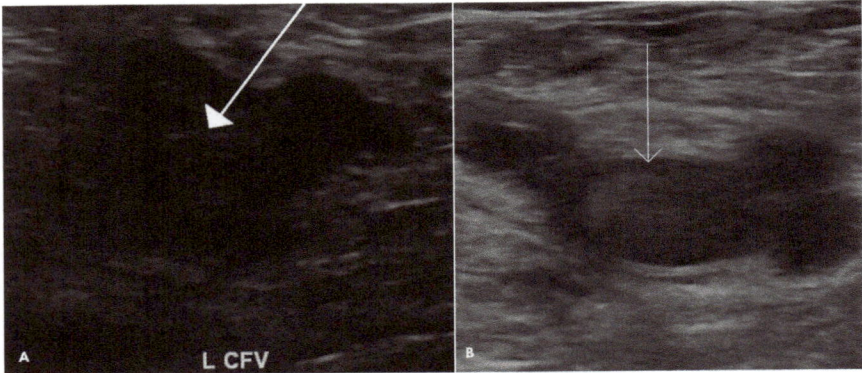

Fig.2.37.9. Direct Clot Visualisation of the left CFV

With time, the thrombi age and evolve from anechoic/hypoechoic to echogenic and retract from the edge of the lumen, rendering it more visible.

When scanning for clots, do not solely rely on direct visualisation, ensure to perform the compression technique to not miss any acute DVTs.

Non-compressibility with ultrasound

Applying gentle pressure with the probe until the artery compresses slightly and the vein compresses totally, is suggestive of DVT at that region. Applying sufficiently to compress the artery while the vein remains not fully compressed is called a "non-compressible" vein and it is suggestive of a clot in that area.

Augmentation with Colour Doppler

Squeezing the leg distal to where you are scanning may increase the venous flow. If Colour Doppler displays a homogenous increase in venous flow, this indicates the absence of an occlusive thrombus between where you are pressing and scanning. The absence of a raised venous flow could suggest a DVT.

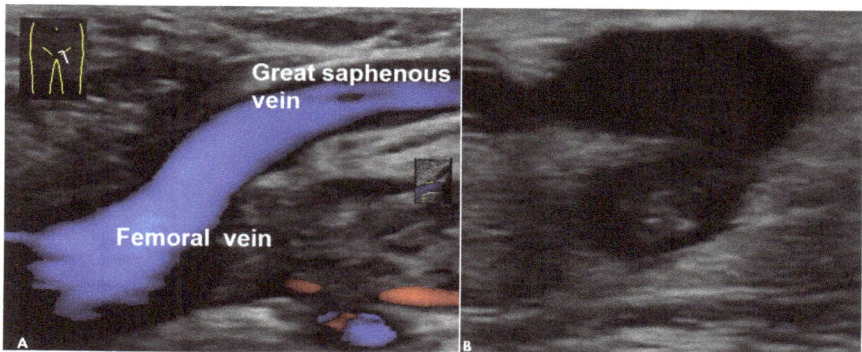

Fig.2.37.10. (A) Colour Doppler displays a homogenous increase in venous flow and (B) Ultrasound imaging of a superficial thrombophlebitis
Credit - Mikael Häggström

Superficial Thrombophlebitis

A clot in a superficial vein will exhibit similar characteristics with a deep vein on ultrasound: an echogenic mass with direct visualisation, non-compressibility, and reduced or lacking colour flow. Let's note that those superficial veins are not adjacent to arteries while deep veins are (Naringrekar et al., 2019).

Baker's cyst

Popliteal cysts can show similar characteristics with DVT (sharp knee pain, calf swelling, and occasionally erythema). On ultrasound, a Baker's cyst is a circular anechoic mass with sharply demarcated boundaries in both the longitudinal and transverse views (Zitek et al., 2016). On Colour Doppler, there should be no flow.

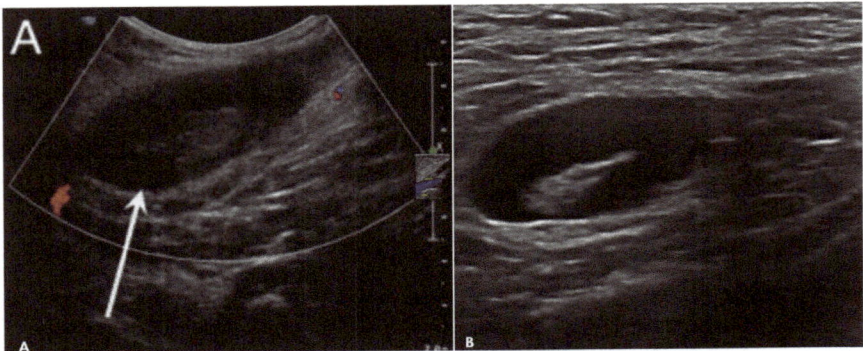

Fig.2.37.11. Baker's Cyst on Ultrasound (Naringrekar et al., 2019) and Ultrasound imaging demonstrate the appearance of a lymph node, which can sometimes be mistaken as thrombus.

Lymph nodes

On ultrasound, a lymph node appears like a clot (hypoechoic oval structure with a hyperechoic centre). Scanning the lymph node in the longitudinal view, it appears circumscribed and not tubular like a vein (Zitek et al., 2016). Unlike an artery or vein that will be a continuous structure, a lymph node quickly disappears when tracked down.

Pseudoaneurysms

On ultrasound, pseudoaneurysms appear anechoic or hypoechoic. With Colour Doppler, there is the presence of the **"Yin-Yang Sign"** from the circular motion of blood inside the pseudoaneurysm cavity.

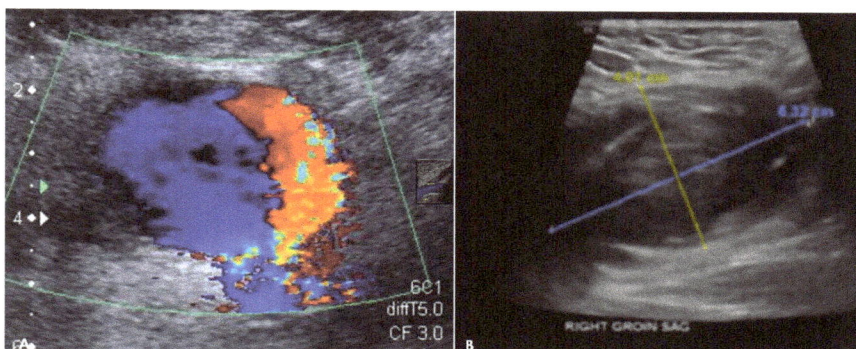

Fig.2.37.12. (A) The Yin Yang Sign and (B) Ultrasound imaging of the groin hematoma

Groin Hematoma

On ultrasound, a groin hematoma is hypoechoic with some anechoic areas scattered throughout.

Unlike an artery or vein that will be a tubular structure, the longitudinal view of a hematoma will show a circumscribed structure.

Further reading

Baker M, Anjum F, dela Cruz J. Deep Venous Thrombosis Ultrasound Evaluation. StatPearls Publishing: https://www.ncbi.nlm.nih.gov/books/NBK470453/

Ultrasound Tutorial: DVT / Lower Limb Veins | Radiology Nation: https://www.youtube.com/watch?v=oo0hPKdtFSQ

References

Ahn, J., & Dinh, V. (2021). DVT Ultrasound Made Easy: Step-By-Step Guide. POCUS 101. Retrieved 28 Dec. 2021 from https://www.pocus101.com/dvt-ultrasound-made-easy-step-by-step-guide/

Burnside, P. R., Brown, M. D., & Kline, J. A. (2008). Systematic Review of Emergency Physician–performed Ultrasonography for Lower-Extremity Deep Vein Thrombosis. Academic Emergency Medicine, 15(6), 493-498. https://doi.org/https://doi.org/10.1111/j.1553-2712.2008.00101.x

Gaillard, F., & Knipe, H. (2021). Deep vein thrombosis. Radiopaedia.org. Retrieved 28 Dec. 2021 from https://doi.org/10.53347/rID-1204

Lockhart, M. E., Sheldon, H. I., & Robbin, M. L. (2005). Augmentation in Lower Extremity Sonography for the Detection of Deep Venous Thrombosis. American Journal of Roentgenology, 184(2), 419-422. https://doi.org/10.2214/ajr.184.2.01840419

Naringrekar, H., Sun, J., Ko, C., & Rodgers, S. K. (2019). It's Not All Deep Vein Thrombosis: Sonography of the Painful Lower Extremity With Multimodality Correlation. J Ultrasound Med, 38(4), 1075-1089. https://doi.org/10.1002/jum.14776

Needleman, L., Cronan, J. J., Lilly, M. P., Merli, G. J., Adhikari, S., Hertzberg, B. S., . . . Meissner, M. H. (2018). Ultrasound for Lower Extremity Deep Venous Thrombosis. Circulation, 137(14), 1505-1515. https://doi.org/doi:10.1161/CIRCULATIONAHA.117.030687

Zitek, T., Baydoun, J., Yepez, S., Forred, W., & Slattery, D. E. (2016). Mistakes and Pitfalls Associated with Two-Point Compression Ultrasound for Deep Vein Thrombosis. West J Emerg Med, 17(2), 201-208. https://doi.org/10.5811/westjem.2016.1.29335

| 38 |

Echo in Life Support

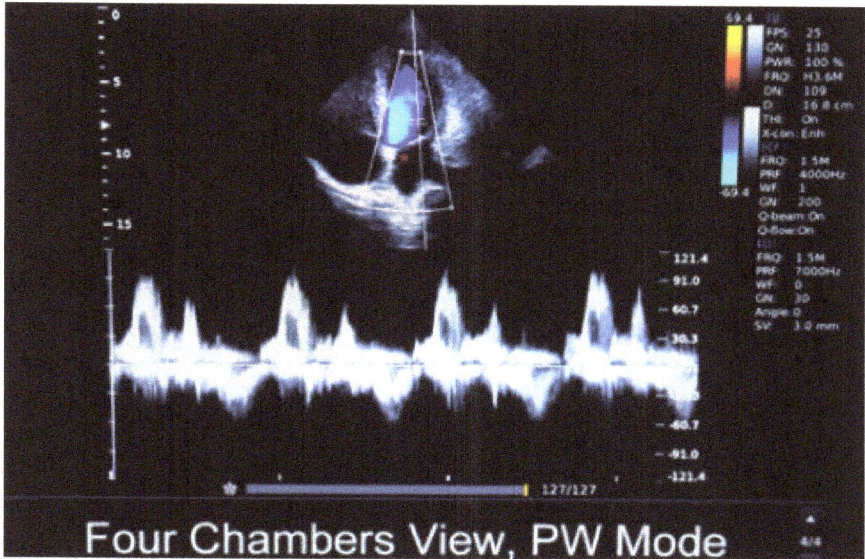

Four Chambers View, PW Mode

Overview

The examination sequence proposed to answer these questions begins with the lung views to rule out pneumothorax and identify the lung profile, followed by the subcostal window (four-chamber view and IVC assessment) to rule out tamponade, estimate fluid status and assess qualitative cardiac function. At this point, the clinician will often be able to confidently estimate the volume status of the shock patient. The next step of the ultrasound examination depends on whether the patient is deemed hypovolemic or not.

In cases of hypovolemic shock, one should expect clear lungs (e.g., no B-lines) associated with a hyperdynamic LV and a collapsible IVC. If this is the case, only limited additional crucial information can be gained from a complete cardiac examination, and a search for potential aetiologies of hypovolemic shock is warranted. Hence, an EFAST examination could be considered at this point.

1. EGLS ALGORITHM

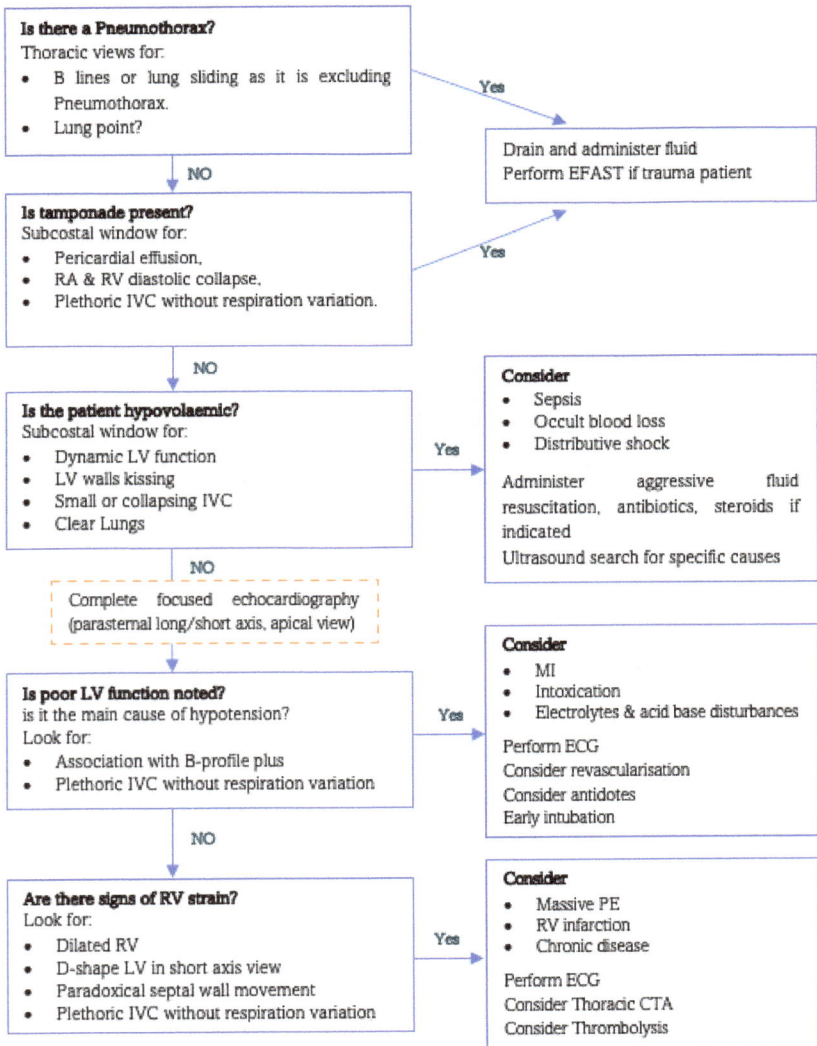

Is there a Pneumothorax?
Thoracic views for:
- B lines or lung sliding as it is excluding Pneumothorax.
- Lung point?

→ Yes

Drain and administer fluid
Perform EFAST if trauma patient

NO

Is tamponade present?
Subcostal window for:
- Pericardial effusion,
- RA & RV diastolic collapse,
- Plethoric IVC without respiration variation.

→ Yes

NO

Is the patient hypovolaemic?
Subcostal window for:
- Dynamic LV function
- LV walls kissing
- Small or collapsing IVC
- Clear Lungs

→ Yes

Consider
- Sepsis
- Occult blood loss
- Distributive shock

Administer aggressive fluid resuscitation, antibiotics, steroids if indicated
Ultrasound search for specific causes

NO

Complete focused echocardiography (parasternal long/short axis, apical view)

Is poor LV function noted?
is it the main cause of hypotension?
Look for:
- Association with B-profile plus
- Plethoric IVC without respiration variation

→ Yes

Consider
- MI
- Intoxication
- Electrolytes & acid base disturbances

Perform ECG
Consider revascularisation
Consider antidotes
Early intubation

NO

Are there signs of RV strain?
Look for:
- Dilated RV
- D-shape LV in short axis view
- Paradoxical septal wall movement
- Plethoric IVC without respiration variation

→ Yes

Consider
- Massive PE
- RV infarction
- Chronic disease

Perform ECG
Consider Thoracic CTA
Consider Thrombolysis

Table 2.38.1. Aetiologies of Shock and Associated Ultrasound Findings

Diagnosis	Associated ultrasound findings
Tension pneumothorax	Abolished lung sliding, No B-lines
Tamponade	Pericardial effusion with RV and RA diastolic collapse, plethoric IVC, dynamic LV
Hypovolemia	Hyperdynamic LV, IVC collapse, clear lungs
Massive pulmonary embolism	Dilated RV, "D-shape left ventricle, paradoxical septal wall movement, plethoric IVC
Myocardial infarction	Poor LV function associated with B-profile and plethoric IVC if cardiogenic shock
Toxicological, electrolyte abnormalities, acid-base disorders	Could be associated with depressed cardiac function

2. LUNG ULTRASONOGRAPHY

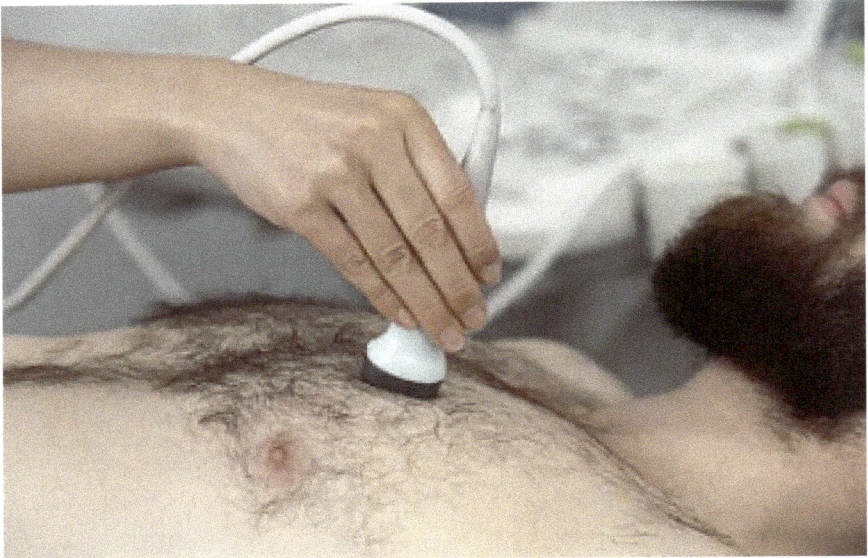

Indications

- Evaluation of respiratory failure and insufficiency due to pneumothorax, pleural effusion, pulmonary oedema, acute respiratory distress syndrome (ARDS), and alveolar consolidation (atelectasis, pneumonia, aspiration)
- Monitoring progress of diseases such as pulmonary oedema and pneumothorax
- Procedural guidance during pleural fluid removal or pneumothorax treatment
- Procedural guidance for chest tube placement for complex pleural effusions, haemothorax, pneumothorax, and other pleural diseases

Materials

- Ultrasound equipment/machine, gel

- Microconvex or phased-array cardiac probe for sufficient evaluation of lung artefact (use abdominal pre-set). Linear array probes, or vascular probes, can be used for a more detailed evaluation of the pleura, although this is insufficient for penetration to deeper structures.
- Sterile materials and equipment where appropriate

Procedure

Probe position

Start examination at the mid-clavicular level at the space between the second and the third ribs. Probe positioning should be perpendicular to the ribs (longitudinal positioning) with the ultrasound marker pointed cephalad.

This should place the most superficial structures at the top, with deeper structures at the bottom of the monitor.

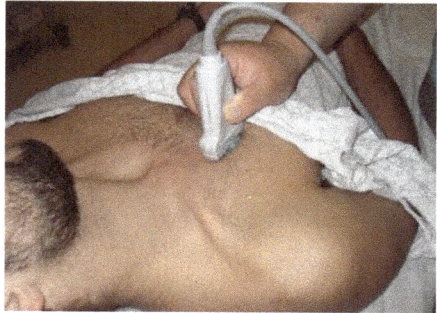

Fig.2.38.1. Longitudinal probe position for Lung ultrasound
Credit - Medscape

Upon completion, probe positioning can be mapped to evaluate three or four additional areas, typically between the anterior and the posterior axillary lines. Lateral views with the probe should be most posterior, typically along the posterior axillary line, tracking caudad toward the diaphragm.

- PLAPS (posterolateral alveolar and/or pleural syndrome) pointed posteriorly should also be evaluated, specifically in supine patients.
- PLAPS is lateral to the scapula and typically requires that the patient be lifted off the bed from one side.

1. BAT SIGN

The initial view observed should be a window of lung flanked by two rib shadows. This view termed the **"bat sign,"** should now allow evaluation of the parietal and visceral pleura, seen most superficial as echogenic line (approximately 0.5 cm below the start of rib shadows), subsequent lung sliding, and other findings such as "A" and "B" lines, as well as abnormal lung tissue.

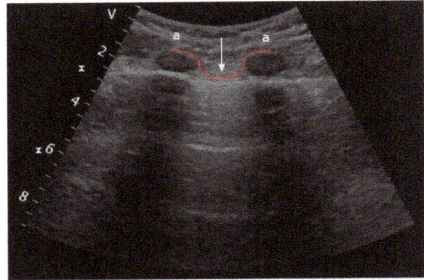
Fig.2.38.2. Bat sign

2. A LINES

A line indicates air. These are multiple echogenic lines appearing horizontally in sequence deep to the pleural line. This artefact represents reverberations of the pleura and can be found in aerated lungs, which can be normal or abnormal (e.g., pulmonary embolism, COPD). The first true A-line denoted "A1," is found equidistant from the chest wall to the pleural line. Many other A-lines might be seen and are denoted "A'" lines. Subsequent equidistant A-lines are "A2, A3," and so on.

3. B LINES

These artefacts appear in well-aerated lungs and are vertical echogenic lines (ray, flashlight, lung rockets) transmitted from the pleura to the deeper parts of the lung on the ultrasound monitor field. They are due to thickened interlobular septa and represent alveolar fluid surrounded by air. True B lines arise from the pleural line and shoot all the way down to the far lung fields, whereas **"comet tails"** are seen only close to the pleural and are sometimes referred to as **"shim-mering"** or **"glimmering"** during movement of the pleural line.

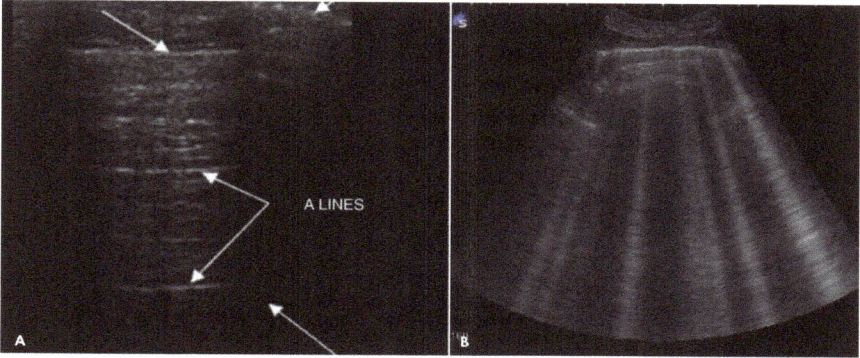

Fig.2.38.3. (A) A-lines and (B) B-lines

When multiple B lines are seen in a patient, it is sometimes referred to as "lung rockets" or "flashlights" because many rays are shooting from the pleura.

- **Characteristics of B-lines are:**
    - They arise from the pleural line.
    - They are long, vertical hyperechoic lines that continue to the depths of the image. They look like comet tails (an old name for them).
    - They erase A-lines
    - They move with lung sliding.

Even though most of the time B lines represent pulmonary oedema, they can be seen in other conditions such as aspiration, pulmonary fibrosis, acute respiratory distress syndrome (ARDS), and pneumonia.

4. LUNG SLIDING

The presence of lung sliding excludes a pneumothorax under the probe with certainty and requires minimal training to recognise. While not specific, its absence in the appropriate context can be highly suggestive of a pneumothorax. M-mode can be used to show a timed clip of this through a still image and should only be used as a method of reporting or saving for documentation purposes.

5. LUNG POINT

The "lung point", which is pathognomonic for a pneumothorax, is observed when lung sliding is intermittently absent from the ultrasound field at expiration. A lung point might not be observed in the case of tension pneumothorax because the lung is expected to be completely collapsed. The more rib spaces found to have absent lung sliding, the larger the pneumothorax.

Lung sliding can be evaluated with M-mode, which can help identify a normal parietal-visceral interface at that level. Obtain an adequate two-dimensional view ("bat sign") and press the "M-mode" option on the equipment. A normal interface appears as multiple hyperechoic lines, the pleura (termed "seashore"), followed by a sand-like pattern, the lung tissue. This pattern together is termed a "**seashore sign.**"

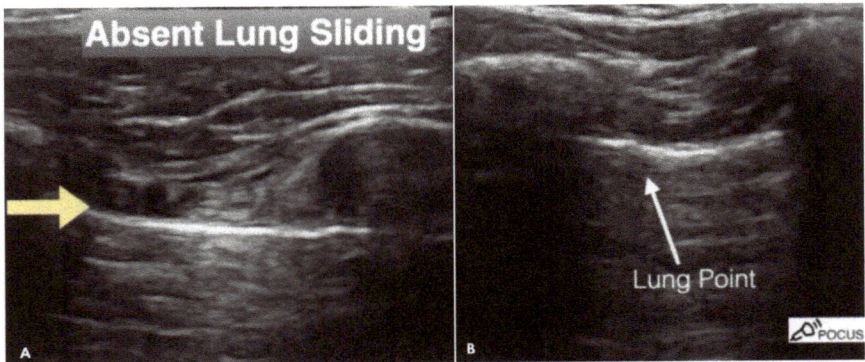

Fig.2.38.4. (A) Absence of lung sliding, suggestive of Pneumothorax and (B) The Lung point, suggestive of pneumothorax
Credit - POCUS 101

Air that disrupts the parietal-visceral interface, as found within a pneumothorax, is identified as horizontal repeating echogenic lines, like a barcode and is termed as "**Barcode sign**" or "**stratosphere sign.**"

M-mode can be discontinued.

Lung sliding can be absent in conditions other than pneumothorax: apnoea, right or left bronchial intubation, lung collapse (blebs), pneumonia, and pulmonary fibrosis.

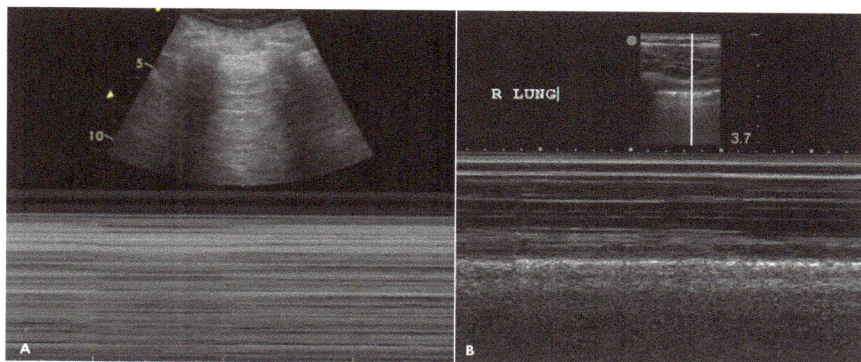

Fig.2.38.5. (A) The stratosphere or barcode sign. Absent lung sliding on M-mode in a patient with a pneumothorax. Notice the absence of T lines (the lung pulse) and (B) The seashore sign confirms active lung sliding

6. LUNG PULSE

This appears as a shimmering of the pleural line due to cardiac activity. This is most apparent on the left side of the chest, closest to the heart. This helps to exclude pneumothorax as well.

Move posteriorly: over the ultrasound probe laterally and posteriorly to the PLAPS point. The transducer can be directed toward the centre of the patient's body in supine patients. Pleural effusions and consolidations are found in the dependent areas of the lung.

Move caudally: With the marker still pointing cephalad, move along the posterior axillary line in two or three additional rib spaces. Identification of pleural disease and other pathology requires multiple views and will aid in evaluating the extent of the disease. This will also allow for the identification of boundaries of the lung, such as the diaphragm. Identification of the diaphragm is most critical to determining the location of fluid. Along the posterior axillary line or the posterior chest wall, move the probe caudad to identify the diaphragm. This appears as an echogenic curvilinear structure, with the liver or spleen being sub-diaphragmatic and typically of different echogenicity than the lung.

Many times, the diaphragm is very high in the supine critically ill patient. Massive oedema and obesity may also degrade image quality in this location. Always identify the diaphragm.

Hypoechoic fluid surrounding the liver or spleen can appear as pleural effusion and must not be mistaken as such. In addition, lung tissue may mimic hepatic tissue in certain diseases such as dense consolidations termed **"hepatisation"** of the lung.

Proper probe positioning, clear identification of the diaphragm, subdiaphragmatic structures, and lung are crucial. This is a common error in novice operators owing to the confusion of the hepatorenal or splenorenal recess for the diaphragm. Identifying the diaphragm can be technically difficult depending on patient position, size, and clinical condition.

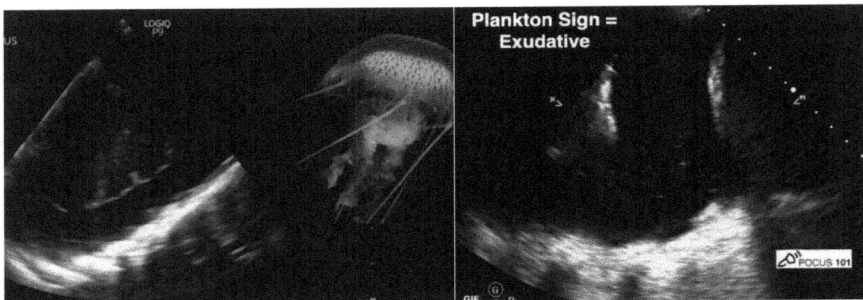

Fig.2.38.6. (A) Jellyfish Sign for Pleural Effusion and (B) The plankton sign shows an effusion with swirling, hyperechoic debris.
Credit - (A) NeproPocus and (B) POCUS 101

Identify pleural effusions

- Confirming the presence of pleural effusions requires identifying anechoic material between the pleura and the lung.
- This can be seen as lung movement in an undulating pattern, which typically is facilitated by cardiac activity and respiration.

- This is termed the **"jellyfish sign,"** where the lung flaps as it freely floats in the effusion. Floating debris can also confirm effusion, termed **"plankton sign."**

- It is also important to identify the depth of the chest wall to the pleural fluid to determine the best location/depth of needle insertion when attempting thoracentesis or chest tube insertion.

Identify consolidations

- Compressed lung appears with alveolar consolidation pattern (tissue-like sign).

- Alveolar consolidations are devoid typically of air and appear as tissue density; these can be atelectasis, pneumonia, aspiration, or another diseased lung.

7. Hepatisation of the lung

It is typical, where the images mimic liver tissue. Images may also have hyperechoic foci representing air bronchograms, which would indicate pneumonia. Probe location should be correlated with an anatomical lobular or segmental area.

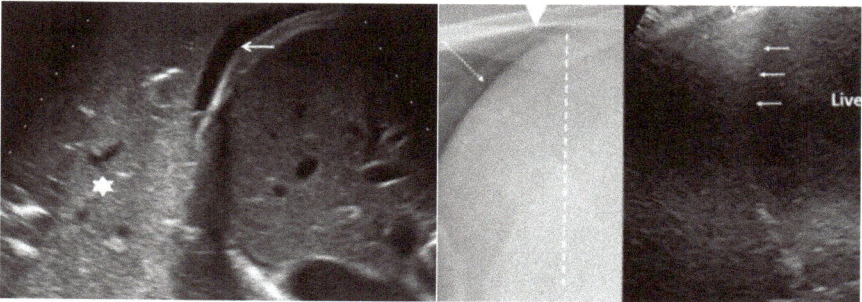

Fig.2.38.7. (A) Hepatization of the lung, suggestive of lung consolidations and (B) The Curtain sign in lung ultrasound

The lung may slide into the effusion during the respiratory cycle and can be problematic during needle insertion, causing pneumothorax or abnormal wire placement during the performance of pigtail chest tube catheters. This is called a **"curtain sign."**

8. Sinusoid sign

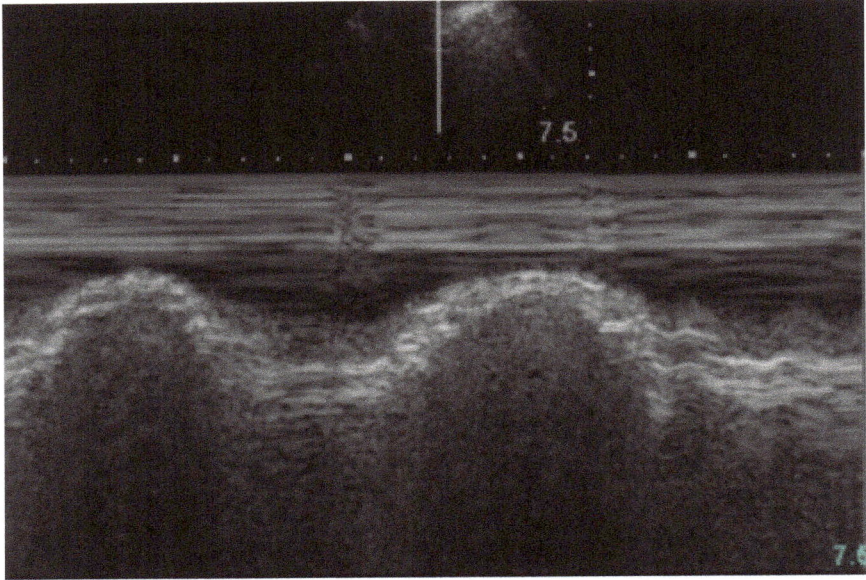

Fig.2.38.8. In M-mode, identification of pleural effusion becomes evident with the sinusoidal sign

M-mode is placed in the centre of the visible lung when a large amount of pleural fluid is seen. A **sinusoid sign** strengthens the operator's determination that pleural fluid is present and that the pleural fluid is not necessarily compromising lung dynamics. If the sinusoid sign is absent, it may indicate a "trapped" lung dynamic.

Assessment and clinical decision making. Upon completion of ultrasonography of bilateral lung fields, clinical decision-making tools may be of benefit, especially in undifferentiated respiratory failure. A protocol has been developed to organise the exam of a respiratory failure patient (on non-invasive or invasive ventilation only). The BLUE protocol assesses patients based on findings (e.g., A-lines, B lines, lung sliding) of both lungs and incorporates them into an algorithm.

With acceptable sensitivities and specificities, practitioners can diagnose pulmonary oedema, pneumonia, pneumothorax, and COPD/asthma with the BLUE protocol.

Potential causes of abolished lung sliding other than pneumothorax:

Pneumonia
Acute respiratory distress syndrome (ARDS)
Pleurodesis, pleural scarring
Severe emphysema
Bronchial obstruction
Mainstem intubation
Apnoea

3. CARDIAC ULTRASONOGRAPHY

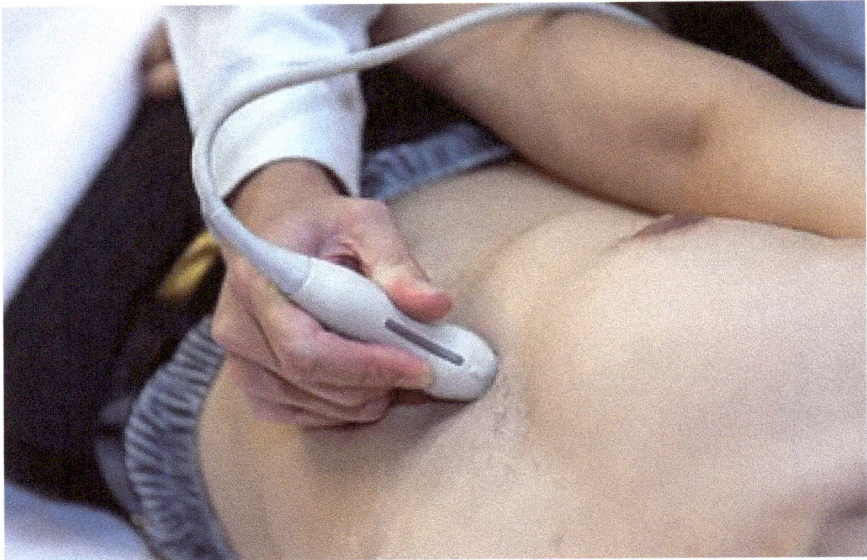

While the familiar curvilinear transducer can give good subxiphoid views, it is difficult to achieve the other cardiac views using this transducer. Therefore, a phased array transducer is required. The key benefit of the phased array transducer is its small footprint. A cardiac pre-set also optimises the machine settings to give you the best possible image production, particularly for moving vascular structures. This transducer typically has a frequency range of between 1-5 MHz. The evolutionary pathway of echocardiography has been different from conventional ultrasound. When the cardiac pre-set is selected, the default marker position is to the left, e.g., the marker on the probe should be orientated to the patient's left side, and the marker indicator on the screen image will be opposite to what you would typically expect.

Cardiac Ultrasonographic views

1. SubXiphoid View

The initial view should be a transverse subxiphoid (SX) four-chamber view. This requires increasing the machine depth to around 20cm and holding the transducer almost flat against the indented epigastrium. Remember that the heart is an anterior structure and too deep at probe angulation is a common mistake. This answers four key questions:

1. Is there coordinated cardiac activity?
2. Is there a pericardial effusion?
3. What are the relative right and left ventricular chamber sizes?
4. What is the overall LV function like?

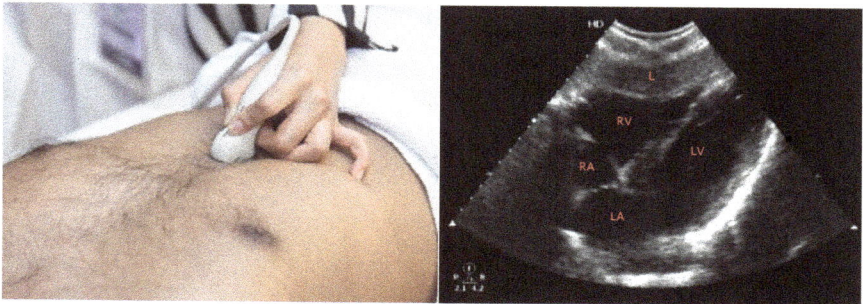

Fig.2.38.9. Cardiac US- (A) Subxiphoid probe placement and (B) Normal subxiphoid view

This view is obtained with the phased array transducer (marker at 3 o'clock). If you do not have the benefit of a phased array transducer then a traditional FAST subxiphoid view with a curvilinear transducer can be obtained. The key to obtaining a good view is to place the handle of the probe flat on the skin under the xiphisternum, with the probe pointing towards the patient's chin and then press the flattened probe down gently towards the bed at maximal inspiration.

An increased depth, often over 20cm, is required initially to appreciate the correct angle followed by optimal adjustment of depth.

2. Parasternal Long Axis View (PLAX)

The machine depth settings should be around 14-16cm for this. Ideally, this requires a phased array transducer. To obtain the PLAX view the dot on the transducer points along the axis of the heart, which is towards the patient's right shoulder. In fact, the axis is probably more towards the right mid-clavicular line. The transducer is placed tightly against the sternum in the third of the fourth intercostal space (try both). The image produced is a slice through the left ventricle, from apex to base (the valve annulus region). At the base, the image plane intersects the mitral and aortic valves as well as the left atrium and aorta.

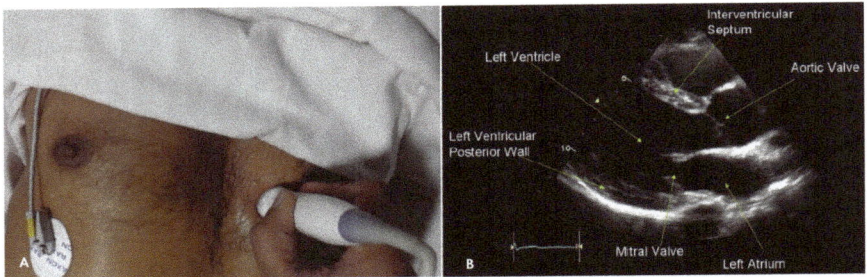

Fig.2.38.10. Cardiac US- (A) Parasternal Long Axis probe placement and (B) Normal Parasternal long Axis View (PLAX)

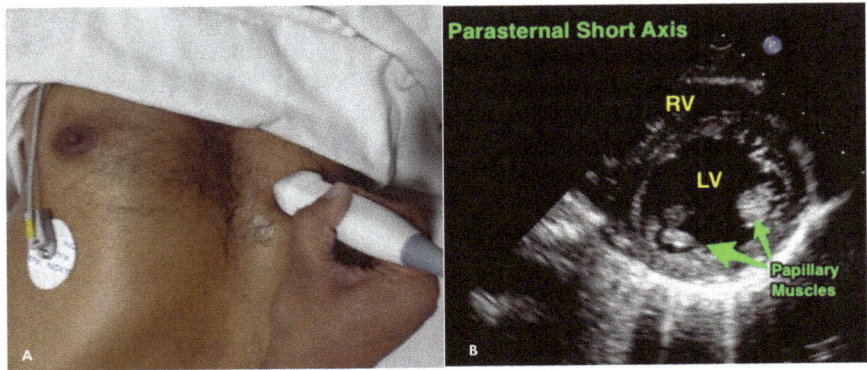

Fig.2.38.11. Cardiac US- (A) Parasternal Short Axis probe placement and (B) Normal Parasternal Short Axis View (PSAX)

3. Parasternal Short Axis View (PSAX)

Can be obtained, using similar depth settings.

4. Apical 4 Chamber View

It is an alternative second view but is possibly more difficult in a supine patient and often requires rotating the patient onto their left side by 45 degrees. The marker is to the patients left and the probe axis attempts to follow the cardiac axis.

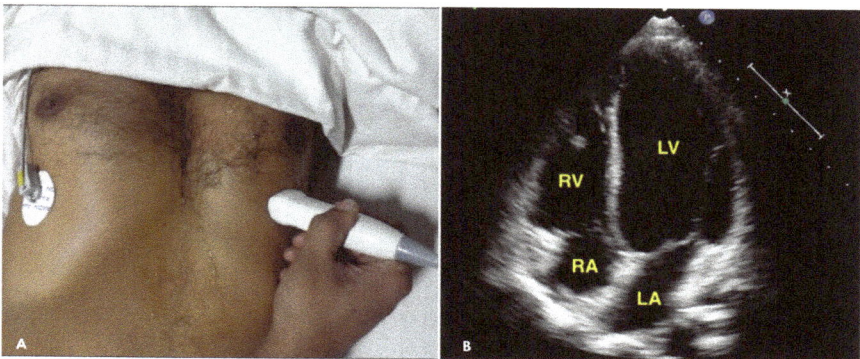

Fig.2.38.12. Cardiac US- (A) Apical 4 Chamber view probe placement and (B) Normal Apical 4 Chamber View

5. IVC View

Must be visualised for collapse as it is an ultrasonic CVP. An inferior vena cava (IVC) view is very similar to the longitudinal aortic view but lies to its right, and the transducer needs to look more into the chest. With a curvilinear transducer, the marker faces cranially, as in the aortic view. Using a phased array transducer (in a cardiac pre-set) the marker faces caudally. This longitudinal Subxiphoid window views the IVC as it passes posterior to the liver and into the heart.

The IVC is identified lying posterior to the liver receiving hepatic veins anteriorly before it passes through the diaphragm and into the right atrium. The point to identify for interpretation (more later) is 2cm distal to the atrio-caval junction.

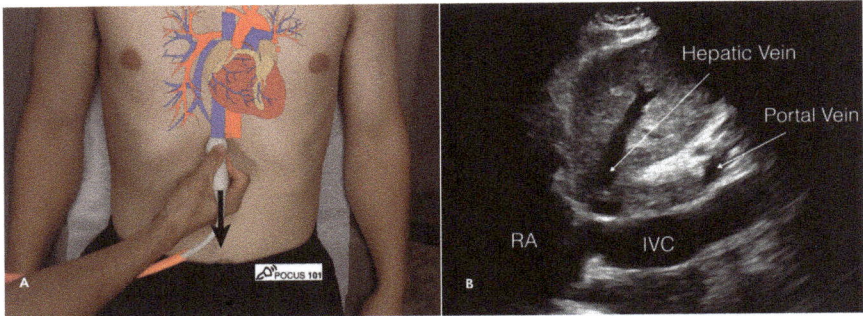

Fig.2.38.13. (A) IVC Ultrasound Probe Position and (B) Ultrasonographic view of the IVC
Credit - POCUS 101

INTERPRETATION OF THE VIEWS OBTAINED

Interpretation of the Subxiphoid view

In this view, the right ventricle (RV) is seen as the closest chamber through the window of the left lobe of the liver. Beyond is the left ventricle (LV) and more distant are both atria.

This view is excellent for pulse check imaging as it shows global motility, the possibility of a pericardial effusion, the RV/LV ratio and basic LV function. The end-systolic RV/LV ratio should be around 0.5, with the LV indenting the RV into a bean shape, or a letter D. If this D is reversed with the RV indenting the LV it is strongly indicative of high right-sided pressures. In the acute setting, this may suggest pulmonary embolus. In this case, it is important to quickly look at the IVC for signs of distension.

RV/LV ratios > 1 are associated with adverse clinical outcomes.

The RV/LV ratio correlates with pulmonary artery pressure and the normal should be around 0.5. Ratios above 1 are associated with adverse clinical outcomes

Interpretation of the parasternal long-axis view

The parasternal long-axis view (PLAX) is excellent for assessing the posterior pericardium, where very early effusions will be identified. The left atrium (LA), mitral valve (MV), left ventricle (LV), left ventricular outflow tract (LVOT) and aortic valve (AV) are all seen very clearly. The right ventricular outflow tract (RVOT) is closest to the transducer.

The movement of the mitral valve leaflets should be dynamic and energetic, and the anterior leaflet should almost touch the interventricular septum in the diastole. If not, the myocardial motility is sub-optimal.

Similarly, if the movement of the mitral valve leaflets are hyper-dynamic and the left ventricle completely collapses each cycle, then this suggests the patient is hypovolaemic and would benefit from an urgent fluid challenge.

Interpretation of the parasternal short-axis view

The parasternal short axis view (PSAX) enables the assessment of the concentricity of LV motility. This is particularly useful in the ischaemic heart. At the level below the mitral valve, the left ventricle should be contracting in a concentric fashion and if a finger is placed in the ventricular cavity, the walls should all thicken and move towards the finger.

The indented right ventricle (RV) is clearly seen. In addition, the posterior pericardium is seen (for early effusion).

Interpretation of the collapsing IVC view

As already stated, the point of assessment (POA) is 2cm distal to the atrio-caval junction. In a haemodynamically normal, spontaneously ventilating patient, the IVC collapses slightly on inspiration. In fact, in such patients, a pronounced 'sniff' results in the walls at the POA just touching, so-called 'kissing contact'.

This is reversed in a mechanically ventilated patient where there is an increased diameter in the abdominal IVC during inspiration.

Interpretation of the distended IVC view

The IVC view is of great value in the acute assessment of shock and shortness of breath. As an example, in healthy blood donors, the measurement of the IVC diameter is a reliable indicator of blood loss, with even small amounts (450 ml) causing a mean decrease in IVC diameter of 5 mm.

Conversely, a distended IVC suggests a high preload. Changes in diameter correlate with changes in intrathoracic and intra-abdominal pressure. A collapse index is calculated as the change in diameter between inspiration and expiration divided by the maximal diameter. It may be more useful to measure trends of IVC diameter and collapsibility in response to fluid resuscitation; however, there is evidence for cut-off values which can indicate an underfilled or overfilled status. A maximal IVC diameter of 2 cm with a collapse of 40-50% suggests a pressure of >10 mm Hg.

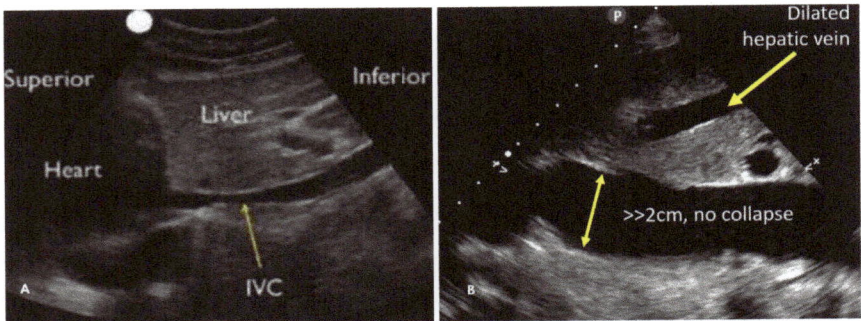

Fig.2.38.14. (A) IVC Kissing Contact and (B) Distended IVC

Interpretation of the M Mode IVC view

Most EPs do not calculate the collapse index, as a more qualitative approach is equally useful in the acute setting. A dilated non-collapsing IVC implies that the patient is well filled or overfilled, or that there is an obstructive aetiology, whereas a narrow fully collapsing IVC suggests an under-filled patient where aggressive fluid resuscitation is required, and points towards hypovolaemia as the likely cause. It is important to remember that these rules about the IVC are rules of thumb and that there are circumstances where they will not apply. In a fit, healthy person, the IVC collapse can be greater than half due to the mechanics of respiration on the thorax. Patients with right-sided heart failure can have a fixed & dilated IVC despite being hypovolaemic. If it is required to calculate the collapse index, this is best carried out using M mode. M stands for measurement (B for brightness). Using M mode calculations at the POA of minimal and maximal diameter can be made across the proximal IVC. A dilated non-collapsing IVC implies that the patient is well filled or overfilled, or that there is an obstructive aetiology, whereas a narrow fully collapsing IVC suggests an under-filled patient

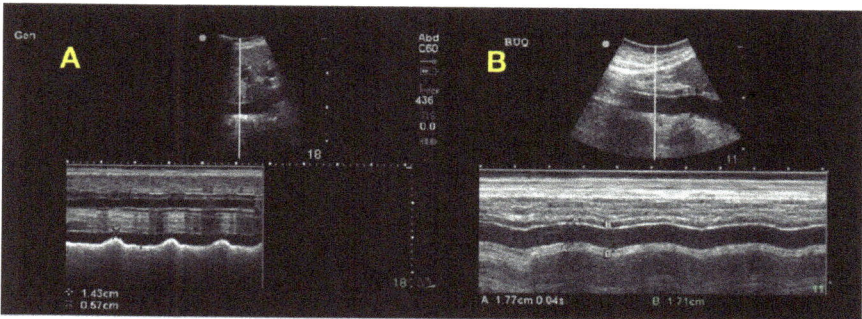

Fig.2.38.15. IVC imaged in M-mode. (A) Demonstrates small and collapsible IVC with a respiratory variation. (B) Demonstrates plethoric IVC with minimal respiratory variation, which, in the right clinical setting, could suggest that the patient is volume overloaded.

4. ULTRASOUND EVALUATION OF PULMONARY EMBOLISM & HEART STRAIN

Indications
- Undifferentiated respiratory distress
- Unexplained hypotension
- Evaluation for cardiac tamponade, pericardial effusion

Contraindications
- **Relative**
  - Morbidly obese patients
  - Patients with chest wall deformities
  - Patient with subcutaneous emphysema, pneumopericardium
  - Combative or altered patients

Procedure

Begin with the parasternal long-axis view. If possible, have the patient turn to the left decubitus side (that helps "move" the heart closer the chest wall). Find the phased array probe, select the "cardiac examination" on the machine, and make sure the orientation marker is pointed toward the right shoulder of the patient. Place the probe along the left side of the sternum over the fourth to sixth intercostal space. This should produce the image shown below:

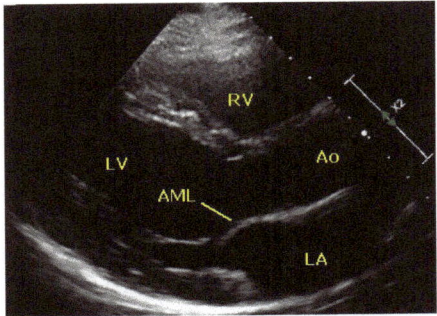

Fig.2.38.16. The aortic Mitral valve (AML) is seen in a nearly closed position. The left ventricular outflow tract anterior to AML is seen as very wide. Aortic leaflets are not visible as they are thin and in the fully open position, almost merging with the aortic wall echoes.

Measure the diameter of the ventricle during the end of diastole (normal values, 21 mm ± 1 mm; any measurement >25–30 mm is abnormal). Using the aorta as a landmark, evaluate the structures starting with the pericardium (bright white line around the heart), making sure there is no fluid around it.

- *Fluid above the aorta indicates a pericardial effusion.*
- *Fluid below the aorta indicates a pleural effusion.*
- *If a hypoechoic or anechoic stripe appears in the anterior side of the heart, it is most likely a fat pad.*
- *Fluid seen "all-around" categorises it as an effusion*

While keeping the probe in the same place, rotate the probe marker 90° clockwise toward the left shoulder to obtain the parasternal short-axis view. The parasternal short-axis view will give information on the contractility of the heart. The right ventricle should be anterior and to the left and the left ventricle to the right. The normal position of the septum bows slightly toward the right ventricle.

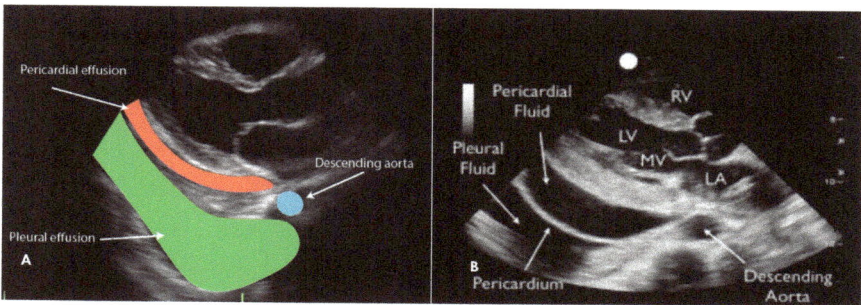

Fig.2.38.17. Pericardial and pleural effusion

Obtain a four-chamber view.

Place the orientation marker to the patient's left. Palpate for the point of maximum impulse (PMI) and place the transducer. All four chambers should appear in one view

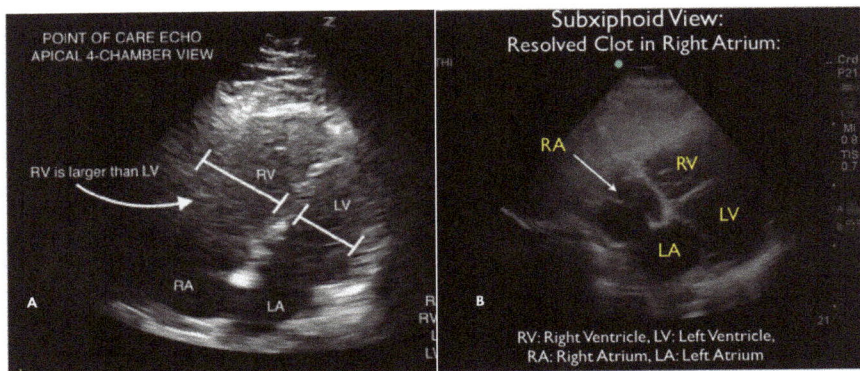

Fig.2.38.18. (A) Point-of-care echocardiogram in apical 4-chamber view demonstrates significant right ventricle dilation and (B) Subxiphoid view demonstrating thrombi in RA. LA, left atrium; LV, left ventricle; RA, right atrium; RV, right ventricle

Compare the sizes of the ventricles and note any difference. Also, notice the interventricular septum. The normal right-to-left ventricular ratio is less than 0.5. A Subxiphoid approach is also possible. Make sure the orientation marker is toward the right side of the patient

Use the liver for orientation. The right side of the heart will be nearest to the liver (think that the liver is on the right of the body); again, note for any differences in the size ratio. Next look at the inferior vena cava (IVC) by placing the curved array transducer just inferior to the xiphoid in a longitudinal fashion. (Switch from the Subxiphoid view to the IVC by rotating the probe counterclockwise until the IVC is seen.) Evaluate the IVC. During normal physiological inspiration, the drop in intrathoracic pressure "pulls" blood into the heart, thus decreasing the relative IVC size. If something is preventing venous return, such as a massive PE, the collapse will not be as evident and the suspicion for PE increases (fluid overload and increased central venous pressure [CVP] will also account for this finding). Normal IVC diameter is 1.2–2.3 cm, and total collapse and greater than 50 % collapse are normally visualised. An increase in IVC size and less than 50 % or no change has been correlated with increased right atrial pressures (11 to >20 cm Hg).

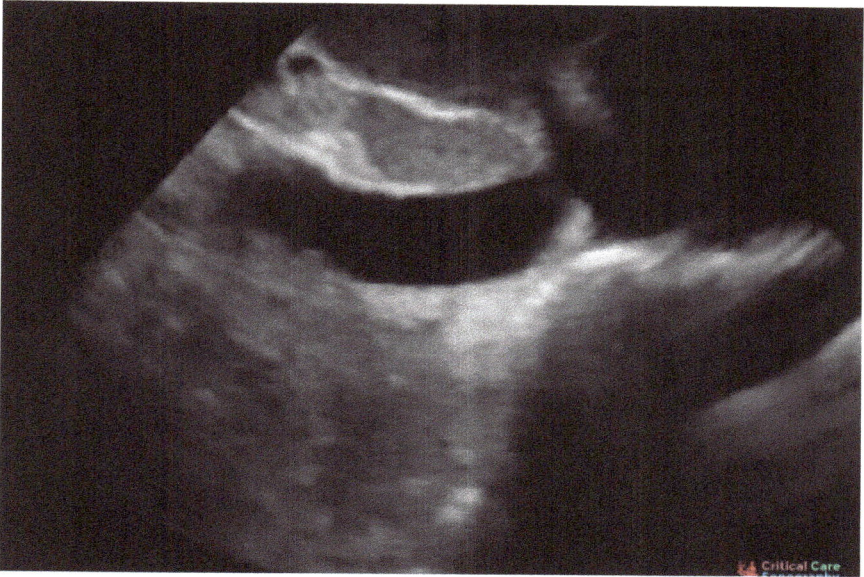

Fig.2.38.19. Subcostal view demonstrating long axis of the dilated inferior vena cava, (IVC) with no collapse on inspiration consistent with elevated right heart pressures.

Findings

A right heart that is "strained" or pumping against a higher resistance owing to a PE will show some or all these changes:

1. Right ventricular dilation
2. Right ventricular hypokinesis (especially of the middle segment), McConnell's sign but the normal motion of the apex.
3. Tricuspid regurgitation.
4. Abnormal septal motion: deviated toward the left ventricle (normally it relaxes during diastole toward the RV); as pressure increases, the right ventricle will not empty properly and septal flattening can be seen.
5. Dilated IVC with little or complete loss of changes in diameter with respiration (variability); the IVC collapses less than 50 % during inspiration.

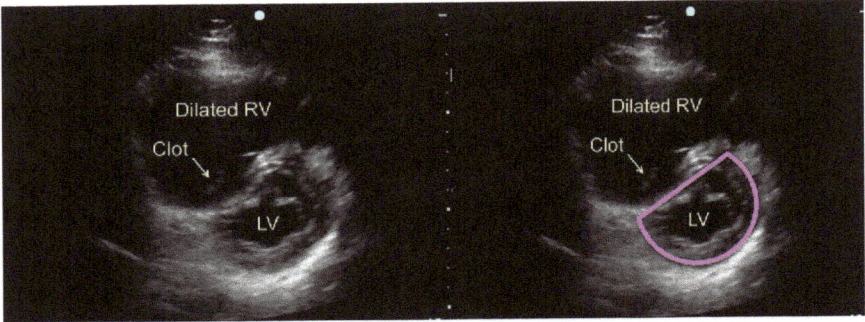

Fig.2.38.20. Septal bowing into the LV, otherwise known as the D-sign, on the parasternal short-axis view of the heart.

- **McConnell's Sign:** if a reduction in RV free wall motility with sparing of the apex is present (specificity for PE is 96%, but sensitivity is 16%).
- The **"D Sign"** on the parasternal short-axis view occurs when the increased pressure of the RV pushes the interventricular septum into the LV.

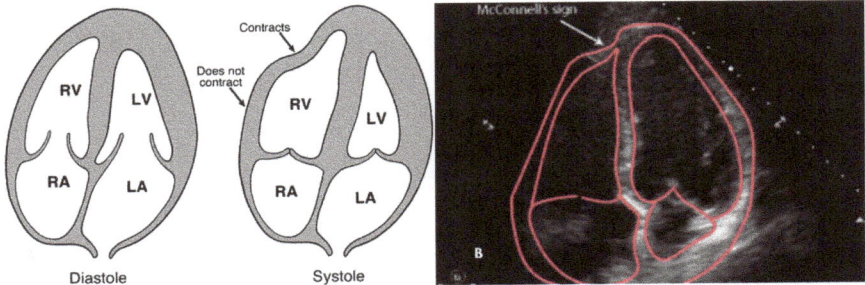

Fig.2.38.21. McConnell's sign

Complications

Ultrasound per se has been shown to cause no direct complications with proper use unless it is interfering with advanced airway or life-saving procedures.

| 39 |

RUSH Protocol

PUMP   **TANK**   **PIPES**

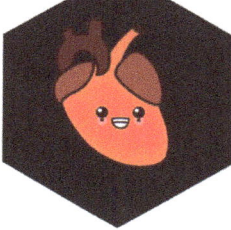
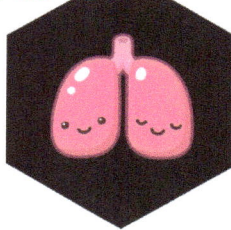
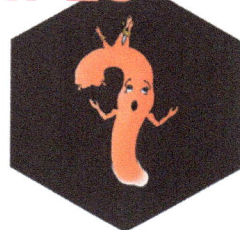

HEART

LUNGS
IVC
ABDOMEN

AORTA
DEEP VEINS

Overview

Point-of-care ultrasound is rapidly transforming the assessment approach of critically ill patients in shock and has evolved as an essential tool in the emergency and critical care departments. Undifferentiated shock is a familiar patient presentation in our emergency departments, but narrowing the precise aetiology can be challenging (Reim et al., 2021). The mortality rate of hypotensive or shocked patients remains high, standard physical exam techniques cannot always be accurate (Rezaie, 2013), and traditional laboratory testing and imaging are time-consuming. In addition, they may not differentiate between the different types of shock (cardiogenic, hypovolemic, obstructive, and distributive) (Reim et al., 2021). Early recognition and appropriate management of shock have been shown to decrease mortality (Rivers et al., 2001). Therefore, the introduction of bedside ultrasound in patients with undifferentiated shock allows for rapid evaluation of reversible causes of shock and enhances the diagnosis accuracy in undifferentiated hypotension (Jones et al., 2004). The "RUSH Exam" (Rapid Ultrasound for Shock and Hypotension), first introduced in 2006 by Weingart SD et al., was conceived to be an easy way to perform a quick bedside assessment of a patient with undifferentiated shock (Ghane et al., 2015; Reim et al., 2021; Rezaie, 2013). The **rapid ultrasound in shock (RUSH)** is more complex and prolonged than the FAST scan. Therefore, it is always executed by a trained clinician (hacking). This protocol involves a 3-part bedside physiologic assessment simplified as (Perera et al., 2010): The pump, the tank and the pipes.

Indications
- To quickly assess any patient with undifferentiated Shock and Hypotension.

The RUSH Ultrasound Exam
- Patient position: supine.
- Transducer: The phased array probe is preferred. Switch to the linear probe if DVT is suspected.
- **Pre-set:** eFAST Exam or Abdominal Exam Mode.
- **US Machine position**: Place the ultrasound machine on the patient's right to allow the clinician's right hand to manoeuvre the probe and the left hand to adjust settings.

The RUSH Protocol: "Pump-Tank-Pipe"

Protocol 1 includes assessment of the 'pump, tank and pipes' (Perera et al., 2010):

- **The pump: the heart**
  - Pericardial effusion
  - Signs of tamponade
  - Left ventricular (LV) contractility
  - Symptoms of right ventricular (RV) strain

- **The tank: the lungs**
  - ○ Inferior vena cava (IVC) volume and collapse with inspiration
  - ○ Internal jugular vein (IJV) volume
  - ○ Free fluid in pleural or peritoneal spaces
  - ○ Pulmonary oedema
  - ○ Tension pneumothorax
- **The pipe: the vessels**
  - ○ Abdominal aortic aneurysm (AAA) or dissection
  - ○ Thoracic aortic aneurysm or dissection
  - ○ Lower limb deep vein thrombosis (DVT) (as a source of pulmonary embolus (PE))

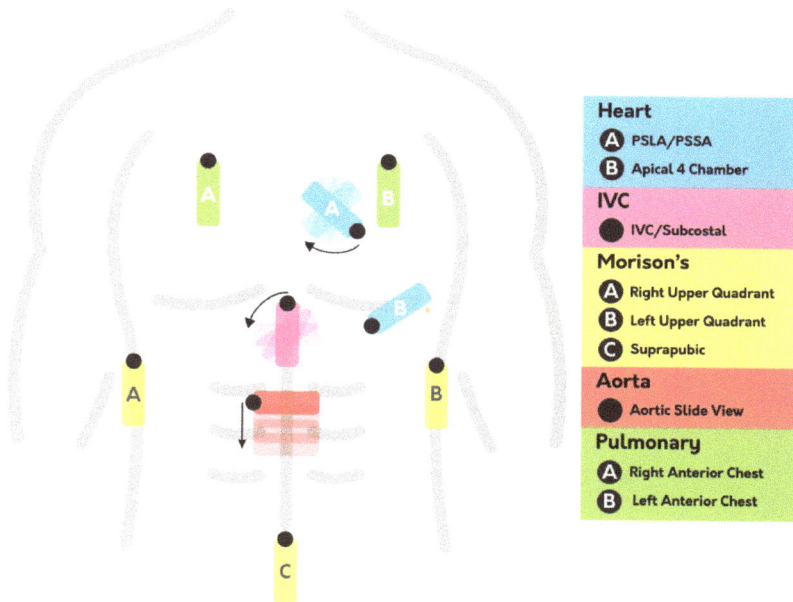

The RUSH Protocol Scan Locations

Heart
- Ⓐ PSLA/PSSA
- Ⓑ Apical 4 Chamber

IVC
- ● IVC/Subcostal

Morison's
- Ⓐ Right Upper Quadrant
- Ⓑ Left Upper Quadrant
- Ⓒ Suprapubic

Aorta
- ● Aortic Slide View

Pulmonary
- Ⓐ Right Anterior Chest
- Ⓑ Left Anterior Chest

*Probe orientation is based on a single dot location set to the left-upper screen. For this reason, cardiac imaging probe orientation is based on emergency medicine preference.

Fig.2.39.1. Scanning Locations and Probe Orientation for the RUSH Exam
Credit - The POCUS Atlas

Using the RUSH protocol to diagnose the type of shock

Adapted from Dina Seif's (Seif et al., 2012)

- Pump
  - **Step 1: Pericardial effusion:**
    - Effusion present?
    - Signs of tamponade? The diastolic collapse of R Vent +/− R Atrium?
  - **Step 2: Left ventricular contractility:**
    - Hyperdynamic?
    - Normal?
    - Decreased?
  - **Step 3: Right ventricular strain:**
    - Increased size of RV?
    - Septal displacement from right to left?
- Tank
  - **Step 1: Tank volume:**
    - Inferior vena cava:
      - Large size/small Insp collapse? -CVP high
      - Small size/large Insp collapse? -CVP Low
    - Internal jugular veins:
      - Small or large?
  - **Step 2: Tank leakiness:**
    - E-FAST exam:
      - Free fluid Abd/Pelvis?
    - Free fluid thoracic cavity?
      - Pulmonary oedema: Lung rockets?
  - **Step 3: Tank compromise:**
    - Tension pneumothorax?
      - Absent lung sliding?
      - Absent comet tails
- Pipes
  - **Step 1: Abdominal aorta aneurysm:**

- Abd aorta > 3 cm?
  - ○ **Step 2: Thoracic aorta aneurysm/dissection:**
    - Aortic root > 3.8 cm?
    - Intimal flap?
    - Thoracic aorta > 5 cm?
  - ○ **Step 3: DVT:**
    - Femoral vein DVT? Non-compressible vessel?
    - Popliteal vein DVT? Non-compressible vessel?

The RUSH Protocol – "HI MAP" Approach

The RUSH Exam Ultrasound Protocol (Reim et al., 2021).

- **H: Heart:**
  - ○ Ejection Fraction (Reduced): Systolic Heart Failure
  - ○ Ejection Fraction (Hyperdynamic): Distributive or Hypo-volemic Shock
  - ○ Pericardial Effusion: Tamponade
  - ○ Right Ventricular (RV) Strain: Pulmonary Embolism (PE)
  - ○ Regional Wall Motion Abnormality: Myocardial Infarction
  - ○ Low Cardiac Output: Cardiogenic, Hypovolemic, or Obstructive Shock
  - ○ High Cardiac Output: Distributive Shock
- **I: IVC**
  - ○ IVC Collapsible: Hypovolemic or Distributive Shock
  - ○ IVC Non-collapsible: Obstructive or Cardiogenic Shock
- **M: Morison's/eFAST**
  - ○ Hemoperitoneum/Haemothorax: Haemorrhagic Shock
- **A: Aorta**
  - ○ Abdominal Aortic Aneurysm
  - ○ Aortic Dissection
- **P: Pulmonary**
  - ○ Pneumothorax

Step 1: Evaluation of the PUMP

The first step in assessing the patient in shock is determining cardiac status, termed for simplicity "the pump" (Seif et al., 2012). Imaging of the heart usually involves four classical views: parasternal long and short axis, subxiphoid, and Apical 4 Chamber view (See Section 6 on US-Guided Echo life Support). In addition, clinicians caring for the patient in shock should look for three specific findings (Pericardial effusion and tamponade, left ventricular contractility and right ventricular strain for pulmonary embolism).

1. Pericardial effusion and tamponade

Look at the border of the heart. Is there a significant anechoic border surrounding it? If so, pericardial effusion is likely. Be sure to distinguish a pericardial effusion from a pleural effusion by identifying the location of the fluid with help from the descending aorta: *Anechoic fluid anterior to the descending aorta is a pericardial effusion, whereas fluid posterior to the descending aorta is a pleural effusion.*

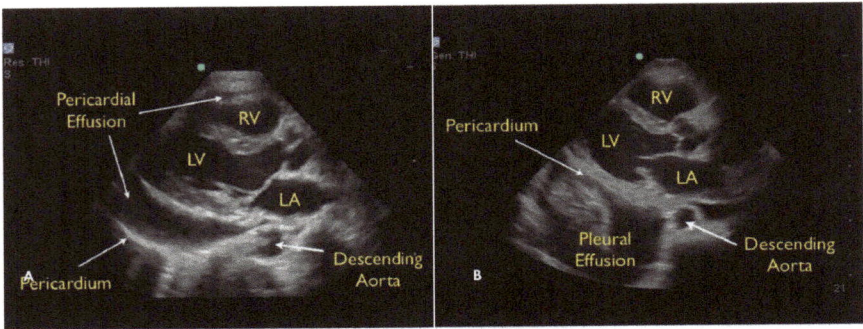

Fig.2.39.2. Pericardial effusion and Pleural effusion, parasternal long axis view RV
(Seif et al., 2012)

2. Left ventricular ejection fraction estimation

Look if the left ventricle is hyperdynamic or hypodynamic? If it squeezes uniformly? Then, does the anterior leaflet of the mitral valve move freely and approach the interventricular septum with each diastolic filling? If not, the heart's contractile function may be impaired, and the patient may be experiencing an exacerbation of systolic heart failure resulting in hypotension (Reim et al., 2021). If the heart appears hyperdynamic, sepsis or hypovolaemia might be the source of hypotension.

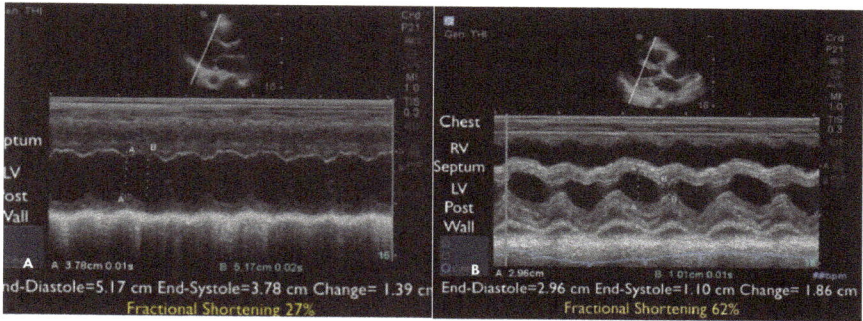

Fig.2.39.3. M mode showing contractility- (A) Poor contractility and (B) excellent contractility
(Seif et al., 2012)

Look at the anterior leaflet of the mitral valve, which should generally touch the septum. If a <30% difference in LV size between systole and diastole indicates severely decreased LV function (Rezaie, 2013).

3. Right ventricular strain for pulmonary embolism.

The RV chamber typically size should be about 60% the size of the LV chamber. If RV size equates to the LV, this is abnormal. Any increase in this ratio or twisting the interventricular septum towards the left side of the heart means RV strain: the right seat is struggling to eject. Hence, the RV chamber enlarges and infringes on the LV as pressure builds.

- Look out for **McConnell's Sign:** if a reduction in RV free wall motility with sparing of the apex is present (specificity for PE is 96%, but sensitivity is 16%) (Rezaie, 2013).
- Look for the **"D Sign"** on the parasternal short-axis view, which occurs when the increased pressure of the RV pushes the inter-ventricular septum into the LV.

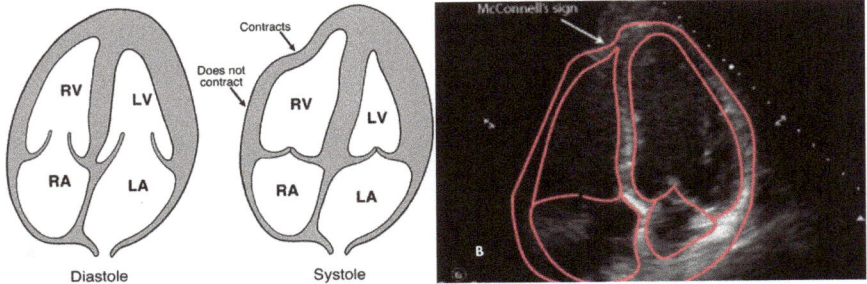

Fig.2.39.4. McConnell's sign: reduction in RV free wall motility with sparing of the apex

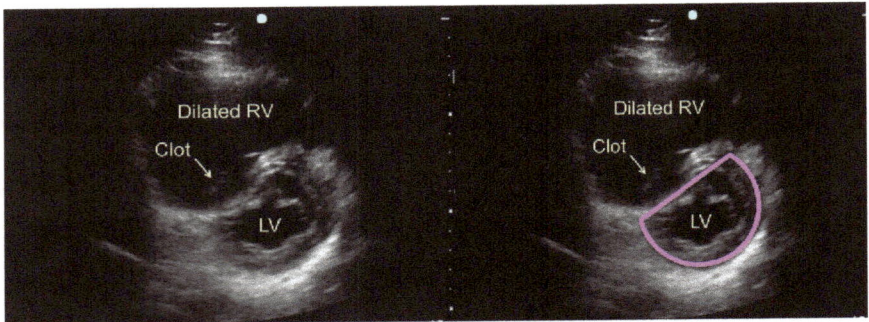

Fig.2.39.5. D Sign suggestive of right ventricular strain

*The signs mentioned above are indicative of RV strain and **not specific to PE**. If RV strain is found on ultrasound, the clinician should proceed with evaluating the legs for potential deep vein thrombosis by looking for a non-compressible vein. Findings of DVT in the setting of RV strain will significantly increase the possibility of a significant pulmonary embolism (Reim et al., 2021).*

Step 2: Evaluation of the TANK

The second part of the RUSH protocol concentrates on evaluating the adequate intravascular volume status, referred to as "the tank" (Seif et al., 2012). The clinician should look for three components:

1. The fullness of the Tank: Inferior Vena Cava and Internal Jugular Veins.
2. The Leakiness of the Tank: FAST and Thoracic Ultrasound
3. The Compromise of the Tank: Pneumothorax

1. The fullness of the Tank: IVC and Internal Jugular Veins.

Now, look at the Inferior Vena Cava (IVC) to evaluate the patient's central venous pressure (or right atrial pressure). Then, check if there is any leak causing hypotension or a fluid overload that is causing the heart not to pump adequately. Finally, check if CVP is high or low to categorize the likely type of shock further.

- IVC >2 cm in diameter and inspiratory collapse less than 50% approximates CVP >10 cmH20
- Not applicable for intubated patients. Spontaneously breathing patients create negative intrathoracic pressure. Ventilated patients create positive intrathoracic pressure (Rezaie, 2013).
- A high CVP suggested by a dilated and non-collapsible IVC may hint towards an obstructive or cardiogenic aetiology.
- A low CVP suggested by a small and collapsible IVC may hint towards a distributive or hypovolemic aetiology.

The IVC measurement is mainly used to assess fluid tolerance rather than fluid responsiveness. Using the IVC collapsibility Index (below), the diameter and collapsibility during inspiration or with a sniff test can be used to esti-

mate CVP. Limitations include body habitus, increased intraabdominal pressure, etc. (Reim et al., 2021).

Table 2.39.1. The IVC collapsibility Index. Adapted from Kircher et al.

IVC Diameter (cm)	Percent Collapsible (%)	Estimated CVP (mmHg)
<1.5	>50	0-5
1.5-2.5	>50	6-10
1.5-2.5	<50	11-15
>2.5	<50	16-20

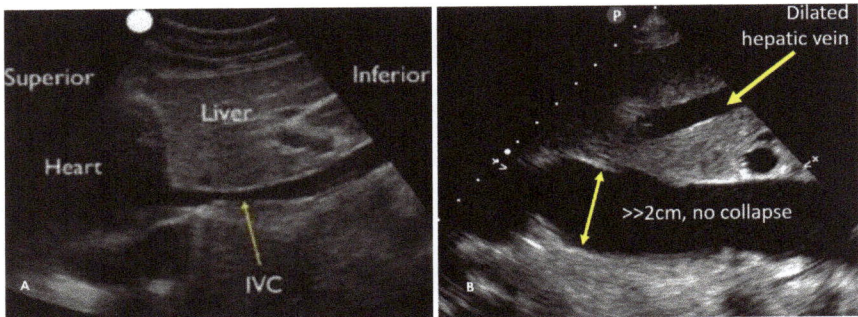

Fig.2.39.6. (A) Collapsible IVC – Suggesting LOW CVP and (B)Dilated and Non-collapsible IVC – Suggesting HIGH CVP

2. The Leakiness of the Tank: FAST and Thoracic Ultrasound

The "leakiness of the tank" refers to hemodynamic compromise due to a loss of critical fluids from the core vascular circuit.

- In the context of trauma: ensure if hemoperitoneum or haemothorax is present.

- In non-traumatic settings: accumulation of excess fluid into the abdominal and chest cavities often signifies "tank overload," think effusions and ascites that may build up with failure of the heart, kidneys, and/or liver.
- In a female patient of childbearing age: think ruptured ectopic pregnancy.

A. Hemoperitoneum

- The three standard locations for free fluid to accumulate in the RUQ of the eFAST scan are the:
  - ○ Hepatorenal Space or "Morison's Pouch"
  - ○ Caudal Tip of the Liver
  - ○ Suprahepatic Space
- The three standard locations for free fluid to accumulate in the LUQ of the eFAST scan are the:
  - ○ Perisplenic Space
  - ○ Spleen Tip
  - ○ Splenorenal Recess

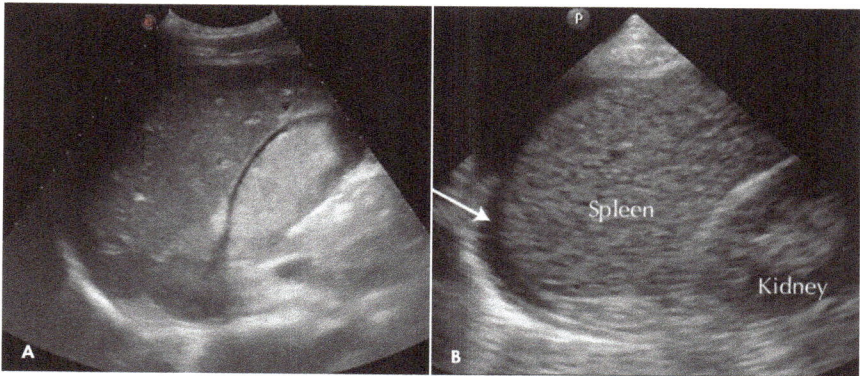

Fig.2.39.7. (A) eFAST RUQ Morison's Pouch with free fluid and (B) Positive left upper quadrant view (free fluid between spleen and diaphragm)

In the male pelvis, free fluid can be found in the rectovesical pouch/space. In the female pelvis, free fluid can be found in the Pouch of Douglas (Rectouterine Pouch).

B. Haemothorax

After assessing the RUQ or LUQ, try to move the probe superiorly to examine the thorax for fluid accumulation. Since the aerated lung reflects all the ultrasound waves, it usually is impossible to see the spine going above the diaphragm due to the **mirror Image Artifact**.

Any visualization of the patient's spine beyond the diaphragm suggests free fluid (e.g., blood) in the thorax as the ultrasound waves can readily pass through the free fluid in the chest cavity, allowing you to see the spine. This phenomenon is called a **Positive Spine Sign** (Reim et al., 2021).

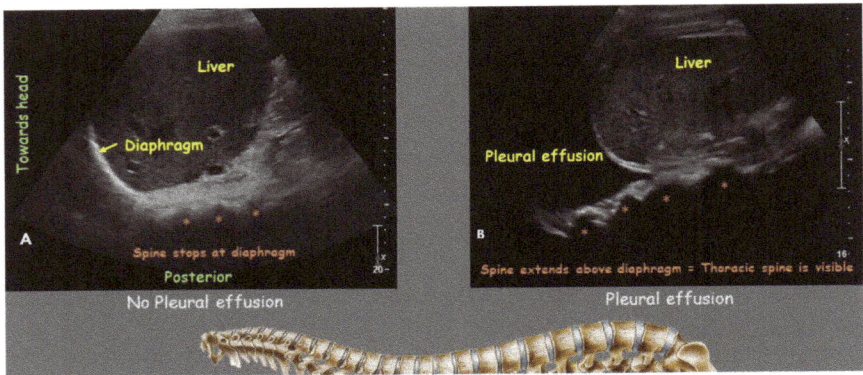

Fig.2.39.8. (A) Absence of Spine above Diaphragm (Mirror image effect = Normal Finding) and (B) Presence of Spine above Diaphragm (Positive spine sign=Pathologic Finding).
Credit - Nephro POCUS

3. The Compromise of the Tank: Pneumothorax

The third component of the evaluation of the tank is to consider "tank compromise." This usually transpires because of a tension pneumothorax.

A. Pneumothorax

There are three crucial steps to assessing for pneumothorax:

- **Lung sliding present**

- If lung sliding is present, rule *out* pneumothorax with 100% accuracy at that ultrasound point.
- The presence of lung sliding only rules out pneumothorax at that specific point you are scanning. Enhance your sensitivity by scanning multiple points on the chest.

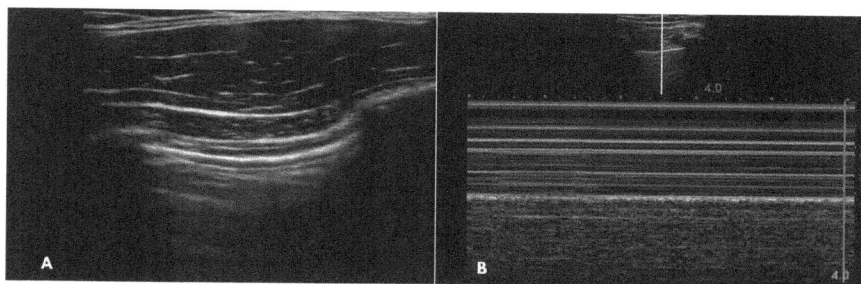

Fig.2.39.9. (A) Normal Lung Sliding (B-mode) and (B) Normal Lung Sliding with Seashore sign (M-mode): Rule out pneumothorax

- **Lung sliding absent**
  - If lung sliding is ABSENT, do *not automatically presume that pneumothorax is present.*
  - Refer to the Echo-guided life support chapter to recall other causes of reduced/absent lung sliding.

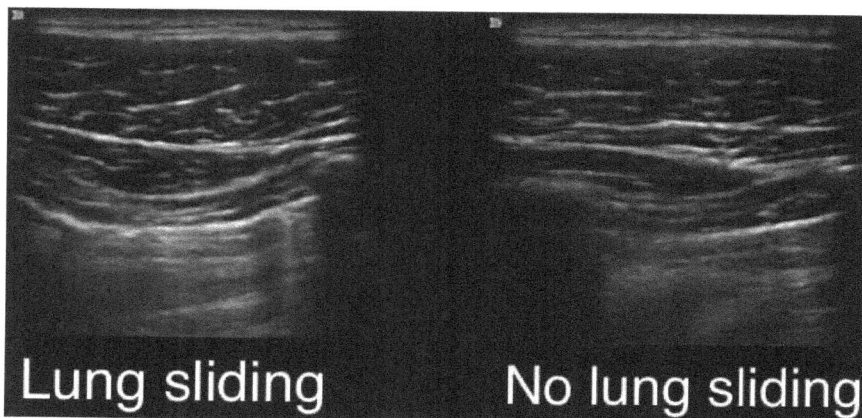

Fig.2.39.10. Presence and Absence of Lung Sliding (B-mode)

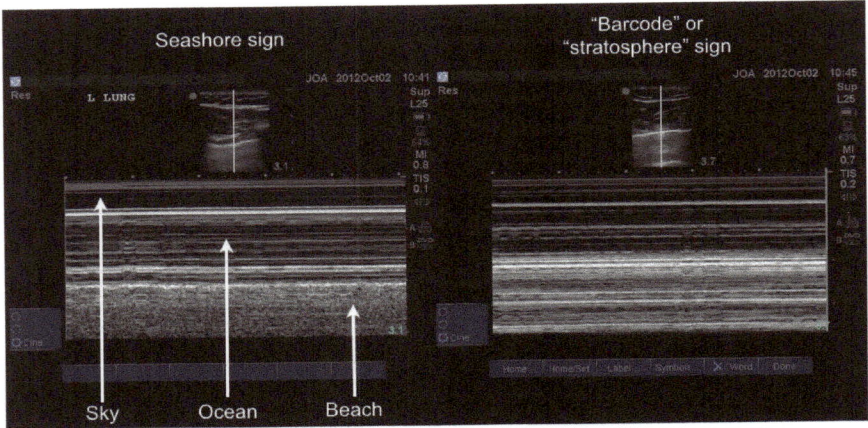

Fig.2.39.11. M-Mode views of (A) the presence of lung sliding (Seashore sign) and (B) the absence of Lung Sliding (Barcode Sign)

- **Lung point present**
  - The presence of **lung point** can definitively *rule in* pneumothorax with 100% accuracy.

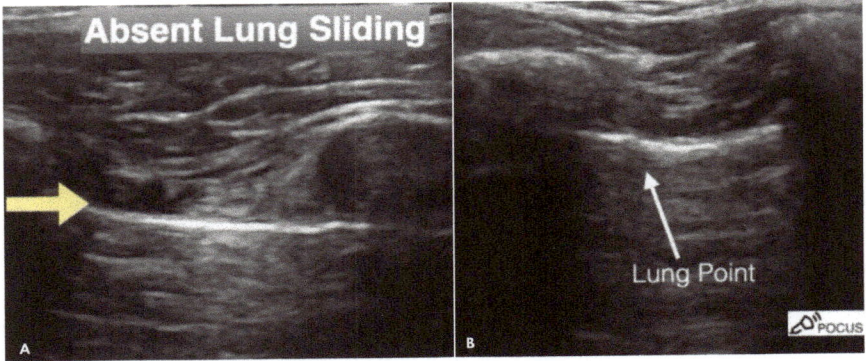

Fig.2.39.12. (A) Absence of lung sliding and (B) Lung Point Sign suggestive of pneumothorax

Step 3: Evaluation of the PIPES

The third and last phase in the RUSH exam is to examine "the pipes," looking first at the arterial side of the circulatory system and secondly at the venous side. Vascular catastrophes, such as a ruptured abdominal aortic aneurysm (AAA) or an aortic dissection, are life-threatening causes of hypotension. The survival of such patients may often be measured in minutes, and the ability to quickly diagnose these diseases is crucial (Seif et al., 2012). Therefore, clinicians should look for the:

1. Rupture of the Pipes: Aortic Aneurysm and Dissection.
2. Obstruction of the Pipes: DVT

1. Aorta

At this stage, we evaluate if the Abdominal Aortic Aneurysm (AAA) or Aortic Dissection are the causes of hypotension in the RUSH Exam.

A. Abdominal Aortic Aneurysm

- A normal aorta is usually ~**2.0cm** in diameter. Consider AAA if:
  - ≥ **3cm diameter for** the **abdominal aorta** or a **> 50% increase** in the aortic diameter.
  - ≥ **1.5cm diameter** for the **iliac arteries**.
  - Anytime a patient presents with a AAA of >/= 5cm and hypotension, assume a rupture until proven otherwise.
- Ensure to measure "**Outer wall to Outer wall**" for accurate aorta measurements.

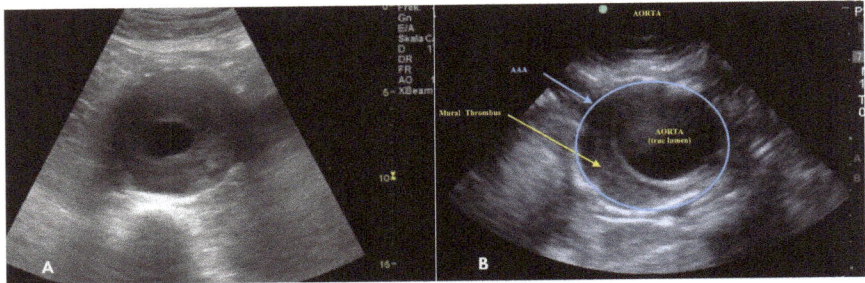

Fig.2.39.13. A and B: Abdominal Aortic Aneurysm with Mural Thrombus

B. Aortic Dissection

An aortic dissection may present as a free flap in the aortic lumen of either the descending abdominal aorta, ascending aorta, and/or the aortic arch. Aortic dissections in the ascending aorta can also cause aortic regurgitation and a diastolic murmur (Reim et al., 2021).

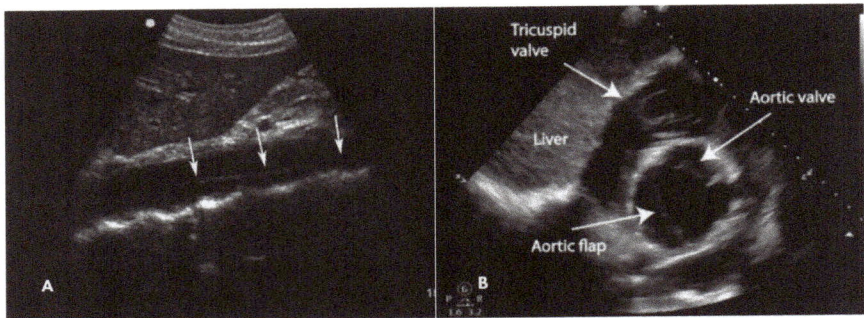

Fig.1.39.14. (A) Extensive aortic dissection and (B) Stanford type A aortic dissection ultrasound ultrasound

2. DVT

Refer to the section Deep vein thrombosis ultrasound above.

Further reading

Medstar Emergency Physicians – RUSH Protocol - Rapid Ultrasound for Shock and Hypotension: https://www.youtube.com/watch?v=Udh7bBij52Q

References

Ghane, M. R., Gharib, M., Ebrahimi, A., Saeedi, M., Akbari-Kamrani, M., Rezaee, M., & Rasouli, H. (2015). Accuracy of early rapid ultrasound in shock (RUSH) examination performed by emergency physician for diagnosis of shock etiology in critically ill patients. Journal of emergencies, trauma, and shock, 8(1), 5-10. https://doi.org/10.4103/0974-2700.145406

Jones, A. E., Tayal, V. S., Sullivan, D. M., & Kline, J. A. (2004). Randomized, controlled trial of immediate versus delayed goal-directed ultrasound to identify the cause of nontraumatic hypotension in emergency department patients. Crit Care Med, 32(8), 1703-1708. https://doi.org/10.1097/01.ccm.0000133017.34137.82

Perera, P., Mailhot, T., Riley, D., & Mandavia, D. (2010). The RUSH Exam: Rapid Ultrasound in Shock in evaluating the Critically Ill. Emergency Medicine Clinics of North America, 28(1), 29-56. https://doi.org/https://doi.org/10.1016/j.emc.2009.09.010

Reim, P., Moore, L., Minalyan, A., & Dinh, V. (2021). RUSH Exam Ultrasound Protocol: Step-By-Step Guide. POCUS 101. Retrieved 28 Dec. 2021 from https://www.pocus101.com/rush-exam-ultrasound-protocol-step-by-step-guide/

Rezaie, S. (2013). RUSH protocol: Rapid Ultrasound for Shock and Hypotension. ALiEM. Retrieved 28 Dec. 2021 from https://www.aliem.com/rush-protocol-rapid-ultrasound-shock-hypotension/

Rivers, E., Nguyen, B., Havstad, S., Ressler, J., Muzzin, A., Knoblich, B., . . . Tomlanovich, M. (2001). Early goal-directed therapy in the treatment of severe sepsis and septic shock. N Engl J Med, 345(19), 1368-1377. https://doi.org/10.1056/NEJMoa010307

Seif, D., Perera, P., Mailhot, T., Riley, D., & Mandavia, D. (2012). Bedside ultrasound in resuscitation and the rapid ultrasound in shock protocol. Crit Care Res Pract, 2012, 503254. https://doi.org/10.1155/2012/503254

www.ingramcontent.com/pod-product-compliance
Lightning Source LLC
Chambersburg PA
CBHW040844210326
41597CB00029B/4725